BIOSTATISTICS IN HEALTH

Yevhen Tarasov

ALLIED
HEALTH
PRESS

Biostatistics in Health

Author: **Yevhen Tarasov**

Allied Health Press
4164 Lakeshore Road
Burlington ON L7L 1A4
Canada
www.alliedhealthpress.com
Email: orders@arclereducation.com

ISBN: 978-1-77956-250-0

Allied Health Press publishes wide variety of books and eBooks. For more information about Allied Health Press and its products, visit our website at www.alliedhealthpress.com

ABOUT THE AUTHOR

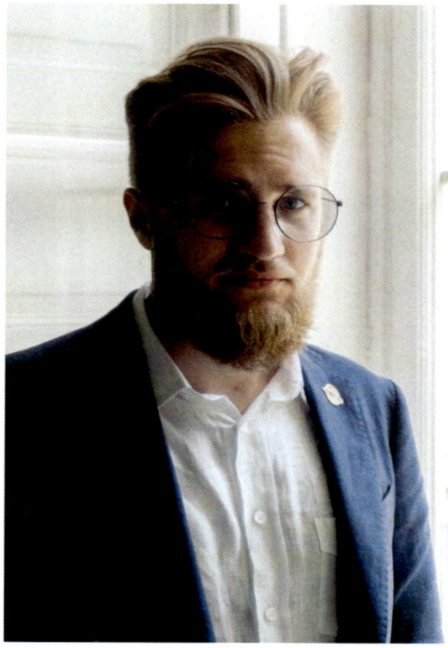

Yevhen Tarasov, MD, EuSpLM is an assistant professor at the Department of General and Clinical Epidemiology and Biosafety with course on Microbiology and Virology at Odesa National Medical University. Yevhen Tarasov received his MD in 2018 and got specialization in Medical Laboratory Science in 2019 with residency at The Filatov Institute of Eye Diseases and Tissue Therapy of the National Acadeny if Medical Science of Ukraine. He then joined the at the Department of General and Clinical Epidemiology and Biosafety with course on Microbiology and Virology at Odesa National Medical University, Odesa, Ukraine as an assistant professor. His research interests include epidemiology and diagnostics of autoimmune diseases and allergy. He is a group leader of work group on Ukrainian adaptation of the the International Consensus on Antinuclear Antibody (ANA) Patterns (ICAP).

Word Roots, Prefixes, and Suffixes by Chapter

Chapter 1 Introduction Biostatistics in Health

Bio-: Root word meaning "life" or "living organism."

Stat-: Root word derived from "statistics," referring to the collection, analysis, interpretation, and presentation of data.

-logy: Root word indicating "study" or "science" of a particular subject.

Epi-: Prefix meaning "upon," "on," or "above," is often used in epidemiology to study the distribution and determinants of health-related states or events.

Meta-: Prefix meaning "beyond," "after," or "transcending," is often used to describe meta-analysis, which combines data from multiple studies to generate conclusions.

Multi-:refix indicating "many" or "multiple," often used in multivariate analysis, which involves the analysis of multiple variables simultaneously.

-ics: Suffix indicating "study of" or "knowledge of," commonly used in biostatistics to denote the study of statistical methods applied to biological and health-related data.

-metry: Suffix indicating "measurement" or "process of measuring," used in biometry, which involves the application of statistical methods to biological data.

Chapter 2 Quantifying the Extent of Disease

Adren/o-: Gland

Angi/o-: Blood vessel

Bronch/i-: Bronchus

Carcin/o-: Cancer

Cardi/o-: Heart

Gastr-: Stomach

Hist/o-, Histio-: Tissue

Mamm-, Mast/o:Breast

Muscul/o-: Muscle

Nephr/o-: Kidney

Onco-: Tumor; Bulk; Volume

-pathy, Path/o-: Disease

Chapter 3 Summarizing Data Collected in the Sample

Popul: People, Population

Range: Extent, Scope

-able: Biodegradable

-ible: Irreversible

-osis: Condition, Disease

-metry: the process of measuring

Chapter 4 Basic Probability

probābilis: possibility

post-: after/ following

-sect: to cut or divide

bene-: good, well

bi-: two

-ial: of or relating to

Chapter 5 Confidence Interval Estimates

Uni-: one

Bi-: two

Poly-: many

Hetero-: Other; Different

Iso-: Equal; Like

Chapter 6 Hypothesis Testing Procedures

Auto-: Autocrine

Bio- : Biology

Chem/o-: Chemotherapy

Contra-: Contraception

Cyt/o-: Cytokine

Dys-: Dyspnea

Eu-: Good; Well

Fibr/o-: Fibrosis

Gluco-,: Glucose; Sugar Glycogen

Chapter 7 Power and Sample Size Determination

Gyn/o-: Gynecology

Hydr/o-: Hydrocephalus

Idio-: Self; One's own

Necr/o-: Necrosis

Neo-: Neonate

Oxy-: Oxytocin

Pan-, Pant/o-: Pancytopenia

Chapter 8 Multivariable Methods

Multi-: many or multiple

Variable: Root refers to something that can vary or change

-analysis: the process of examining or analyzing something

Method: systematic procedure or approach

-dimensional: multiple dimensions or aspects

Chapter 9 Nonparametric Tests

dis-: not; opposite of

en-, em-: cause to

pre-: before

-able, -ible: is; can be

-al, -ial: having characteristics of

-ed: past tense verbs; adjectives

-en: made of

Chapter 10 Survival Analysis and Data Visualization

anti-: against

gram: thing written

graph: writing

logy: study of

de-: opposite

Table of Contents

List of Figures xi
List of Tables xiii
Preface xvii

1 Introduction: Biostatistics in Health 1

Introduction 2
1.1. Biostatistics 4
1.1.1. Bio-statistical Issues 4
1.1.2. Extent of Disease in a Group or Region Quantified 4
1.1.3. Rate of Development of a New Disease Estimated 5
1.1.4. Risk Factors or Characteristics That Might Be Related to the Development or Progression of Disease Identified 6
1.1.5. Effectiveness of a New Drug Determined 6
1.1.6. Contradictory Results between Different Studies of the Same Disease 7
1.2. Observational Study Designs 7
1.2.1. The Case Report/Case Series 7
1.2.2. The Cross-Sectional Survey 8
1.2.3. The Cohort Study 8
1.2.4. The Case-Control Study 11
1.2.5. The Nested Case-Control Study 13
1.3. Randomized Study Designs 14
1.3.1. The Randomized Controlled Trial (RCT) or Clinical Trial 14
1.3.2. The Crossover Trial 16
1.4. The Framingham Heart Study 18
1.5. More on Clinical Trials 18
1.6. Significance of Biostatistics in Improving Public Health Services 23
1.6.1. Data Collection Methods 23
1.6.2. Significance of Health Information in Improving Public Health Services 24
1.6.3. Significance of Biostatistics in Clinical Research 24
1.6.4. Six Ways Biostatistics is Transforming Healthcare 25
1.7. The Role of Biostatistics in Public Health 27
1.7.1. Data Collection and Interpretation 27
1.7.2. The National Healthcare Problem 28
1.7.3. Bio-statistical Lessons from the COVID-19 Pandemic 29
1.8. The Evolution and Future of Biostatistics in Public Health 31
1.8.1. Significant Progress Thus Far 31
1.8.2. The Influence of Technology in the Years Ahead 31
Summary 33
References 33

2 Quantifying the Extent of Disease 35

Introduction 35
2.1. Absence of Disease and Infirmity 37

2.1.1. The Biomedical Paradigm in Global Health and Disease 37
2.1.2. Disease (and Condition) Causation 37
2.2. Common Diseases and Conditions 38
2.3. Classification of Diseases and Conditions 40
2.3.1. A Comment on Mental Health/Neurological Diseases and Conditions 41
2.4. Epidemiology 41
2.4.1. Health-Related States or Events 42
2.4.2. Specified Populations 42
2.4.3. Application 42
2.4.4. Uses and Functions of Epidemiology 42
2.4.5. Public Health Surveillance 43
2.4.6. Types of Epidemiology 44
2.5. Disability-Adjusted Life Years 47
2.5.1. Data Needs 47
2.5.2. DALY as a Summary Measure of Population Health 48
2.5.3. Years of Life Lost (YLL), Years Lived with Disability (YLD), and Their Sum, the DALY 49
2.6. Prevalence 50
2.7. Incidence 50
2.7.1. Problems Estimating the Cumulative Incidence 51
2.7.2. Person-Time Data 51
2.7.3. Incidence Rate 52
2.8. Comparing the Extent of Disease Between Groups 54
2.8.1. Difference Measures: Risk Difference and Population Attributable Risk 55
2.8.2. Ratios: Relative Risk, Odds Ratio, and Rate Ratio 56
2.8.3. Issues with Person-Time Data 58
Summary 61
References 61

3 Summarizing Data Collected in the Sample 63

Introduction 64
3.1. Data Collection Methods 66
3.1.1. Choosing a Method of Data Collection 68
3.1.2. Types of Questions 69
3.1.3. Steps in Designing a Questionnaire 70
3.1.4. Methods of Data Organization and Presentation 72
3.2. Why Select a Sample? 83
3.2.1. Simple Random Sampling 84
3.2.2. Convenience Sampling 84
3.2.3. Systematic Sampling 85
3.2.4. Stratified Random Sampling 86
3.2.5. Cluster Sampling 86
3.2.6. Bootstrap Sampling 87
3.3. Types of Variables 87
3.3.1. Frequency Distribution Tables for Dichotomous Variables 88
3.3.2. Frequency Distribution Tables for Categorical Variables 89
3.3.3. Frequency Distribution Tables for Ordinal Variables 89
3.3.4. Descriptive Statistics for Continuous Variables 91
Summary 97
References 97

4 Basic Probability 99

Introduction 99
4.1. Elementary Sets as Events and their Complements 103
4.2. Independent and Disjoint Events 103
4.3. Probability Rules 105
4.3.1. Product (Multiplication) Rule for Independent Events 105
4.3.2. Addition Rule for Mutually Exclusive Events 105
4.4. Permutations and Combinations 107
4.5. Probability Distribution 109
4.6. The Binomial Distribution 114
4.7. The Monty Hall Problem 115
4.8. A Quality Assurance Problem 117
4.9. Improved Diagnostic Accuracy Through Probability-Based Diagnosis 119
4.9.1. Reasons to Refocus Training on Probability 120
4.9.2. Methods to Teach and Inform Probability for Diagnostic Decision-Making 121

Summary 124
References 124

5 Confidence Interval Estimates 127

Introduction 127
5.1. Understanding Estimation 129
5.1.1. Common Sources of Bias 129
5.1.2. Types of Modelling 130
5.1.3. Uses 130
5.1.4. Statistical Modelling 132
5.1.5. Uses of Statistical Modelling 133
5.1.6. Model Frameworks and Validation 134
5.1.7. Presenting Results 134
5.2. Choosing Effect Measures and Computing Estimates of Effect 137
5.2.1. Types of Data and Effect Measures 137
5.2.2. Study Designs and Identifying the Unit of Analysis 139
5.2.3. Extracting Estimates of Effect Directly 140
5.2.4. Dichotomous Outcome Data 142
5.2.5. Continuous Outcome Data 147
5.2.6. Ordinal Outcome Data and Measurement Scales 154
5.2.7. Count and Rate Data 155
5.2.8. Time-to-event Data 156
Summary 160
References 161

6 Hypothesis Testing Procedures 163

Introduction 163
6.1. Hypothesis Testing 166
6.1.1. Steps for Hypothesis Testing 166
6.1.2. Potential Errors 168
6.1.3. Hypothesis Testing Works 169
6.1.4. Null Hypothesis and Alternate Hypothesis 169
6.1.5. Hypothesis Testing Calculation with Examples 170
6.1.6. Steps of Hypothesis Testing 170
6.1.7. Types of Hypothesis Testing 171
6.1.8. Hypothesis Testing and Confidence Intervals 171
6.1.9. Simple and Composite Hypothesis Testing 171
6.1.10. Type 1 and Type 2 Error 172
6.1.11. Level of Significance 173
6.1.12. P-Value 173
6.1.13. Why is Hypothesis Testing Important in Research Methodology? 173
6.1.14. Limitations of Hypothesis Testing 173
6.2. Hypothesis Testing: P Values, Confidence Intervals, and Significance 174
6.2.1. Process of Hypothesis Testing 174
6.2.2. Significance 175
6.2.3. P Values 175
6.2.4. Confidence Intervals 176
6.2.5. Clinical Significance 177
6.2.6. Hypothesis Testing to Improve Patient Outcomes 177
6.3. Chi-Square (X^2) Test 178
6.3.1. The X^2 Distribution 180
6.3.2. X^2 Test As A Test of Goodness of Fit 180
6.3.3. Chi-Square Test for Independence 180
6.4. Reliability of the Estimates 183
6.4.1. Sampling Errors 183
6.4.2. Steps in Testing of Statistical Hypothesis 184
6.4.3. Non-Sampling Errors 185
Summary 191
References 191

7 Power and Sample Size Determination 193

Introduction 194
7.1. Issues in Estimating Sample Size for Confidence Intervals Estimates 196
7.1.1. Sample Size for One Sample, Continuous Outcome 197
7.1.2. Sample Size for One Sample, Dichotomous Outcome 198

7.1.3. Sample Sizes for Two Independent Samples, Continuous Outcome 200
7.1.4. Sample Size for Matched Samples, Continuous Outcome 202
7.1.5. Sample Sizes for Two Independent Samples, Dichotomous Outcome 203
7.2. Issues in Estimating Sample Size for Hypothesis Testing 204
7.2.1. Ensuring That a Test Has High Power 207
7.2.2. Sample Size for One Sample, Continuous Outcome 207
7.2.3. Sample Size for One Sample, Dichotomous Outcome 208
7.2.4. Sample Sizes for Two Independent Samples, Continuous Outcome 209
7.2.5. Sample Size for Matched Samples, Continuous Outcome 211
7.2.6. Sample Sizes for Two Independent Samples, Dichotomous Outcomes 212
Summary 215
References 215

8 Multivariable Methods 217

Introduction 217
8.1. Correlation and Regression 219
8.1.1. Scatter Diagram 219
8.1.2. Correlation 219
8.1.3. Regression 223
8.2. Sensitivity to Outliers, Outlier Rejection, and Robust Regression 228
8.3. Multiple Linear Regression 234
8.3.1. Multiple Linear Regression Formula 235
8.3.2. Assumptions of Multiple Linear Regression 236
8.4. Logistic Regression 236
8.4.1. How Does Multiple Logistic Regression Work? 238
Summary 241
References 241

9 Nonparametric Tests 243

Introduction 244
9.1. Parametric and Nonparametric Tests 246
9.2. Nonparametric Testing 249
9.3. Tests with Two Independent Samples 251
9.4. Tests with Matched Samples 257
9.5. Tests with More than Two Independent Samples 268
Summary 275
References 275

10 Survival Analysis and Data Visualization 277

Introduction 277
10.1. Survival Analysis 279
10.1.1. Survival Data 282
10.1.2. Estimating the Survival Function 283
10.1.3. Issues of Concern 291
10.1.4. Clinical Significance 293
10.2. Data Visualization 293
10.2.1. Design Principles 294
10.2.2. When and How to Use Text, Tables, and Figures 296
10.2.3. Resenting Data and Statistical Results in Tables 301
Summary 316
References 316

Index 319

LIST OF FIGURES

Figure 1.1. The cross-sectional survey
Figure 1.2. The prospective cohort study
Figure 1.3. The retrospective cohort study
Figure 1.4. The case-control study
Figure 1.5. The randomized controlled trial
Figure 1.6. The crossover trial
Figure 1.7. Data collection and interpretation biostatistics in public health
Figure 1.8. Biostatistics scientific, historical data and results
Figure 1.9. Data collection related to immunization and vaccination against smallpox, polio, influenza, SARS-CoV-2 and other viruses
Figure 2.1. Epidemiologic Triad Model. One model shows the agent, host, and environment as having equal influence. The other model shows agent and host as variables dependent on each other and the environment
Figure 2.2. Surveillance information flows from public and health care providers such as clinicians, laboratories, hospitals, and health departments. Feedback flows from health departments back to public and health care providers
Figure 2.3. Course of follow-up for six participants
Figure 3.1. Immunization status of children (Simple Bar Chart)
Figure 3.2. TT Immunization status by marital status of women 15-49 years (Multiple Bar Chart)
Figure 3.3. TT Immunization status by marital status of women 15-49 years (Actual Component Bar Diagram)
Figure 3.4. TT Immunization status by marital status of women 15-49 years (Percentage Component Bar Diagram)
Figure 3.5. Immunization status of children (Pie Chart)
Figure 3.6. Histogram for the amount of time college students devoted to leisure activities
Figure 3.7. Frequency polygon curve on time spent for leisure activities by students
Figure 4.1. Intersection
Figure 4.2. Union
Figure 4.3. Decomposition of AU B into disjoint sets
Figure 4.4. Continuous probability densities
Figure 7.1. Distribution of Under H0: $\mu = 90$
Figure 7.2. Rejection Region for Test H0: $\mu = 90$ versus H1: $\mu \neq 90$ at $\alpha = 0.05$

Figure 7.3. Distribution of Under H0: $\mu = 90$ and Under H1: $\mu = 94$
Figure 7.4. Distribution of Under H0: $\mu = 90$ and Under H1: $\mu = 98$
Figure 8.1. Scatter diagram for ln urea and age
Figure 8.2. Correlation coefficient (r) = +0.9. Positive linear relationship
Figure 8.3. Correlation coefficient (r) = –0.9. Negative linear relationship
Figure 8.4. Correlation coefficient (r) = 0.04. No relationship
Figure 8.5. Correlation coefficient (r) = –0.03. Nonlinear relationship
Figure 8.6. Subgroups in the data resulting in a misleading correlation. All data: r = 0.57; males: r = -0.41; females: r = -0.26
Figure 8.7. Regression line for ln urea and age: ln urea = 0.72 + (0.017 × age)
Figure 8.8. Regression line obtained by minimizing the sums of squares of all of the deviations
Figure 8.9. Total, explained and unexplained deviations for a point
Figure 8.10. Regression line, its 95% confidence interval and the 95% prediction interval for individual patients
Figure 8.11. Scatter diagram with outliers
Figure 8.12. A scatterplot of the votes for Bush versus the votes for Buchanan. Florida presidential votes (all counties).
Figure 8.13. Votes for Gore to votes for Buchanan. Florida presidential votes (all counties).
Figure 8.14. Votes for Nader to votes for Buchanan. Florida presidential votes (all counties).
Figure 8.15. Florida presidential vote (Palm Beach county omitted)
Figure 8.16. Florida presidential vote (Palm Beach county omitted)
Figure 8.17. Multiple linear regression model predictions for individual observations
Figure 9.1. Distribution of symptom severity in total sample
Figure 9.2. Distribution of days in the hospital following transplant
Figure 9.3. Visual pain scales
Figure 9.4. Number of episodes of shortness of breath
Figure 10.1. Participants' experiences in a 10-year study of myocardial infarction
Figure 10.2. Sample survival curve
Figure 10.3. Survival function
Figure 10.4. Kaplan-Meier Survival Curve for Data in Example 10.2
Figure 10.5. Kaplan–Meier survival curve with confidence intervals for data in example 10.2
Figure 10.6. Cumulative incidence curve for data in example 10.2
Figure 10.7. Mean change in pain intensity over 4 weeks
Figure 10.8. Response to treatment by group and time
Figure 10.9. Components of a table
Figure 10.10. Exponential cure rate model with cure rate p = 0.20 and exponential rate parameter $\lambda = 1$

LIST OF TABLES

Table 2.1. Top 20 global health diseases 2019
Table 2.2. Global health disease classifications and some examples
Table 2.3. Men and women with diagnosed CVD
Table 2.4. Smoking and diagnosed CVD
Table 2.5. Men and women who develop CVD
Table 2.6. Total disease-free time in men and women
Table 2.7. Prevalent hypertension and prevalent CVD
Table 2.8. Smoking and cancer
Table 2.9. Summary of key formulas
Table 3.1. Distribution of the data collected
Table 3.2. Overall immunization status of children
Table 3.3. TT immunization by marital status of the women of childbearing age
Table 3.4. Distribution of health professionals by sex and residence
Table 3.5. Frequency distribution table for sex
Table 3.6. Frequency distribution table for treatment with antihypertensive medication
Table 3.7. Treatment with antihypertensive medication in men and women
Table 3.8. Frequency distribution table for marital status
Table 3.9. Frequency distribution for blood pressure category
Table 3.10. Data values for a small sample
Table 3.11. Means and medians of variables in subsample of size n=10
Table 3.12. Ranges of variables in subsample of size n=10
Table 4.1. The probability distribution for the number of heads in three coin tosses
Table 5.1. Results of a two-group randomized trial with a dichotomous outcome
Table 6.1. Possible results for any hypothesis test
Table 6.2. Phenomena of voting preferences
Table 8.1. Age and ln urea for 20 patients attending an accident and emergency unit
Table 8.2. 5% and 1% points for the distribution of the correlation coefficient under the null hypothesis that the population correlation is 0 in a two-tailed test

Table 8.3. Regression parameter estimates, P values, and confidence intervals for the accident and emergency unit data

Table 8.4. Small data set with the fitted values from the regression, the deviations, and their sums of squares

Table 8.5. Analysis of variance for a small data set

Table 8.6. Analysis of variance for the accident and emergency unit data

Table 8.7. 2000 Presidential vote by county in Florida

Table 8.8. Relation of death (a dichotomous outcome) with (a) treatment given (variceal ligation versus sclerotherapy), (b) prior beta-blocker therapy, and (c) both treatment given and prior beta-blocker therapy

Table 8.9. Different methods of representing results of a multivariate logistic analysis: (a) As a table showing regression coefficients and significance levels, (b) as an equation for log (odds) containing regression coefficients for each variable, and (c) as an equation for odds using coefficients (or anti-loge) of regression coefficients (which represents adjusted odds ratios) for each variable

Table 9.1. Assigning ranks

Table 9.2. Assigning ranks

Table 9.3. Assigning ranks

Table 9.4. Repetitive behavior before and after treatment

Table 9.5. Differences in repetitive behavior

Table 9.6. Signs of the differences

Table 9.7. Probabilities based on the binomial distribution model

Table 9.8. Quality of life before and after chemotherapy treatment

Table 9.9. Differences in quality of life before and after chemotherapy treatment

Table 9.10. Signs of the differences

Table 9.11. Repetitive behavior before and after treatment

Table 9.12. Differences in repetitive behavior

Table 9.13. Ranking the absolute values of the differences

Table 9.14. Attaching signs to the ranks

Table 9.15. Systolic blood pressure before and after exercise program

Table 9.16. Differences in systolic blood pressure before and after exercise program

Table 9.17. Ranking the absolute values of the differences

Table 9.18. Attaching signs to the ranks

Table 9.19. Albumin levels in three different diets

Table 9.20. Assigning ranks

Table 9.21. Anaerobic thresholds

Table 9.22. Ordering the anaerobic thresholds

Table 9.23. Assigning ranks

Table 10.1. Year of death or year of last contact

Table 10.2. Number alive, number of deaths, and number censored in each interval
Table 10.3. Constructing the life table—first interval
Table 10.4. Constructing the life table—second interval
Table 10.5. Life table for data in example 10.2
Table 10.6. Life table for data in example 10.2 using the Kaplan–Meier approach
Table 10.7. Standard errors of survival estimate for the data in example 10.2
Table 10.8. Life table with cumulative failure probabilities for data in example 10.2
Table 10.9. Association between BMI categories and incident cardiovascular disease after adjustment for clinical risk factors
Table 10.10. Example of a table shell
Table 10.11. Impact of high intake of grains and incident cardiovascular disease and cancer
Table 10.12. Background characteristics of study participants by intervention group
Table 10.13. Numbers of men and women by BMI category
Table 10.14. Distribution of men and women in normal, overweight, and obese categories of BMI
Table 10.15. Distribution of BMI categories in men and women
Table 10.16. Characteristics of participants at baseline
Table 10.17. Association between racial/ethnic background, maternal age, gestational age, and birth weight
Table 10.18. Association between racial/ethnic background, maternal age, and preterm birth
Table 10.19. Association between moderate to heavy drinking and hypertension

PREFACE

Every year, substantial public and private funding is allocated to research, heavily relying on accurate methodology definition, data analysis, and result interpretation. The current era is characterized by "big data," which refers to enormous datasets from government databases and large healthcare entities using new algorithms and powerful computers. This process requires expertise in modeling, computing, and statistics. One solution that has been proposed to improve access to healthcare services is the use of artificial intelligence (AI). This solution has a wide range of applications, including detecting diseases such as COVID-19 and issuing diagnostic reports. The use of artificial intelligence by healthcare providers also includes the decision-making process regarding surgical procedures, the auditing of medical bills, and the identification of individuals who should be included in chronic patient programs or require closer monitoring. The overarching goal of these applications is to improve services. Because of these developments, it is more important than ever to alter people's perceptions of biostatistics from the beginning of their educational experience. Biostatistics has occasionally been subjected to a negative reputation, which can be partially attributed to the absence of engaging instructional strategies. Even though there have been efforts made to improve statistical education at the primary and secondary levels, there has been a recent surge in the number of studies that address this issue in higher education. Students in healthcare-related fields have been the focus of recent efforts to develop techniques and tools that are engaging for them.

The field of biostatistics is not merely a collection of tools; rather, it is a well-established scientific field in its own right. To perform biostatistical work effectively, one must have a strong understanding of mathematics, probability, and the sources of bias that are the foundation of statistical theory and methods. Additionally, it necessitates the possession of increasingly complex technical skills, including the ability to use computers effectively. It is essential to receive comprehensive training to develop these skills, as well as the understanding that is required to frame problems and navigate the complexities that exist between advanced techniques and real-world health inquiries.

One example that illustrates this point is the shifting perspectives on the risk of cardiovascular disease that is associated with postmenopausal estrogen therapy among women. It is becoming increasingly important for decision-makers and researchers to have expertise in biostatistics because of the advent of big data. This is because more and more people are looking to gain insights from complex datasets.

The purpose of this book is to provide readers with the resources they need to comprehend, interpret, and apply statistical methods to data about health, such as clinical trials, epidemiological studies, and public health research. It aims to improve the reader's capacity to critically evaluate and conduct research in the health sciences by providing clear explanations and practical examples. This will ultimately contribute to evidence-based decision-making and outcomes that are more favorable for health.

Its content bridges the gap between statistical theory and practical application in health sciences, making it indispensable for epidemiologists, public health professionals, and clinicians. The emphasis on cutting-edge statistical methods and their relevance to health research ensures its appeal to a wide audience, from students seeking foundational knowledge to seasoned professionals seeking to stay abreast of the latest advancements. Biostatistics in Health is a vital resource for anyone interested in leveraging statistics to enhance health-related decision-making and advance scientific knowledge in the field.

Chapter

1

INTRODUCTION: BIOSTATISTICS IN HEALTH

Contents

Introduction 2
1.1. Biostatistics 4
1.2. Observational Study Designs 7
1.3. Randomized Study Designs 14
1.4. The Framingham Heart Study 18
1.5. More on Clinical Trials 18
1.6. Significance of Biostatistics in Improving Public Health Services 23
1.7. The Role of Biostatistics in Public Health 27
1.8. The Evolution and Future of Biostatistics in Public Health 31
Summary 33
References 33

Introduction

The study of biostatistics, which comprises a set of methods and ideas that enable us to infer important conclusions from information or data, is essential to public health education and practice. Applying and comprehending bio-statistical applications requires both science and art. Given that we deal with statistics daily, having a proper understanding of them is crucial for both professional and personal relationships.

For instance, the leading cause of death in the US for both men and women is cardiovascular disease. According to the American Heart Association, cardiovascular disease claims the lives of over 2600 Americans every day, or one person every 34 seconds. More than 70 million adult Americans suffer from cardiovascular disease; the yearly incidence rates are estimated to be 7 cases per 1000 for men in the 35–44 age group and 68 cases per 1000 for men in the 85–94 age group. In general, women's rates are approximately ten years behind those of men. Numerous risk factors for cardiovascular disease, such as blood pressure, cholesterol, diabetes, smoking, and weight, have been identified by researchers. In the US, smoking and weight—more especially, being overweight or obese—are regarded as the leading and second-leading preventable causes of death from cardiovascular disease. Significant risk factors for cardiovascular disease also include diet, physical activity, and family history.

Although cardiovascular disease is the focus of the example, statistics about many other illnesses, such as cancer, diabetes, asthma, and arthritis, are also comparable. We get a lot of information about cardiovascular and many other diseases from the Internet, newspapers, and news reports. Every day, reporters write or describe research studies. There is nearly always a report on at least one research study on nightly newscasts. Certain research findings are readily apparent, like the health benefits of exercise, while other studies report on novel drugs that either prevent or treat illness. Contradictory or conflicting findings from medical research can make a topic interesting. A new medical treatment may be beneficial in one study but ineffective in another; similarly, vitamin supplements that were previously thought to be beneficial may turn out to be harmful or ineffective in other studies. A drug may be shown to be beneficial in one study, but years later it may be found to be harmful due to a serious side effect. It takes statistical thinking and an understanding of statistical principles to comprehend and interpret these results.

The essence of biostatistics is the ability to answer questions such as how to quantify the extent of disease in a group or region, estimate the rate of development of new diseases, identify risk factors or characteristics that may be related to the development or progression of diseases, determine the effectiveness of new drugs, and explain contradictory results.

Orientation and Directional Terms

Term	Definition	Illustration
Biostatistics	Biostatistics is a branch of statistics that applies statistical methods to biological topics, including the design, collection, analysis, and interpretation of biological experiments.	
Public health	Public health is the science and art of preventing disease, prolonging life, and promoting health through the efforts of individuals, communities, organizations, and society.	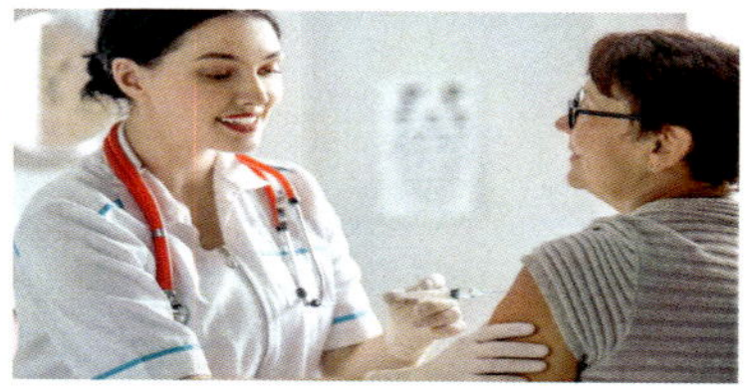
Statistical modelling	Statistical modelling is a data science technique that uses statistical analysis to apply mathematical models to datasets to generate sample data and make predictions.	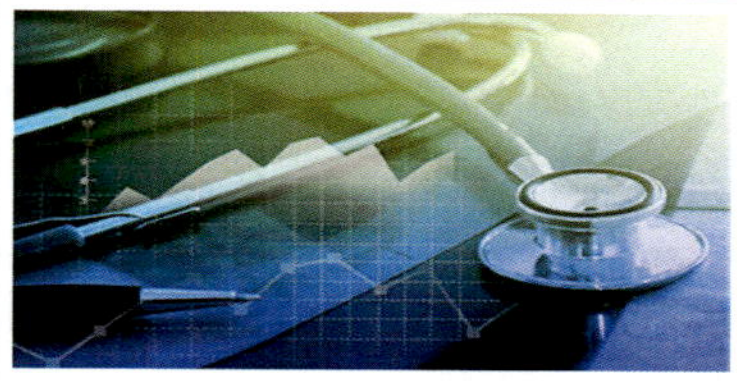
Statistical analysis	Statistical analysis means investigating trends, patterns, and relationships using quantitative data.	
Clinical Trial	Clinical trials are a type of research that studies new tests and treatments and evaluates their effects on human health outcomes.	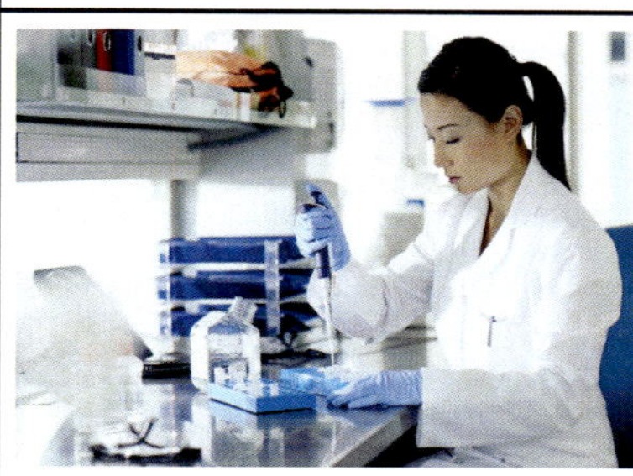

1.1. Biostatistics

The use of statistical concepts in public health, biology, or medicine is known as biostatistics. Applied mathematics forms the foundation of statistical principles, encompassing methods and instruments for gathering data and compiling, evaluating, and interpreting the findings. These guidelines also apply to inferring and drawing conclusions that suitably account for uncertainty.

All of the above questions can be answered with the help of bio-statistical techniques. Making an inference about a particular population is typically the goal of applied biostatistics. Everyone we want to say something about is collectively referred to as this population. Either all adults residing in the United States or all adults residing in Boston could be the population of interest. The goal of the analysis, the investigator's study question, determines the definition of the population. Assume that all adult Americans comprise the population of interest and that we wish to calculate the percentage of adults who have cardiovascular disease. To fully address this question, we would evaluate the prevalence of cardiovascular disease in every adult in the United States. To estimate the desired proportion, a statistical analysis would be a better and more practical approach, as this would be an impossible task.

We examine samples or subsets of the relevant population in biostatistics. In this example, we take a sample of American adults and determine if they have cardiovascular disease or not. The percentage of adults in the sample who have cardiovascular disease should be a good indicator of the percentage of adults in the population who have the same condition if the sample is representative of the population. In biostatistics, conclusions about the population are drawn from sample analysis and sample analysis. This conclusion is fairly sweeping, particularly in the case of a sizable population (e.g., the 300 million people that make up the US population) and the sample size is modest (5000, for instance). When we read about studies or hear news reports, we frequently consider how the findings might relate to us individually. Most of us have never taken part in a research study before. When we or anyone we know has never taken part in a research study, we frequently question whether we should accept the findings.

1.1.1. Bio-statistical Issues

Appropriately conducting and interpreting bio-statistical applications requires attention to many important issues. These include, but are not limited to, the following:

- Clearly defining the objective or research question
- Choosing an appropriate study design (i.e., how data are collected)
- Selecting a representative sample, and ensuring that the sample is of sufficient size
- Carefully collecting and analyzing the data
- Producing appropriate summary measures or statistics
- Generating appropriate measures of effect or association
- Quantifying uncertainty
- Appropriately accounting for relationships among characteristics
- Limiting inferences to the appropriate population

1.1.2. Extent of Disease in a Group or Region Quantified

The best-case scenario is to choose a sample of people from the group or area of interest. For the analysis of the sample to yield sufficiently precise, the sample size must be sufficient. Larger samples are generally better for analysis; that being said, for ethical and budgetary reasons, we should never sample more participants than necessary. Additionally, the sample needs to be typical of the population. For instance, we would prefer the sample to contain roughly 60% women if the population is 60% female. Following the selection of the sample, the disease status of each participant is evaluated. The ratio of the number of sick to the total sample size is used to calculate the percentage of the sample that is diseased. This percentage represents the approximate percentage of the population that is ill. Assume that the sample proportion is determined to be 0.17 (i.e., 17% of individuals surveyed have the illness). We calculate that the percentage of the population that is ill is roughly 0.17, or 17 percent. We must take uncertainty into account because this is an estimate based on a single sample, and the result is what is known as a margin of error. Because of this, we may estimate the percentage of the population that is ill to be between 0.13 and 0.21, or 13 and 21 percent.

This kind of study, known as a cross-sectional study, would probably be carried out at a single point in time. Our assessment of the disease's scope is limited to the study period. Concluding this study regarding the severity of the disease at any time in the future would be inappropriate. It would also be incorrect to assume that the level of disease in other cities or regions of Massachusetts would be comparable to that seen in a sample of Bostonians if we had chosen adults residing in Boston as our population. Estimating the disease burden in a region or group appears to be a simple task at first glance. But there are a lot of problems that make things more difficult. For instance, how do we choose who is included in the sample, where can we find a list of the population, and how can we make sure that particular groups are represented (e.g., women) in the sample, and how do we locate the individuals we designate for the sample and persuade them to take part? All of these issues need to be properly addressed to produce reliable data and accurate conclusions.

1.1.3. Rate of Development of a New Disease Estimated

We require a particular sampling strategy in order to estimate the rate of development of a new disease, such as cardiovascular disease. We would only sample people who were free of cardiovascular disease for this analysis, and we would track them prospectively—that is, going forward in time—to gauge the progression of the illness. The follow-up period is a crucial consideration in these kinds of studies; the researcher must choose whether to monitor participants for the onset of the disease for 1, 5, 10 or any other length of time. It is necessary to track each sample member for ten years to ascertain their disease status if it is of interest to estimate the development of disease over that time. The percentage of cumulative incidence of new disease over the predetermined follow-up period is indicated by the ratio of the number of new cases to the total sample size. Let's say we track each member of our sample for five years and discover that 24.4% of them get sick. Once more, it is usually useful to give a range of reasonable values for the percentage of new cases of illness; this is accomplished by adding a margin of error to account for the accuracy of our estimate. An estimate of the cumulative incidence of disease over 5 years that takes the margin of error into account could range from 1.2 percent to 3.6 percent.

The study of health and illness in human populations, patterns of health or disease, and the variables influencing these patterns are the main topics of epidemiology. An illustration of an epidemiological study is this one.

1.1.4. Risk Factors or Characteristics That Might Be Related to the Development or Progression of Disease Identified

Let's say we have a hypothesis that links a specific exposure or risk factor to the onset of a disease. There exist multiple study designs or methods by which data can be gathered to evaluate the correlation between a putative risk factor and the onset of a disease. The distribution of the risk factor and the outcome in the population of interest determines the most suitable study design, among other factors (e.g., as to the proportion of participants who are likely to have a specific risk factor or not). Every sample member needs to have both the risk factor and the outcome measured, regardless of the exact design that is employed. Should we be intrigued by the correlation between the risk factor and the emergence of illness, we would enlist individuals who were disease-free at the onset of the study and monitor every participant for the emergence of illness. To determine whether a risk factor and the outcome are related, we calculate the percentage (or proportion) of participants who have the risk factor and compare it to the percentage (or proportion) of participants who do not have the risk factor and develop the disease. This comparison can be based on a ratio of proportions or a difference in proportions, among other methods.

Assume 12 percent of individuals with the risk factor and 6 percent of those without it get sick over the course of the follow-up period. Relative risk, defined as the ratio of the proportions, is equal to 0.12 / 0.06 = 2.0 in this case. According to the interpretation, individuals with the risk factor are twice as likely to get sick as those who do not have it. The question then becomes whether this estimate, found in a single study sample, represents a higher risk within the population as a whole. When uncertainty is taken into account, an estimate of the relative risk for those who have the risk factor may be anywhere between one and three times higher. Since a value of 1 indicates no increased risk, the data show an increased risk because the range contains risk values greater than 1.

Understanding the intricate relationships between risk factors is another challenge when evaluating the relationship between a specific risk factor and disease status. Individuals who have the risk factor may differ from those who do not; for instance, they may be older and more likely to have additional risk factors. The impact of the other risk factors can be considered when evaluating the relationship between the proposed risk factor and disease status using certain techniques. These methods make use of statistical modelling.

1.1.5. Effectiveness of a New Drug Determined

From a statistical perspective, the randomized controlled trial, also known as a clinical trial, is the ideal study design. (The word "clinical" denotes that subjects participate in the study. Let's say, for instance, that we wish to evaluate the efficacy of a novel medication intended to reduce cholesterol. The majority of clinical trials have predetermined inclusion and exclusion standards. For instance, since the new drug would probably work best in people with elevated cholesterol, we might want to restrict the sample to those whose total cholesterol is more than 200 or 220. People with a history of cardiovascular disease may also be excluded. We begin the participant recruitment process after deciding on the inclusion and exclusion criteria. Random assignments are made to give each participant a control drug or the new experimental medication. The important aspect of these studies is the randomization component. Theoretically, randomization encourages equilibrium between the comparison groups. A placebo, or inert substance, or the current standard of care—a cholesterol-lowering medication—could be used as the control drug.

The type of disease determines which comparator is most appropriate. For instance, it would be unethical to stop treatment for a life-threatening illness; hence, a placebo comparator would never be suitable. In this case, a placebo might be suitable if the subjects' cholesterol levels were not high enough to require medical attention. Participants are not informed which treatment they are assigned when they are enrolled and randomized to receive the comparator or the experimental treatment. We refer to this as masking or blinding. Following instructions on appropriate dosage, participants' cholesterol levels are measured and compared between groups after a predetermined amount of time. Due to the random assignment of participants to treatment groups, all characteristics of the groups should be comparable, except the treatment received. Should we discover that the cholesterol levels differ amongst groups, the treatment is most likely to blame.

Once more, after taking uncertainty or chance into account, we must interpret the observed difference. A significant difference in cholesterol levels between subjects taking the experimental medication and those receiving the comparator suggests that the experimental medication is working. However, conclusions regarding the drug's impact can only be applied to the population that the participants are selected from—that is, to the population that is defined by the inclusion and exclusion criteria. Clinical trial designs and analyses need to be done with great care.

In the news, clinical trials are a hot topic, especially lately. The Food and Drug Administration (FDA) in the US has strict regulations on them. Studies involving medications that were approved for particular purposes but later taken off the market owing to safety concerns are covered in recent news reports. We go over these studies, evaluate the methodology, and—above all—examine the rationale behind the revaluation. Randomized controlled trials are the gold standard for assessing medications. However, they may spark debate. Studies that don't involve clinical trials are less ideal and frequently involve greater controversy.

1.1.6. Contradictory Results between Different Studies of the Same Disease

Analyzing a sample from the population of interest is the foundation of all statistical research. There are instances when research designs are inadequate, leading to potentially dubious outcomes. Too few participants are enrolled at times, which may produce results that are imprecise or even erroneous. There are also cases where research designs are sound, but two distinct replications yield disparate findings. We shall talk about how and when this could happen throughout the book.

1.2. Observational Study Designs

Numerous designs exist for observational studies. From the most basic to the most intricate, we outline some of the most well-liked designs.

1.2.1. The Case Report/Case Series

A case report is an extremely thorough account of the unique characteristics of a given subject or case. A case series is an organized examination of the intriguing and typical elements found in a short run of cases, or series of cases. Because these kinds of studies have historically helped to identify new diseases, they are significant in the medical field. There is no control or comparison group (e.g., in the case series). A group of individuals free from illness. These studies can be criticized for being unplanned, uncontrolled, and not intended to address a specific research question, despite being reasonably simple to conduct. They are frequently employed to produce targeted hypotheses that are subsequently investigated in more extensive research. Gottlieb et al.'s 1981 publication serves as an illustration of a significant case series., who wrote about five young gay men who went to the doctor for uncommon infections and a rare kind of pneumonia. More series with similar presentations followed the original report, and in 1982 the condition being described was named acquired immune deficiency syndrome (AIDS).

1.2.2. The Cross-Sectional Survey

A cross-sectional survey is done all at once. When the research question is centered on the prevalence of a disease, an existing practice, or an opinion, the cross-sectional survey design is suitable. A group of participants in the non-randomized study are identified at a specific point in time, and data is gathered at that point. For determining the prevalence of a disease at a particular moment in time or of particular risk factors, cross-sectional surveys are helpful. Comparing groups of participants can be interesting in certain situations (e.g., between participants who are under 40 and those who are over 40, between men and women). Nevertheless, conclusions drawn from the cross-sectional survey are restricted to the period of data collection and do not extend to subsequent periods.

Cross-sectional surveys are typically large in size, ethical, and simple to conduct (i.e., involve a large number of participants) to enable the estimation of risk factors, illnesses, behavior or viewpoints in various interest subgroups. Nevertheless, a significant drawback of cross-sectional surveys is that both the emergencies or exposure to a risk factor (e.g., hypertension) and the result has materialized. It is not possible to evaluate temporal relationships, specifically whether the exposure or risk factor occurred before the outcome of interest, because the study is done at a specific point in time (see **Figure 1.1**). Non-response is a further problem. Even though a sizable sample size may be the goal, occasionally only a small percentage of those contacted consent to take part in and finish the survey. The absence of a response may introduce bias or restrict generalizability, contingent on the characteristics of both participants and non-participants.

About one-third of the participants in **Figure 1.1**. have the risk factor, while the other two-thirds do not. In comparison to a much smaller fraction of those without the risk factor, nearly half of those with the risk factor also have the disease.

1.2.3. The Cohort Study

In a cohort study, participants are typically those who initially satisfy a predetermined set of inclusion criteria. A risk factor and a disease are linked while the cohort is being monitored. Enrolling a cohort of people who are free of cardiovascular disease at the beginning of the study is ideal if, for instance, we are researching risk factors for cardiovascular disease. Participants in a prospective cohort study are enrolled and tracked over time. A cohort may be assembled in some circumstances, or it may be drawn from the general population in others. For instance, a cohort selected from the general population will probably contain a sufficient number of people who have and do not have the risk factor of interest when researching the relationship between a relatively common risk factor and an outcome (see **Figure 1.2**).

When studying the relationship between a rare risk factor and a particular outcome, it is important to carefully design the cohort group.

In such cases, researchers may create a cohort that includes individuals with the risk factor, known as a special exposure cohort.

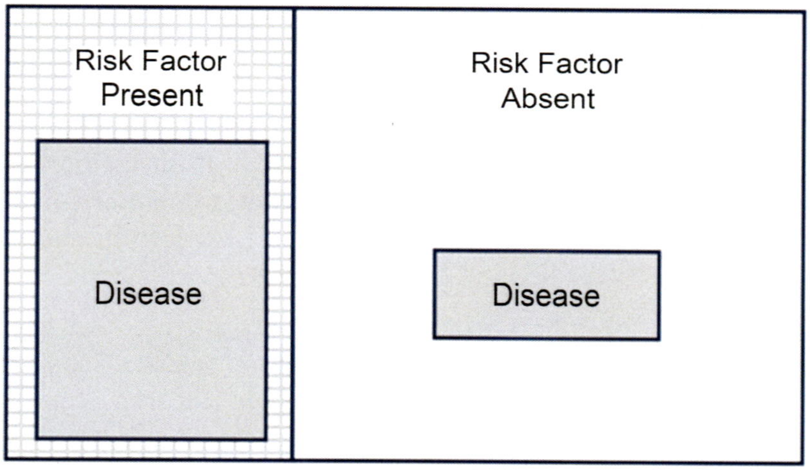

Figure 1.1. *The cross-sectional survey.*

Source: Lisa M. Sullivan, Essentials of Biostatistics in Public Health Third Edition, ISBN 9781284108194.

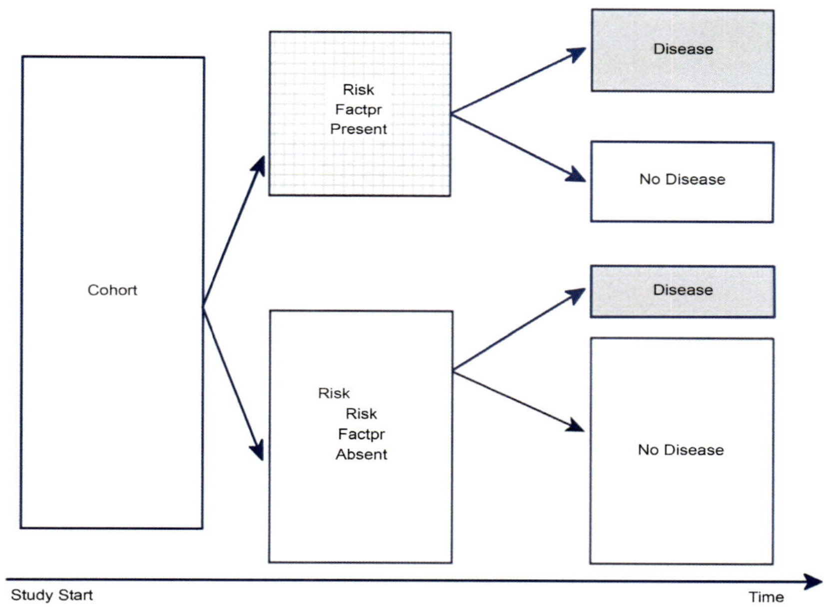

Figure 1.2. *The prospective cohort study.*

Source: Lisa M. Sullivan, Essentials of Biostatistics in Public Health Third Edition, ISBN 9781284108194.

It is also essential to include a comparison cohort consisting of individuals without the risk factor but similar in other important characteristics to the exposed group. In a retrospective cohort study, the participants' exposure or risk factor status is determined by looking back in time. For example, if we want to study the connection between multivitamin use and neural tube defects in new born, we could enrol a group of women who have given birth to healthy babies and ask them to recall their multivitamin usage before pregnancy. Based on this information, we can divide the cohort into exposed and unexposed groups and then analyze the pregnancy outcomes for each woman.

Retrospective cohort studies often rely on data collected from medical records where both risk factors and outcomes have already occurred and been recorded. Researchers conduct a study by reviewing these records to determine the status of the risk factors and outcomes that have already manifested.

The more popular design for cohort studies is the prospective cohort study. One big benefit of cohort studies is that they let researchers evaluate temporal relationships. Additionally, one can calculate a disease's incidence (i.e., the rate at which individuals free of a disease contract that illness). Comparing incidence rates across groups is another option (see **Figure 1.3**).

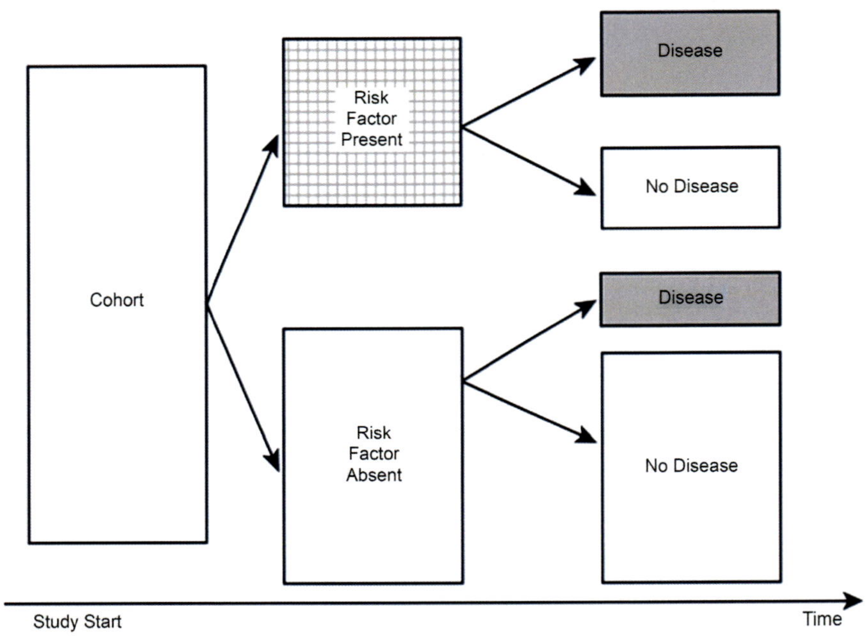

Figure 1.3. *The retrospective cohort study.*

Source: Lisa M. Sullivan, Essentials of Biostatistics in Public Health Third Edition, ISBN 9781284108194.

To quantify the relationship between smoking and cardiovascular disease, we could, for instance, compare the incidence of cardiovascular disease between participants who smoke and participants who do not. If the disease or outcome being studied is uncommon, or if there is a lengthy latency period (i.e., the disease takes a long time to manifest or develop). In cases where the disease is uncommon, it is necessary to have a large enough cohort to ensure a sufficient number of events, or disease cases, are recorded. By "adequate numbers," we specifically mean that there are enough occurrences to allow meaningful statistical analyses to yield precise, stable conclusions. When a disease is being studied that has a lengthy latency period, the study needs to last long enough to capture a sufficient number of events. But for a longer study period, this may lead to another problem: participant follow-up loss.

Confounding is another issue that can complicate cohort studies. Confounding occurs when other characteristics distort how an exposure or risk factor affects the result. Let's say we want to evaluate the link between smoking and cardiovascular disease, for instance. Smokers in our cohort may have a significantly higher risk of cardiovascular disease. It's also possible that smokers have higher cholesterol, are less likely to exercise, and have other health issues. The intricate relationships between the variables need to be balanced through statistical analysis.

1.2.4. The Case-Control Study

When conducting epidemiologic research, the case-control study is frequently employed to investigate the possibility of an association between a specific risk factor or exposure and an outcome. Studies using case-control methodology are especially helpful when the desired outcome is uncommon. Cohort studies, as previously mentioned, are ineffective when the desired outcome is uncommon because a significant number of participants must be enrolled in the study to achieve a sufficient number of outcome events. Participants in a case-control study are identified according to the status of their outcome. To be more precise, we choose a group of cases or individuals with the desired result. Next, we designate a group of controls, which are individuals who are comparable to the cases but devoid of the outcome of interest (see **Figure 1.4**).

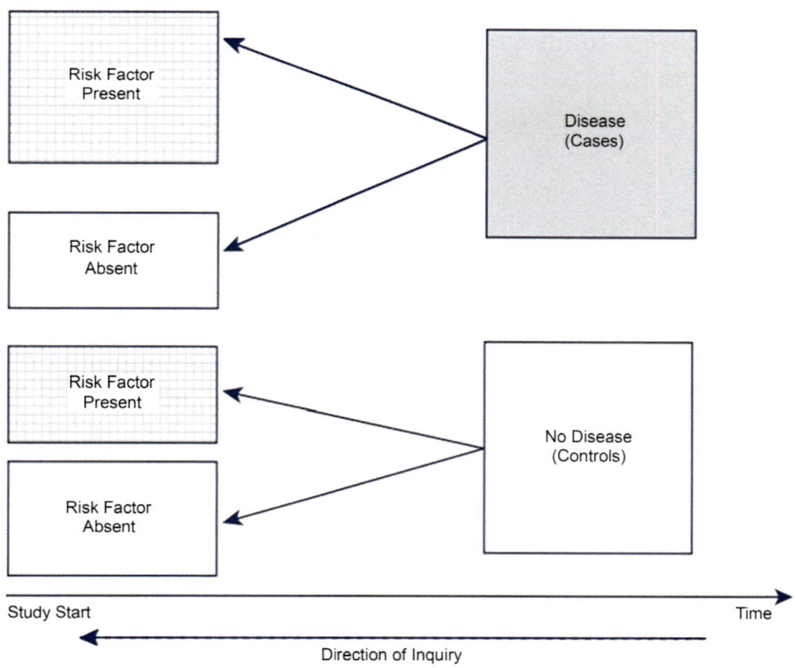

Figure 1.4. *The case-control study.*

Source: Lisa M. Sullivan, Essentials of Bio-statistics in Public Health Third Edition, ISBN 9781284108194.

Next, we evaluate exposure or risk factor status after the fact. We make assumptions about the association between exposure or risk factor status and disease by comparing the proportions of exposure in the cases and controls. This allows us to assess our hypothesis that exposure or risk factor is related to the disease. While creating case control studies, several crucial considerations need to be made. We go over a few of the more significant ones.

First, cases need to be carefully chosen. To identify cases and make them as homogeneous as possible, a clear definition is required. It is necessary to define a case precisely before choosing participants or gathering data. Whenever possible, diagnostic tests to confirm the status of the disease should be included in order to reduce the chance of an incorrect classification.

Care must also be taken when choosing controls. Except not having the relevant disease, the controls ought to be identical to the cases in every way. The controls ought to be participants who were not afflicted with the disease and who, had they been, would have been counted as cases. To verify the controls' lack of disease, the same diagnostic procedures that were utilized to determine the cases' disease status ought to be used on them as well.

It is frequently possible to choose multiple controls for each case, increasing the sample size for analysis, as there are typically far more controls available for inclusion in a study than cases. Researchers have demonstrated that adding more than four controls to a case does not significantly increase the analysis's precision. This outcome will be covered in the chapters that follow. A 2:1 ("two to one") control-to-case ratio is used when there are two controls chosen for each case.

The assessment of exposure or risk factor status is the next concern, and it is carried out after the fact. Studies that can determine risk factor status based on documentation or records are preferred over those that rely on a participant's recollection of past events because the exposure or risk factor may have occurred in the past. Participants are sometimes asked about their status about risk factors even though such data are not recorded. All participants, regardless of their outcome status, must have this done carefully and consistently; exposure and risk factor status assessments must be carried out in accordance with the same protocols or procedures for cases and controls. Furthermore, the person gathering exposure data shouldn't know the participant's outcome status (i.e., they ought to be unaware of the participant's status as a case or a control.

Case-control studies have several advantageous aspects. They are time- and money-effective for researching uncommon illnesses. An investigator can make sure that a sufficient number of cases are included by using case-control studies. Case-control studies are useful for researching diseases with protracted latency periods as well. Researchers are not waiting for the disease to manifest during the study period because the investigation begins after the illness has been diagnosed. When multiple potentially harmful exposures are being considered, case-control studies can be helpful because data can be gathered and assessed for each exposure.

Bias is the primary issue with the case-control study. Although we address some of the more prevalent sources of bias here, there are still additional sources to take into account. When an incorrect outcome status (case or control) or exposure status is classified, it can lead to misclassification bias, which can be problematic in case-control studies. The correlation between the exposure and the result may be weakened (underestimated) if misclassification happens at random, that if both groups misclassify to a comparable degree. The association may be overstated (overestimated) if misclassification is not random, such as when more cases are mistakenly identified as having the exposure or risk factor. Selection bias is another type of bias that can lead to an under- or over-estimation of the true association between exposure and outcome status as a result of how cases and controls are chosen. In particular, people who opted to participate in the study may have a different relationship between exposure status and disease than people who did not. Recall bias is an additional source of bias that can distort the relationship between exposure and outcome. When cases or controls remember exposure status differently, it happens. People who are ill (cases) remember previous exposures more vividly than people who are well. The latter may not be able to recall the same details as easily. Furthermore, it is not always possible to determine a temporal relationship between exposure and outcome in case-control studies. For instance, in the current example, measurements are made of the exposure and the result at the time of data collection. In case-control studies, the method of participant selection (based on their outcome status) precludes us from estimating incidence (i.e., the speed at which an illness spreads).

1.2.5. The Nested Case-Control Study

One particular kind of case-control study typically derived from a cohort study is the nested case-control study. Let's take an example where a cohort study with a sample size of 1000 people is conducted to determine whether smoking is associated with cardiovascular disease. Assume that 20 study participants experience myocardial infarction (MI, i.e., heart attack), and we're curious to see if body mass index (defined as the weight in kilograms divided by the square of the height in meters) and MI are related. Evaluating the association between body mass index and MI would be challenging due to the small number of participants experiencing this specific outcome and the numerous confounding variables that would need to be considered. Large samples are typically needed for this process. To choose appropriate controls for the 20 cases that are comparable to the cases but do not have MI, a nested case-control study could be created. We would carefully choose the controls and possibly match them to cases based on gender, age, and other risk factors—like blood pressure and cholesterol—that are known to affect MI to facilitate the analysis. Confounding can be managed, for example, by matching. The relationship between body mass index and MI would then be the primary focus of the analysis. Nested case-control studies are also employed in the evaluation of costly tests or technologies, as well as in the assessment of novel biomarkers—measures of biological processes. Let's take an example where a sizable cohort study is conducted to evaluate risk factors for unplanned preterm birth. Pregnant women fill out self-administered questionnaires covering demographic, medical, and behavioural data as part of the study. Furthermore, at around 13 weeks of pregnancy, each woman provides a blood sample, which is frozen and kept. Every woman is tracked throughout her pregnancy to determine whether or not she had a spontaneous preterm delivery (e.g., as term delivery, induced preterm delivery, etc.). A novel test is created to quantify a hormone thought to be connected to spontaneous preterm birth in the mother's blood. Women who give birth prematurely and spontaneously (cases) are matched to women who do not (controls) based on maternal age, race/ethnicity, and previous history of preterm delivery in a nested case-control study. Every instance and control are measured for the hormone using the newly developed test on serum samples that have been stored (not frozen). The analysis focuses on the relationship between hormone levels and spontaneous preterm delivery. The nested case-control study is a useful method in this case to assess whether the risk factor (i.e., hormone) is connected to the result (i.e., an unexpected preterm birth). To save costs, the new test is only administered to the women who are chosen for the nested case-control study, not to all of the women enrolled in the cohort. (Altman et al., 1982) (DerSimonian et al., 1982)

1.3. Randomized Study Designs

Studies using cohort and case-control data frequently ask whether there is a link between an exposure or risk factor and a particular result (e.g., an illness). Every one of these observational research designs has benefits and drawbacks. While in the case-control study we compare exposure between individuals with and without a disease, in the cohort studies we compare incidence between the exposed and unexposed groups. Although these are distinct comparisons, we conclude relationships in both cases. As we have discussed, bias and confounding can occur in observational studies. Randomized studies, on the other hand, are regarded as the best study designs because they reduce bias and confounding. The random assignment of participants to the comparison groups is a fundamental characteristic of randomized studies. Theoretically, randomization equalizes the groups in every way save participant treatment (e.g., treated with a placebo, an experimental drug, or neither, and whether or not to receive behavioural treatment therapy). We go into great detail about two common randomized designs.

1.3.1. The Randomized Controlled Trial (RCT) or Clinical Trial

The randomization of participants to one of several comparison treatments or groups is a crucial and unique characteristic of the randomized controlled trial (RCT) design. Two comparison groups are frequently used in pharmaceutical trials; one group receives an experimental drug, while the other receives a control drug. A placebo could be used as the control if it is morally possible. If it is not possible to use a placebo (e.g., Since the participants require medication, it is unethical to use a placebo; instead, a drug that is currently on the market and regarded as the standard of care would be a suitable comparator. Unlike a placebo-controlled trial, this is referred to as an active-controlled trial. Data for clinical trials are gathered in advance.

Randomization aims to create groups with balanced prognostic factors to minimize confounding and ensure that the comparison groups differ only in the treatment they receive. This feature allows for stronger inferences to be made in randomized studies compared to observational studies. In clinical trials, conclusions can be drawn about the effects of treatments on outcomes, while observational studies are limited to identifying associations between risk factors and outcomes.

Concurrent evaluation of the comparison treatments is crucial in clinical trials. The treatments are given simultaneously in the study shown in **Figure 1.5**, creating parallel comparison groups. Think about a clinical study assessing a novel allergy treatment. Since allergies are highly dependent on the season, we may observe very different outcomes if the experimental treatment is given in the spring and the control is given in the winter.

Several study centers should be involved in clinical trials as well; these are known as multi-center trials. To encourage generalizability, several centers are included. There can be doubts about whether other centers would experience the same benefit if a clinical trial is carried out in one and the experimental treatment is proven to be successful. The homogeneity of the effect across centers in multicenter trials can be examined directly.

Ideally, clinical trials should be conducted in a double-blind manner, meaning that both the investigator and the participant are unaware of the treatment assignment. However, there are instances where blinding participants is not feasible or ethical, such as in trials comparing medical and surgical procedures. In such cases, the participant will inevitably know whether they received a surgical intervention. While sham surgeries are occasionally used in rare situations, participant safety is always a top priority, making these practices uncommon. Nevertheless, the outcome assessor must remain blinded to the treatment assignment.

Randomization of clinical trial participants can be done in a variety of ways. By simply flipping a coin, each participant is assigned to either the experimental or control treatment based on the outcome of the coin toss. This is known as simple randomization. Different randomization schedules are typically created for each center in multi-center trials. This prevents the possibility that all patients in one center receive the same treatment and guarantees a balance in the treatments offered within each center.

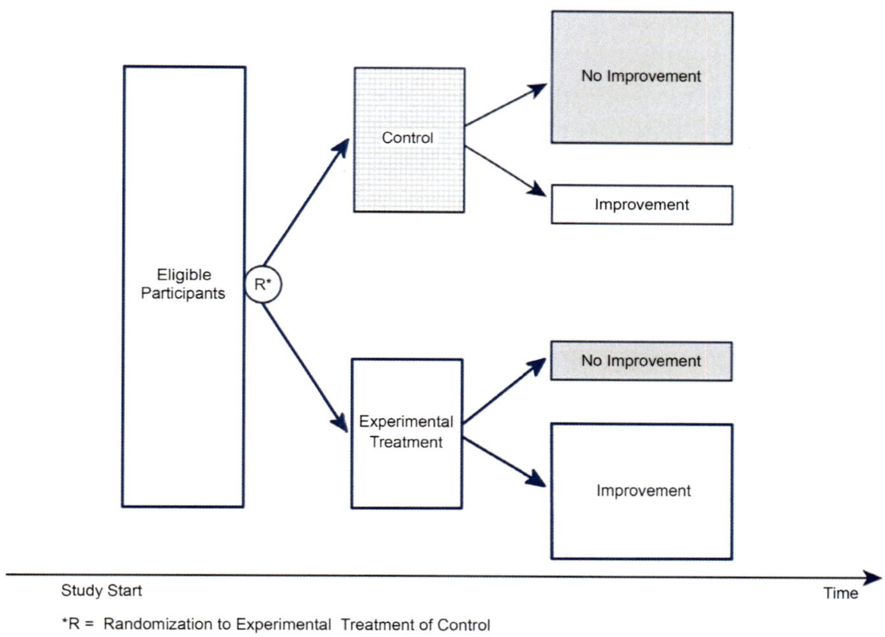

Figure 1.5. *The randomized controlled trial.*

Source: Lisa M. Sullivan, Essentials of Bio-statistics in Public Health Third Edition, ISBN 9781284108194.

Minimizing the disparity in other characteristics between groups can be crucial at times. Let's say, for instance, that we want to guarantee that each comparison group contains participants of a comparable age. Within each center, we could create distinct or stratified randomization schedules for participants under 40 and participants 40 years of age and above. Randomization can be carried out in a variety of ways, and the best method relies on several variables, such as the number of participating centers, the correlation between significant prognostic factors and the outcome, and so forth.

The primary benefit of the clinical trial is that, from an analytical perspective, its design is the cleanest. As randomization reduces bias and confounding, any observed benefit (or harm) can be ascribed to the treatment, in theory. Clinical trials, however, can be highly costly and time-consuming. Numerous participants are needed in clinical trials with outcomes that are considered relatively uncommon to show a meaningful impact. This extends the trial's duration and raises its cost. Clinical trials frequently present a variety of difficulties that must be overcome. First, there may be ethical difficulties with clinical trials. Ethical considerations must be carefully considered when selecting a control group. For instance, using a placebo comparator in cancer trials would never be feasible due to the unnecessary risk this would pose to the participants. Secondly, setting up clinical trials can be challenging. It can be challenging to find centers and participants. People may refuse to take part in a trial, for instance, if they find it intolerable that they could be assigned at random to the control group. Another essential component of clinical trials is the careful observation of participants. For instance, researchers need to confirm that participants are taking the prescribed medication as directed and are not taking any other medications (referred to as concurrent medications) that could conflict with the study medications. For example, participants in most clinical trials must be followed up with every two weeks for twelve weeks. Investigators must minimize follow-up data loss to guarantee the collection of crucial study data at every stage of the investigation. A clinical trial's ability to retain participants and ensure they follow the instructions is crucial to its success. Some clinical trials have strict criteria for who can participate, excluding certain individuals based on specific factors. For instance, when testing a new medication for lowering cholesterol, only those with extremely high cholesterol levels may be allowed to participate to ensure the best chance of proving its effectiveness. However, this may limit the ability to generalize the results to a broader population. Critics often argue that clinical trials are too narrow and restrictive, and investigators must carefully consider the balance between these criteria and the overall impact on the results and their applicability.

Clinical trial design can be extremely difficult. Many issues require careful consideration, such as crafting a clear, concise, and answerable study objective; selecting the right participants for the trial (explicitly defining inclusion and exclusion criteria); choosing the right outcome variable; selecting the right control group; creating and carrying out a stringent monitoring plan; figuring out how many participants to enrol, and specifying the randomization plan. Even though reaching these objectives is difficult, a well-conducted randomized clinical trial is thought to be the most reliable way to determine whether a medical intervention is effective.

1.3.2. The Crossover Trial

In a crossover trial, each participant receives two or more treatments one after the other sequentially. In cases where two treatments (e.g., an experimental group, and a control group), every participant gets both. For instance, randomly assigned participants are divided into two groups: half receive the experimental treatment first, followed by the control, and the other half receive the experimental treatment first, followed by the control. Results are evaluated after each participant receives a course of treatment. In Period 1, participants receive the treatment that is assigned at random. After that, the desired result for the Period 1 treatment is noted. There is typically a "wash-out" period following a crossover trial during which no treatments are administered. To eliminate any potential therapeutic effects of the first treatment before the second treatment is administered in Period 2, a wash-out period is included. Participants who received the control treatment in Period 1 and vice versa receive the experimental treatment in Period 2 of a trial with an experimental and a control treatment (see **Figure 1.6**).

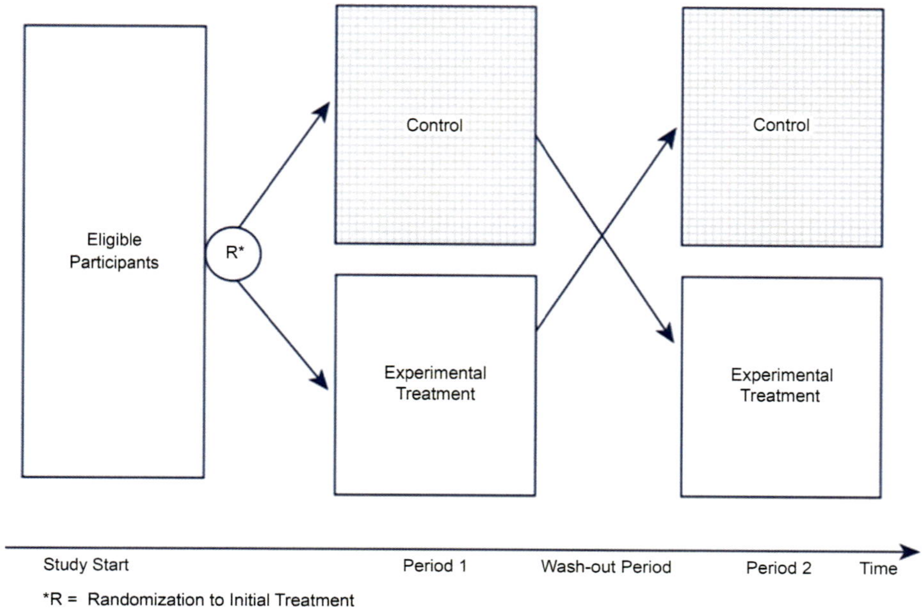

Figure 1.6. *The crossover trial.*

Source: Lisa M. Sullivan, Essentials of Bio-statistics in Public Health Third Edition, ISBN 9781284108194.

In a crossover trial, participants can be assigned to treatments in a variety of ways. The two most widely used strategies are fixed assignment and random assignment. In Period 1, participants are assigned to either the experimental treatment or the control according to the previously mentioned random assignment scheme. In Period 2, participants are then given the other treatment. Every participant in a fixed assignment strategy receives the same treatment regimen. For instance, everyone receives the control treatment after receiving the experimental treatment, or vice versa. The fixed scheme has a drawback in that it requires investigators to assume that the results of the second treatment—and any further treatment if there are any—would be comparable to the results of the treatment given first (i.e., that there are no residual consequences). The researchers can determine whether there is an order effect by arbitrarily switching up the order in which the treatments are administered.

The crossover trial's main benefit is that each participant assumes the role of their control, so we don't have to worry about treatment groups' comparability in terms of baseline characteristics. It takes fewer participants in this study design to show an effect. The possibility of carry-over effects, whereby the first treatment has an impact on the outcome evaluated after the second treatment, is a drawback. Investigators need to take extra care to incorporate a wash-out period that is long enough to reduce carry-over effects. The benefit of the crossover may be nullified if a participant in Period 2 is not at the same baseline as they were in Period 1. Period 1 data may be the only relevant data in this case. The wash-out period must be sufficiently brief to maintain participants' commitment to finishing the trial. A crossover trial's requirement that participants receive every treatment makes the loss to follow-up or dropout crucial since it results in the loss of outcome data for both treatments when one participant leaves.

For the short-term treatment of chronic, relatively stable conditions, crossover trials are most appropriate. For illnesses that experience sudden flare-ups, a crossover trial would not be effective because these events may affect observed outcomes without having any bearing on treatment. Additionally, studies where death or another serious condition is considered the outcome are not appropriate candidates for crossover trials.

Adherence or compliance to the study protocol and study medication is crucial in the crossover trial, just like in the previously mentioned clinical trial. In unpleasant treatments or trials with lengthy or challenging protocols, participants are more likely to stop taking their medications or withdraw from the study. The investigators have to exert every effort to maximize adherence and minimize follow-up loss.

1.4. The Framingham Heart Study

Now, let us discuss one of the most well-known studies of cardiovascular disease risk factors in the world. In 1948, a cohort of slightly more than 5,000 residents of the Massachusetts town of Framingham who were free of cardiovascular disease were enrolled in the Framingham Heart Study. The Framingham Heart Study is a longitudinal cohort study in which participants are reassessed roughly every two years. In 1998, the study commemorated its 50th anniversary is still ongoing. The initial group has undergone more than thirty evaluations. Every assessment involves a thorough physical examination (e.g., participants undergo echocardiograms in addition to other evaluations of cardiovascular functioning, and blood samples are drawn to measure lipid levels and novel risk factors (e.g., vital signs, blood pressure, medication history). The second generation of the original cohort, known as the Framingham Offspring cohort, was made up of about 5000 offspring of the original cohort and their spouses who were enrolled in the early 1970s. These individuals have undergone over nine assessments and have been monitored roughly every four years. A third generation of more than 4,000 participants was enrolled in the early 2000s and is being followed roughly every four years.

Numerous studies from the Framingham Heart Study have been published over the past 50 years, highlighting key risk factors for cardiovascular disease, including diabetes, high blood pressure, cholesterol, smoking, and physical inactivity. Peripheral artery disease, heart failure, and stroke risk factors were also discovered by the Framingham Heart Study. Using data from the Framingham Study spanning three generations, researchers have identified psychosocial risk factors for heart disease. Currently, they are evaluating genetic risk factors for diabetes, obesity, and cardiovascular disease. (DerSimonian et al., 1982; Freiman et al., 1978).

1.5. More on Clinical Trials

Clinical trials are very significant, especially for health-related research described clinical trials from the perspective of their design, but many more facets of clinical trials need to be covered. First and foremost, clinical trials need to be carried out at the appropriate point in history. A clinical trial where some children receive the vaccine and others do not could be started to test the hypothesis, for instance, if the research question is: Is the polio vaccine still necessary today? Withholding the vaccine from some children would be unethical, making the trial impractical today. Nobody would put themselves in danger to investigate if a vaccine is required.

The design of a clinical trial is crucial to guaranteeing the validity and generalizability of the findings, as was previously mentioned. Clinical trials with sound design are relatively simple to analyze, while those with poor design are very challenging, sometimes even impossible. Here is a list of the things to keep in mind when planning clinical trials. Though they have been mentioned before, some are still important to mention.

1. ***The number of treatments involved:*** Statistical analyses are simple when two treatments are involved because only one comparison needs to be made. More complex statistical analyses and attention to the multiple comparison problem are necessary when more than two treatments are involved. Clinical criteria should always determine the number of treatments included in a clinical trial; this number should never be lowered to facilitate statistical analysis.
2. ***The control treatment:*** A control treatment and an experimental (or recently developed) treatment are compared in clinical trials. A placebo may be used as the control treatment, or it may be an existing treatment that is regarded as the standard of care. It is unethical to give patients a placebo when a conventional treatment is readily available, so if one exists, it should be used as the control. (A control group may not always be available, even though clinical trials are the gold standard method for assessing an experimental treatment's efficacy.
3. ***Outcome measures:*** Identifying the desired outcome or outcomes of interest is imperative during the clinical trial's design phase. The planned analysis's primary outcome serves as a guide for calculating the trial's necessary sample size. The main result is typically more objective than subjective. It is appropriate to identify secondary outcomes, and findings that are derived from them ought to be acknowledged as such. Secondary outcome analyses can yield valuable insights and, in certain situations, sufficient proof for a re-examination where the secondary outcomes are elevated to primary status.
4. ***Blinding:*** When patients are blinded, it means they are not aware of the type of treatment they are receiving in a clinical trial—experimental or control. In a single-blind trial, the patient is blind to the treatment they are receiving, but the investigator is aware of it. When neither the patient nor the researcher is aware of which treatment is being assigned, this is referred to as double blinding. In numerous clinical trials, the treatment assigned to each patient is kept a secret by the statistician alone.
5. ***Single-center versus multi-center trials:*** While some clinical trials are carried out at a single location or clinical center, others are carried out—typically concurrently—at multiple locations. Including multiple centers has benefits, including greater generalizability and a larger pool of potential patients. Incorporating

multiple centers has drawbacks as well, including increased resource requirements for trial management and the introduction of center-specific features (e.g., factors that might have an impact on the results that are seen, such as participant characteristics, staff experience, and the availability or state of medical equipment.

6. ***Randomization:*** One essential element of clinical trials is randomization. Several randomization techniques could be used in a particular trial. The specifics of the study protocol will determine the best course of action.

7. ***Sample size:*** The variance in the primary outcome and the anticipated difference in outcomes between the treated and control patients determine how many patients are needed for a clinical trial.

8. ***Population and sampling:*** The investigators of the study should clearly define the study population (patient inclusion and exclusion criteria). Carefully determining a patient recruitment strategy and developing and implementing a system to verify inclusion and exclusion criteria for every prospective enrolee is essential.

9. ***Ethics:*** The design and execution of clinical trials are frequently influenced by ethical considerations. While certain ethical concerns, like the safety of treatment, are universal across all trials, others pertain specifically to individual studies. Institutional review boards (IRBs) are typically tasked with reviewing and approving research protocols, assessing their scientific validity, and weighing the potential risks and advantages for participants. Informed consent, typically granted via IRB-approved forms, is a key requirement for all clinical trial participants.

10. ***Protocols:*** Every clinical trial needs to have a protocol, which is a detailed operational manual that outlines all trial-related details. Every facet of subject enrolment, treatment assignment, data collection, monitoring, data management, and statistical analysis is covered in detail by the protocol. The protocol guarantees uniformity in the trial's execution and is especially crucial when multiple clinical centers (i.e., in a multi-center experiment).

11. ***Monitoring:*** A crucial component of every clinical trial is monitoring. In particular, participants' compliance with every facet of the study protocol, including e. g. completing study assessments, going to all planned appointments, and taking any recommended drugs or treatments). Additionally, participants are closely watched for any negative outcomes or side effects. breach of protocol (e.g., skipping planned appointments) and the frequency of negative outcomes and side effects are compiled at the end of a trial.

12. ***Data management:*** Effective data management is essential to any research project, but it's especially crucial for clinical trials. Data management comprises data entry, quality control (checking data for anomalies or out-of-range values), data cleaning, analytic database construction, and subject tracking (making sure subjects finish every part of the trial on time). The majority of studies designate a data manager to oversee every facet of data management.

    The statistical analysis in a well-designed clinical trial is straightforward. Assuming there are two treatments involved (an experimental treatment and a control), there are essentially three phases of analysis:

- Baseline comparisons, in which the participants assigned to the experimental treatment group are compared to the patients assigned to the control group concerning relevant characteristics measured at baseline. These analyses are used to check that the randomization is successful in generating balanced groups.
- Crude analysis, in which outcomes are compared between patients assigned to the experimental and control treatments. In the case of a continuous outcome (e.g., weight), the difference in means is estimated; in the case of a dichotomous outcome (e.g., development of disease or not), relative risks are estimated; and in the case of time-to-event data (e.g., time to a heart attack), survival curves are estimated.
- Adjusted analyses are then performed, similar to the crude analysis, which incorporates important covariates (i.e., variables that are associated with the outcome) and confounding variables.

When statistically analyzing data from clinical trials, various analytical samples are taken into account. The Intent to Treat (ITT) analysis sample is the first. All of the randomized patients are included in it. Only patients who finished the course of treatment are included in the second sample, which is the Per Protocol analysis sample (i.e., adhered to the prescribed course of treatment). The third sample, known as the Safety analysis sample, consists of all patients who, despite not following the prescribed course of treatment, took at least one dose of the prescribed medication. A clinical trial's planning, execution, and analysis should all be thoroughly documented. Exact and comprehensive documentation of the clinical trial is necessary for submissions to the Food and Drug Administration (FDA).

Safety and efficacy are the main concerns of clinical trials. The kind and severity of unfavorable incidents and side effects are used to evaluate safety. Adverse events may arise from the drug under evaluation, or they may not. Clinicians in most clinical trials indicate whether or not the adverse event is most likely caused by the drug. Improvements in symptoms or other aspects of the indication or disease that the medication is intended to treat are used to gauge an efficacious treatment.

Clinical trials go through several crucial phases. Preclinical investigations examine an agent's safety and effectiveness in animals. Studies on human safety and efficacy are known as clinical studies. Clinical studies are divided into three stages, which are explained here.

13. ***Phase I: First Time in Humans Study:*** A Phase I study's primary goals are to evaluate the treatment's pharmacokinetics—the rate at which a drug enters, passes through, and is secreted from the body—as well as its toxicology and safety about

humans. Safety is usually the main focus of phase I studies rather than efficacy, or how well a treatment works. To evaluate side effects and adverse events, Phase I studies typically involve 10 to 15 patients. Many of these studies are conducted on healthy, normal volunteers. Finding the maximum tolerated dose (MTD) of the suggested medication in humans is one of the objectives of Phase I studies. Researchers begin using extremely low doses and gradually increase them. Typically, investigations begin with three patients, and for every increased dosage, three more patients are added. To evaluate safety, information is gathered at every stage, and some Phase I studies are placebo-controlled. Typically, two or three distinct Phase I studies are carried out.

14. ***Phase II: Feasibility or Dose-Finding Study:*** While safety is still the main focus of a Phase II study, side effects and adverse events—which may or may not be directly related to the drug—are of greater significance. Efficacy is another goal of the Phase II study; however, the efficacy of the medication is determined by descriptive analyses conducted during the Phase II study. Sometimes, researchers are unsure of the precise features of the indication or illness that the medication may impact, nor which outcome measure best reflects this impact. Typically, investigators assess a range of results to identify the optimal result for the subsequent stage. In Phase II trials, researchers ascertain the ideal medication dosage in terms of effectiveness (e.g., smaller dosages might work just as well as the MTD). Phase II studies typically comprise 50–100 patients with the relevant indication or illness. Phase II trials typically compare a standard, commercially available treatment to a placebo-controlled alternative. Studies are typically double-blind and involve randomized subjects. Research returns to Phase I if a Phase II study finds that the medication is safe but ineffective. Based on observed safety and efficacy, the majority of Phase II studies continue on to Phase III.

15. ***Phase III: Confirmatory Clinical Trial:*** The Phase III trial's primary objective is efficacy, but safety monitoring data is also being gathered. Phase III trials are planned and carried out in order to validate the effectiveness of the experimental intervention. An experimental treatment at the established optimal dose and a placebo, or standard of care, are typically used in phase III trials. Three groups are involved in some Phase III trials: standard of care, experimental treatment, and placebo. 200–500 patients may be included in a sample, depending on what is deemed to be a clinically meaningful effect. (Specific calculations, determine the precise figure. Phase III studies must include at least two successful clinical trials conducted by independent researchers at various clinical centers in order to determine whether the treatment's impact can be replicated in at least two distinct participant sets by independent researchers. You can read more about clinical trial design and analysis in Chow and Liu.

To submit a drug approval application to the FDA, researchers must have at least two independent trials with positive results (statistically proven efficacy). In addition, the FDA mandates that two trials have clinical significance, which is defined by clinical investigators during the design stage when subject count is decided.

Results of Phase I, II, and III studies are summarized in the FDA New Drug Application (NDA). Within six months to a year of submission, the FDA reviews an NDA and decides whether to approve it or not. After a drug is approved, the sponsor may carry out post-marketing or Phase IV trials, which can be retrospective (e.g., based on an analysis of medical records) or future (e.g., a large-scale clinical trial to investigate uncommon adverse events). These investigations are frequently carried out to comprehend the drug's long-term effects (safety and efficacy).

1.6. Significance of Biostatistics in Improving Public Health Services

The analysis, interpretation, and conversion of unprocessed research data into usable form is aided by biostatistics. Clinical trials, biomedical research, and biological field studies all depend on them. It assists in tracking its anticipated growth, improving healthcare, and making wise decisions. Establishing a clinical research framework, managing and analyzing data, conducting clinical trials, conducting epidemiological studies, and enhancing patient care are all facilitated by it. The WHO estimates that COVID-19 causes more than 14.9 million deaths worldwide, and numerous public health campaigns have been put in place to stop its spread. Having a certificate in applied biostatistics program will enable you to apply statistical principles to the analysis of research and scientific data, thereby contributing to the resolution of important scientific inquiries. Gain the ability to handle, comprehend, and present the findings of statistical analysis done on scientific data.

Biostatistics helps analyze, interpret, and convert raw research data suitable for practical applications. Statistical analysis and interpretation of results are essential in the following:

- Clinical trials in healthcare
- Biomedical research and biological field studies

It would be ideal if you worked together with the biomedical and biological research team, public health officials, and researchers to create new methods for data analysis and interpretation as well as to design studies, create policies, and train researchers. It has a major impact on developments in biomedical science and public health. Your ability to apply statistical concepts to important scientific questions will improve with an applied biostatistics certificate program. Use a variety of instruments and methods to analyze research and scientific data. Gain the ability to handle, comprehend, and present the findings of statistical analysis done on scientific data. The impact of public and global health initiatives is measured and monitored by biostatisticians. You develop, look into, and compile data from observational studies and clinical trials in collaboration with teams from a variety of fields. You support decisions made to advance well-being, enhance patient care, and raise people's quality of life everywhere by assisting scientists in the analysis and distinction of data.

Understanding the science and statistical principles is essential as it:

- Improves the decision-making process.
- Effectiveness of providing healthcare support.
- Help track the projected growth of healthcare.

1.6.1. Data Collection Methods

Surveys, medical records, surveillance, disease registers, and peer-reviewed literature are various sources that provide health data.

- Medical records provide information on diagnoses, lab tests, doctor appointments, etc.
- Peer-review literature contains data collected using various methods like survey questionnaires and interviews. It provides data on healthcare services utilized by individuals, specific needs, development, and demographics.
- Surveillance is the systematic process of collecting data by the Center for Disease Control and Prevention (CDC), the National Center for Emerging and Zoonotic Infectious Diseases (NCEZID), and the World Health Organization (WHO).
- Diseases registers of government agencies and hospitals have information about people with specific conditions or infectious diseases.

1.6.2. Significance of Health Information in Improving Public Health Services

The collected data helps in developing initiatives, identifying obstacles, and framing policies.

- It helps evaluate the impact of treatment by analyzing the trends with patient follow-ups after surgery, vaccination rates, and improvement in meeting health standards.
- Identify risks and communities that need health care support.
- Identify obstacles in healthcare delivery by getting patient insights.
- Modify policies based on studies.

1.6.3. Significance of Biostatistics in Clinical Research

Clinical researchers can use it to evaluate and comprehend data that has been gathered. Clinical research benefits from biostatistics in several ways.

1.6.3.1. Setting up Clinical Research Frameworks

You assist the development team by giving them the resources they need to set up the study, create objectives, and create techniques for data analysis to enhance the outcome. You assist in selecting an appropriate sample size. The study's sample size is crucial because too small a sample will yield insufficient data, and too large a sample will waste resources.

1.6.3.2. Data Monitoring and Management

Biostatistics aids in the development of data management plans and pinpoints areas of weakness to enhance the caliber of data collection and analysis techniques. It offers concise and insightful data to aid in decision-making.

1.6.3.3. Data Analysis and Reporting

You design and specify the necessary statistical procedures, statistical methodology, kind of analysis, and visual aids following data collection. It links statistics and data from the life sciences and aids in the analysis and interpretation of clinical and health-related data.

1.6.3.4. Clinical Trials

Clinical trials are carried out to assess the efficacy of novel therapies and diagnostic tools. To gather reliable data, you design clinical trials, analyze the data, and compile the findings. Clinical trials aid in the analysis of therapeutic interventions and the creation of potent medications and vaccines that stop the spread of illness.

1.6.3.5. Epidemiological Studies

Data analysis helps the field progress, which is important for creating public health policies. It investigates the relationship between the illness's cause, effects, and contributing variables. It enables scientists to sharpen their focus and get rid of potential hazards.

1.6.3.6. Improving Patient Care

Data analysis reduces the risk of ineffective treatment and patient care while increasing the efficiency of healthcare systems to enhance patient care and treatment outcomes.

1.6.3.7. Trends in Data

In biostatistics, you must analyze previously gathered data from several studies; you do not always work with brand-new data. Examining the information related to a specific illness enables you to comprehend the possibilities, life expectancy, hereditary components, etc. This is in favor of enhancing viable techniques to enhance outcomes.

Linking biostatistics to healthcare helps in making data-driven decisions and advancements in healthcare. It improves:

- Improve treatment outcomes of patients and provide better healthcare
- Effectiveness of healthcare programs
- Public health and drafting suitable policies

1.6.3.8. Public Health Initiatives in Fighting the Covid-19 Pandemic

According to the WHO, global mortality exceeds 14.9 million. The various public health initiatives implemented to curb its spread include:

- Screening incoming visitors at terminals and stations
- Quarantining sick patients
- Identify and locate infected people and those who were in contact with them.
- Conducting diagnostic tests
- Educating and creating awareness on the best practices like frequent washing of hands, maintaining social distancing, and avoiding sick people
- Developing vaccines
- WHO responded by encouraging the scientific community to work jointly to identify critical research areas, and knowledge gaps from data collected from previous outbreaks and speeding up the process

1.6.4. Six Ways Biostatistics is Transforming Healthcare

Huge volumes of data are generated and collected by the healthcare sector, which requires analysis, processing, and interpretation to produce insights that will guide wise decisions. In order to test hypotheses, carry out statistical analyses, and draw reliable conclusions, biostatistics—the application of statistics to data from the life sciences—plays a crucial role in this procedure.

Experts in biostatistics typically have extensive knowledge of statistical software, tools, and applications, including Excel, R, SPSS, SAS, and STATA. They support the development of evidence-based healthcare, clinical trial design, drug efficacy measurement, and public health program evaluation.

Here are six ways biostatistics is changing healthcare research, policy, and delivery.

1.6.4.1. Clinical Trials

The medical field is always coming up with new ideas and developing treatments at breakneck speed. A treatment must first pass a battery of tests and trials to confirm its efficacy and safety before it is made available to the general public. These investigations entail gathering, analyzing, and interpreting data. A biostatistician assists with study design, sample size optimization, appropriate data collection method selection, coincidence removal, and deceptive information extraction from data. Experts in biostatistics arrive at precise conclusions from comparative studies, which determine whether a novel or substitute medication is superior to those already available on the market.

1.6.4.2. Public Health Programs

Experts in biostatistics evaluate the effects of public health projects and programs run by governmental bodies, non-profit organizations, and medical facilities using statistical methods. They create thorough studies and sampling strategies that aid in determining the efficacy of an endeavour and its potential for replication in other contexts. Healthcare social worker Jessica Adams recently used Kolabtree to hire a seasoned scientist who created a statistical model that assisted her in evaluating the effects of an HIV awareness festival in Uganda.

1.6.4.3. Epidemiological Studies

Numerous factors impact the genesis, spread, and dispersal of an illness. By obtaining a variety of disease-related data and establishing a causal relationship, epidemiological studies seek to identify these factors. Public health policies and preventive healthcare initiatives are developed in light of the findings. A biostatistics specialist is skilled in deriving the most significant information from the data, which is necessary to comprehend the correlation between the variables.

Throughout history, statistical evidence has consistently completed the picture. For instance, the results of a study conducted by Richard Doll and Austin Bradford Hill were published in 1954, providing substantial statistical backing for the association between smoking and lung cancer. Utilizing statistical analysis and visualization techniques, statisticians and data analysts also made significant contributions to our understanding of the West African Ebola epidemic.

1.6.4.4. Estimating the Severity of a Disease and Survival Rates

The use of survival statistics in guiding treatment decisions helps determine the prognosis of a patient who is terminally ill. These figures, which are usually presented as five-year relative rates, assist cancer patients in understanding their best course of action, their chances of remission, their chances of survival after remission, and their chances of leading a disease-free life following treatment. Experts in biostatistics can present figures derived from the meticulous analysis of prior research, offering reference data to medical professionals and patients alike.

1.6.4.5. Meta-Analysis and Evidence-Based Medicine

Systematic reviews and meta-analyses of medical data, which are helpful in creating evidence-based healthcare, also heavily rely on biostatistics. A structured study design called a meta-analysis assesses all of the prior published medical research on a given subject. In order to draw conclusions from these studies, individual findings and outcomes must be integrated into trustworthy conclusions that will direct future investigation. For instance, meta-analysis can be used to identify genetic and environmental factors that contribute to a disease, identify risk factors for a disease in an individual, and identify the best course of treatment for a patient. Healthcare professionals can increase their chances of providing effective, data-driven treatment by having a biostatistics expert examine the literature and provide a thorough, quantitative review of it.

1.6.4.6. Genome Sequencing Data Analysis

Large volumes of data produced by genome sequencing can aid in the understanding of complex traits by scientists. Fast sequencing of entire genomes is made possible by sophisticated instruments and software, which also helps identify variants that cause disease. Usually, information from the variant genome is contrasted with the individual's or a control group's reference genome. Experts in biostatistics examine variant frequencies in populations based on particular characteristics like blood type, ethnicity, etc., and make inferences about how a person's or a subpopulation's genetic composition may influence whether they are at risk or susceptible to particular conditions. R and Matlab are commonly utilized for the analysis of genomic data.

Almost every area of healthcare uses biostatistics, which offers a solid foundation for the development of evaluation, assessment, and treatment models. It aids in the improvement of public health policies and initiatives by governments, pharmaceutical companies, and hospitals in terms of the quality and safety of goods and services. It also aids in the implementation of preventive healthcare measures and the development of affordable treatments. Employing a contract biostatistician can give businesses quick access to specialized knowledge. Healthcare practitioners can make data-driven decisions and provide efficient, evidence-based care for easy access to such expertise (Friedman et al., 1981; Glantz et al., 1980).

1.7. The Role of Biostatistics in Public Health

In the biological and medical sciences, biostatistics is applied statistics used in public health practice. Epidemiology, the study of the causes, progression, and control of disease over time and space, provides information about health, morbidity, and mortality in human populations based on the data and models it offers. Together, epidemiology and biostatistics serve as the cornerstone of public health, directing all other decisions pertaining to the prevention and management of diseases that affect populations both locally and worldwide, both communicable and non-communicable.

Essentially, the statistical approach is used to forecast and explain a portion of the health outcomes as well as the course of pandemics and epidemics, and it undoubtedly has an impact on public health decision-makers. Biostatistics data and results are used by those developing, proposing, and advising mitigation strategies in response to contagions to inform public health and other healthcare practitioners about how to manage these diseases. Studies conducted to evaluate the effectiveness of mask wear as a preventative measure against specific viruses and clinical trials conducted to evaluate the safety and efficacy of vaccines, such as those created to prevent SARS-CoV-2, are two excellent examples.

1.7.1. Data Collection and Interpretation

The most crucial thing to remember when discussing biostatistics in public health or any other application is that they are only useful when the study or data collection design is appropriate and well thought out. After that, we can extrapolate and analyze the results in more detail.

Samples are used in most research studies because they are representative of populations. To accurately generalize the results and design appropriate interventions, it is crucial to select a sample that is as representative as possible of the population and the condition under study. Conversely, epidemiologic metrics—like mortality, incidence, and prevalence rates—are derived from each case and are employed to evaluate and provide information regarding the overall health of a community. The County Health Rankings and Roadmaps program opens in new window, created in partnership with the University of Wisconsin Population Health Institute and the Robert Wood Johnson Foundation, is an exemplar of a dependable and enduring source of local health data and its determinants.

Scientific planning and methodology are the foundation of all research in the health sciences and public health, and they always should be. Biostatistics are truly valuable in emergencies, when connecting the strength of the scientific method to provide answers with the reality of panic and uncertainty. How do we plan and structure the data collection, data analysis, and interpretation of the findings, as well as the application of those findings?

Our initial response plans and public health preparedness strategy were not carried out promptly or effectively in the case of the COVID-19 pandemic. Given the history of pandemics in recent memory, a public health surveillance system that tracks test-positive and disease, hospitalizations, and deaths ought to have been prepared for deployment. It should have been easy to use the Health and Human Services Pandemic Influenza Plan, created in 2005 and updated in 2006, 2009, and most recently in 2017. Additionally, following the 2001 Anthrax attack, the emergency preparedness plan and its communication system were enhanced and expanded with the creation of a functional LINCS (Learning Information Network Communication System) that linked New Jersey's state and local departments of health. This could have been used more wisely during the pandemic and should have been extended to more states years ago, better preparing us for COVID-19.

To make meaningful and appropriate decisions and forecasts, collect data for epidemiologists to research and learn about the disease's severity, modes of transmission, incubation period, and a range of symptomatologic and clinical manifestations, and provide evidence to public health and healthcare professionals, a cogent system was required. But the surveillance system was silent at the time, and the data were not available.

Early on, because of the disorganized public health system and surveillance, it was truly difficult. The federal, state, and local governments needed some time to coordinate and come to an agreement. However, there are some excellent instances of a speedy "recovery" from unavoidable setbacks. For instance, the Department of Health and Mental Hygiene and the Office of Chief Medical Examiner's IT Department collaborated to quickly establish a surveillance system with data collection to provide the mortality rates and inform practice in New York City (see **Figure 1.7**).

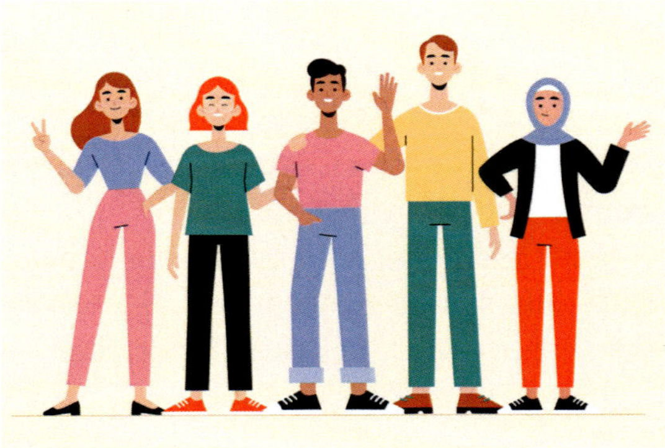

Figure 1.7. *Data collection and interpretation biostatistics in public health.*

Source. https://online.fdu.edu/wp-content/uploads/2021/08/fdu_maph_article_what-role-biostatistics-public-health_image-2.jpg.

1.7.2. The National Healthcare Problem

There is a lack of unity in the so-called US public health and healthcare system. A system is made up of interconnected, cooperative components. That was not demonstrated by the circumstances that existed in this nation at the start of the pandemic. It was very regrettable that there was no efficient communication between federal, state, and local agencies; that would have greatly facilitated and improved the outcome of the pandemic control effort. There was a division between the national and state emergency responses as a result of the federal government assigning the states many public health-related duties without providing enough funding, which became a major issue in the early weeks and months of this health crisis.

Many in the government had the best of intentions following the SARS pandemic. Sadly, the funding was cut off without sufficient explanation after a plan to create these connections and channels of communication between the federal, state, and local governments was developed in 2005. Without funding, services are typically not provided to a sufficient degree, which prevents the plan and strategies from being carried out. The answer, in my opinion, and as I explain to my students in our Foundations and Issues of Public Health course, is to create the missing connections between all tiers of government and to form alliances between public and private entities, such as civil society, non-profits, and academic institutions.

This disconnect has resulted in several issues, one of which is that private pharmaceutical companies began manufacturing test kits at the start of the COVID-19 pandemic, but they were not made available to government agencies for public distribution. Creating solid public-private partnerships would address this problem and improve our system's ability to serve all citizens, which is a guarantee provided by the government.

An example more general is the degree to which social and economic factors, urban planning, and other "non-health" determinants are strongly associated with health outcomes and can obstruct certain populations' access to care, particularly those most in need of it.

1.7.3. Bio-statistical Lessons from the COVID-19 Pandemic

Biostatistics gives us direction for the future by supplying us with historical and scientific data and results. Biostatistics ought to direct us in the proper direction when examining specific diseases or trends in diseases. However, for biostatistics to be able to assist the collaborative efforts of public health and healthcare professionals, the data must be carefully gathered and appropriately interpreted; otherwise, the results could be deceptive, of little value, or even harmful in some circumstances.

While cautiously acknowledging that there may be some limitations when relying solely on surveillance data, public health, and healthcare systems must collaborate for their respective sectors to be effective. For appropriate comparisons between various communities to be made, the surveillance must accurately reflect the state of affairs in that community. Only then can conclusions and recommendations be made. Uneven testing availability or utilization in various localities may have led to improper data comparisons in those areas, which may have contributed to some of last year's lack of coordination in national public health messaging.

A further obstacle that COVID-19 posed to researchers and medical professionals was the diverse range of indications and manifestations that the SARS-CoV-2 virus induces in humans. It was initially very difficult to gather accurate data in order to provide meaningful guidelines and care for mitigation, but it is crucial to time testing and patient onset of symptoms. This was better understood as the pandemic spread, and more precise data were produced to inform healthcare services and public health recommendations.

Developing new vaccines has proven to be successful, which highlights the true value of biostatistics in the fight against COVID-19. This discovery is saving lives and giving us information about the safety and effectiveness of those vaccinations in people, all the while keeping us informed about how the virus spreads in vaccinated vs. unprotected cohorts. For public health and medical professionals, it is energizing information, and the general public can find solace in it. It also provides all of us with a preview of possible future dangers and our capacity to react swiftly to them on a local and international scale (see **Figure 1.8**).

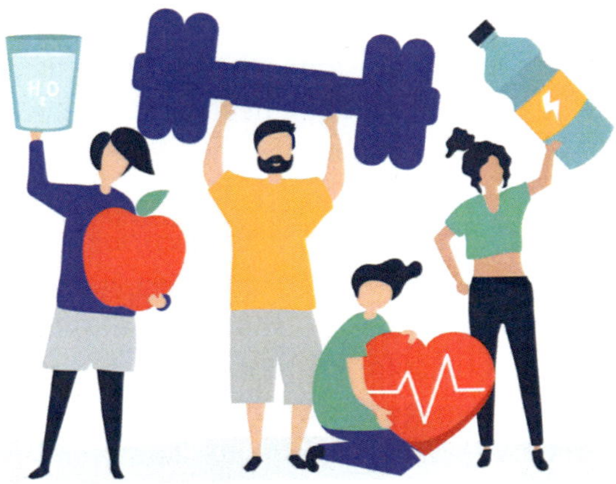

Figure 1.8. *Biostatistics scientific, historical data and results.*

Source.https://online.fdu.edu/wp-content/uploads/2021/08/fdu_maph_article_what-role-biostatistics-public-health_image-3.jpg.

It goes without saying that learning how to read and use data correctly before graduating and entering the field is crucial for aspiring professionals, as biostatistics' significance in public health cannot be overstated. In our Master of Public Health program, the goal of bio-stats is to teach students how to read newspaper and peer-reviewed articles and how to correctly and professionally interpret written material using the knowledge they have learned in other courses, such as epidemiology and health policy. Working in these fields and teaching these subjects require the ability to read, analyze, and present conclusions as reliable proof for suggested policy changes or new policies.

We make sure our students know that in order to provide credible guidance for interventions, they must be able to carefully design studies, suggest appropriate methods of gathering data, and choose statistical analyses to interpret whatever it is they are studying. Our graduates must then be able to communicate this information in an understandable manner to their clients, patients, and the general public—many of whom may not share their level of health literacy or knowledge.

We teach students how to make informed decisions by letting them use accurate, valid, and reliable resources to find the answers to their own questions. This way, they will be ready to successfully complete all of the above objectives and begin working productively the day after graduation. The vaccination and immunization campaigns against smallpox, polio, influenza, SARS-CoV-2, and other viruses, as well as the associated data collection, have been the greatest achievements of biostatistics in the field of public health. It's crucial to keep in mind that models are just that—models—even in the case of pandemics, but they have been helpful in providing guidance on what to do and a clear understanding of how serious some outbreaks were. They have been used to forecast the course and evolution of outbreaks. Regression analysis has also frequently helped us understand how several different variables all contributed to or did not contribute to a particular result. Certain events are explained and described by statistics, without which they would not be understandable or helpful. All of these infectious diseases and the efforts to control them are the best examples, but even in smaller, local epidemics like salmonella, we always turn to biostatistics for information (see **Figure 1.9**).

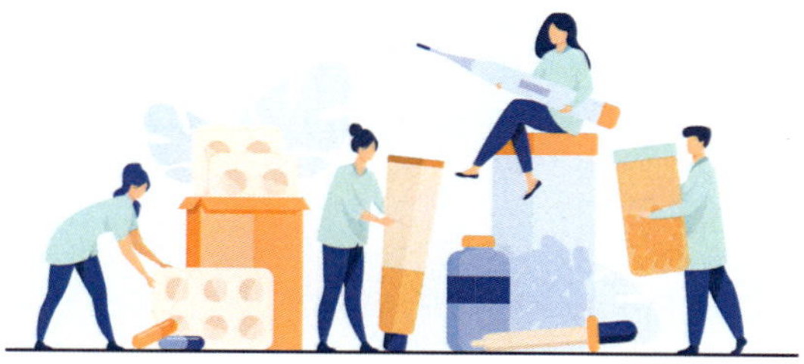

Figure 1.9. *Data collection related to immunization and vaccination against smallpox, polio, influenza, SARS-CoV-2 and other viruses.*

Source.https://online.fdu.edu/wp-content/uploads/2021/08/fdu_maph_article_what-role-biostatistics-public-health_image-4.jpg.

1.8. The Evolution and Future of Biostatistics in Public Health

1.8.1. Significant Progress Thus Far

The field of biostatistics is constantly growing and changing due to its significant role in healthcare. Our use of fundamental mathematical relations and techniques has undoubtedly improved over time, giving us access to more information and more ways to view the same data. We can now recognize trends thanks to these developments, particularly in epidemiology and other research areas concerning diseases. Apart from infectious diseases, biostatistics is enlightening us about cancer and long-term ailments like diabetes and heart disease, resulting in the creation of more effective treatment strategies to manage them.

The development of public health and healthcare has been predicated on biostatistics' capacity to furnish empirical support, and this trajectory is expected to persist in the future. This is the core curriculum for any graduate program in the health sciences.

1.8.2. The Influence of Technology in the Years Ahead

We hope that in the next five to ten years, we will have more knowledge about a wider range of diseases, as well as how to treat and manage those conditions. A significant portion of that is the nexus between biostatistics and artificial intelligence. It's fascinating how IBM uses mathematical models and biostatistics, for example, in their programs. Think about what their supercomputer Watson can do: rather than having to interpret every lab result themselves, scientists and medical professionals can give Watson the patient data it needs, and Watson will diagnose the patient. It is designed to weigh all available options instantly and make decisions in a fraction of the time that humans could ever manage.

This technological innovation and progress are exciting and beneficial for epidemiology, public health, and humanity in general in many ways. This modification gives us access to a tool that was previously unavailable. When applied properly, it can lead to the discovery of novel disease-prevention techniques as well as potential treatments, improving people's health or preventing illness altogether. (Mainland et al., 1982) (O'Brien et al., 1981).

A Closer Look

Experimental Drug

Experimental drugs are substances that have not yet been approved for widespread use by regulatory agencies such as the Food and Drug Administration (FDA) in the United States. These drugs are typically being investigated in clinical trials to determine their safety, efficacy, and potential side effects in treating specific diseases or conditions. Here's an overview in 300 words:

Experimental drugs often emerge from extensive research and development efforts conducted by pharmaceutical companies, academic institutions, or government agencies. These drugs may target a wide range of conditions, including cancer, infectious diseases, neurological disorders, autoimmune diseases, and rare genetic disorders.

Before an experimental drug can be tested in humans, it undergoes rigorous preclinical testing in laboratory and animal studies to assess its safety profile and effectiveness. If the preclinical studies show promising results, the drug may advance to clinical trials, which are conducted in phases.

Phase I trials typically involve a small number of healthy volunteers and focus on evaluating the safety, dosage, and pharmacokinetics of the drug. Phase II trials enrol a larger group of patients with the target condition to further assess safety and efficacy. Phase III trials involve even larger patient populations and compare the experimental drug to standard treatments or a placebo to determine its effectiveness and safety in real-world settings.

Throughout the clinical trial process, researchers closely monitor participants for adverse reactions and collect data on the drug's effects. If a drug demonstrates significant efficacy and an acceptable safety profile in clinical trials, the pharmaceutical company or sponsor may submit a New Drug Application (NDA) to regulatory agencies for approval.

Regulatory agencies review the submitted data to assess the drug's benefits and risks and determine whether it can be approved for commercial distribution. If approved, the drug may become available to patients for treatment.

However, not all experimental drugs complete the clinical trial process or receive regulatory approval. Some may fail to demonstrate sufficient efficacy or safety, leading to discontinuation of development. Additionally, even if a drug receives regulatory approval, ongoing monitoring is necessary to detect any rare or long-term side effects that may emerge with widespread use.

In summary, experimental drugs represent a vital aspect of medical research and innovation, offering hope for improved treatments and potential cures for various diseases. However, their development and approval process require careful evaluation and adherence to regulatory standards to ensure patient safety and efficacy.

Summary

- Biostatistics is defined as the application of statistical principles in medicine, public health, or biology. Statistical principles are based in applied mathematics and include tools and techniques for collecting information or data and then summarizing, analyzing, and interpreting those results.
- Epidemiology is a field of study focused on the study of health and illness in human populations, patterns of health or disease, and the factors that influence these patterns.
- A case report is a very detailed report of the specific features of a particular participant or case. A case series is a systematic review of the interesting and common features of a small collection, or series, of cases.
- A cross-sectional survey is a study conducted at a single point in time. The cross-sectional survey is an appropriate design when the research question is focused on the prevalence of a disease, a present practice, or an opinion.
- A cohort study involves a group of individuals who usually meet a set of inclusion criteria at the start of the study. The cohort is followed and associations are made between a risk factor and a disease.
- The case-control study is used in epidemiologic research where again the question of interest is whether there is an association between a particular risk factor or exposure and an outcome.
- The randomized controlled trial (RCT) is a design with a key and distinguishing feature—the randomization of participants to one of several comparison treatment or groups.
- The crossover trial is a clinical trial where each participant is assigned to two or more treatments sequentially. When there are two treatments (e.g., an experimental and a control), each participant receives both treatments.
- Surveys, medical records, surveillance, disease registers, and peer-reviewed literature are various sources that provide health data.

References

1. Altman, D. G. (1980). Statistics and ethics in medical research. Misuse of statistics is unethical. *British Medical Journal, 281*(6249), 1182–1184.
2. Altman, D. G. (1982). Statistics in medical journals. *Statistics in Medicine, 1*(1), 59–71.
3. DerSimonian, R., Charette, L. J., McPeek, B., & Mosteller, F. (1982). Reporting on methods in clinical trials. *New England Journal of Medicine, 306*(22), 1332–1337.
4. Freiman, J. A., Chalmers, T. C., Smith, H. Jr., & Kuebler, R. R. (1978). The importance of beta, the type II error, and sample size in the design and interpretation of the randomized control trial. Survey of 71 "negative" trials. *New England Journal of Medicine, 299*(13), 690–694.
5. Friedman, S. B., & Phillips, S. (1981). What's the difference? Pediatric residents and their inaccurate concepts regarding statistics. *Pediatrics, 68*(5), 644–646.
6. Glantz, S. A. (1980). Biostatistics: How to detect, correct, and prevent errors in the medical literature. *Circulation, 61*(1), 1–7.

7. Gore, S. M. (1981). Assessing methods—descriptive statistics and graphs. *British Medical Journal (Clinical Research Edition), 283*(6289), 486–488.

8. Gore, S. M. (1981). Statistics in question. Assessing clinical trials--trial size. *British Medical Journal (Clinical Research Edition), 282*(6277), 1687–1689.

9. Mainland, D. (1982). Medical statistics vs arithmetic. *Journal of Chronic Diseases, 35*(6), 413–417.

10. O'Brien, P. C., & Shampo, M. A. (1981). Statistics for clinicians. 2. Graphic displays--histograms, frequency polygons, and cumulative distribution polygons. *Mayo Clinic Proceedings, 56*(2), 126–128.

11. Reed, J. F. III, & Slaichert, W. (1981). Statistical proof in inconclusive 'negative' trials. *Archives of Internal Medicine, 141*(10), 1307–1310.

12. Rothman, K. J. (1978). A show of confidence. *New England Journal of Medicine, 299*(24), 1362–1363.

13. Sackett, D. L. (1979). Bias in analytic research. *Journal of Chronic Diseases, 32*(1-2), 51–63.

14. Schor, S., & Karten, I. (1966). Statistical evaluation of medical journal manuscripts. *JAMA, 195*(13), 1123–1128.

15. Wallenstein, S., Zucker, C. L., & Fleiss, J. L. (1980). Some statistical methods are useful in circulation research. *Circulation Research, 47*(1), 1–9.

Chapter 2

QUANTIFYING THE EXTENT OF DISEASE

Contents

Introduction 35
2.1. Absence of Disease and Infirmity 37
2.2. Common Diseases and Conditions 38
2.3. Classification of Diseases and Conditions 40
2.4. Epidemiology 41
2.5. Disability-Adjusted Life Years 47
2.6. Prevalence 50
2.7. Incidence 50
2.8. Comparing the Extent of Disease Between Groups 54
Summary 61
References 61

Introduction

Diagnostic criteria must be specified in order to measure the frequency of disease in populations. In the context of clinical practice, the term "a case" usually denotes the division of individuals into two distinct groups: those who are afflicted and those who are not. This premise is reasonably effective in the hospital ward, and it was previously believed to be suitable for populations as well. For example, cholera was previously only recognized by an intense bout of watery diarrhoea, which was frequently fatal. However, modern research indicates that the infection can also be subclinical or result in only mild diarrhoea.

A variety of metrics, such as disability-adjusted life years (DALYs), years lived with disability (YLDs), prevalence, incidence, and risk, can be used to quantify the extent of the disease.

Orientation and Directional Terms

Term	Definition	Illustration
Disease burden	Disease burden is the impact of a health problem on a given population, and can be measured using a variety of indicators such as mortality, morbidity or financial costs.	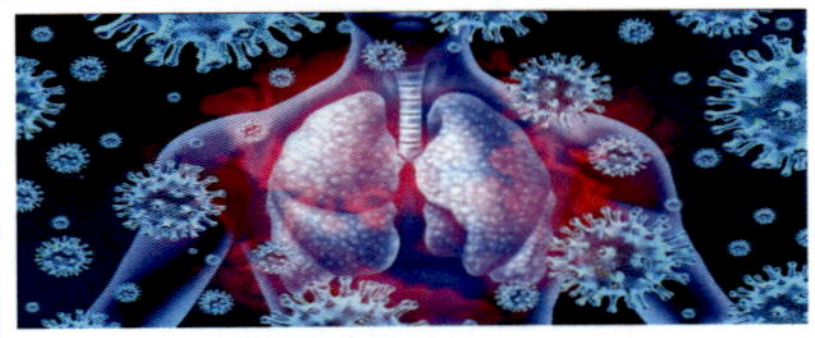
Disability-Adjusted Life Years (DALYs)	A measure of the total burden of disease, which includes years of life lost and years lived with a disability. One DALY is equal to one lost year of healthy life.	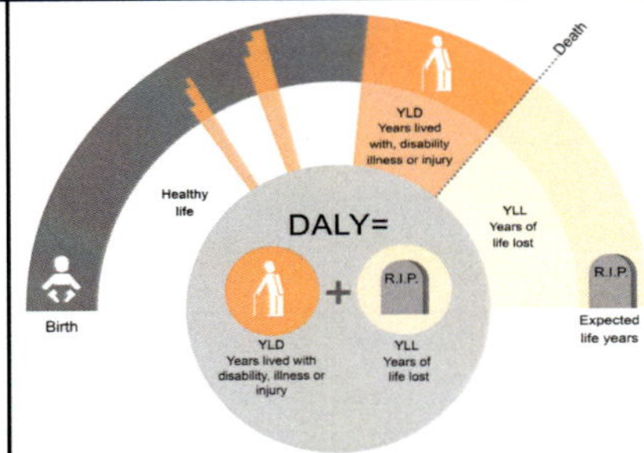
Health policy	Health policy is a collection of decisions, plans, and actions that a society takes to achieve specific healthcare goals.	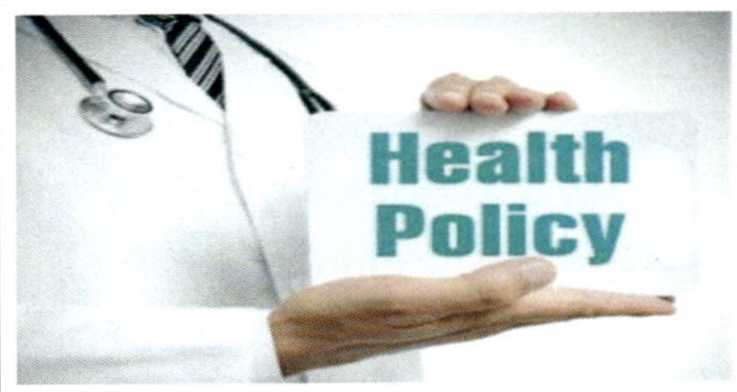
Incidence rate	Incidence rate is a measure of disease that's calculated by dividing the number of new cases of a disease by the number of people at risk for that disease during a specific period of time.	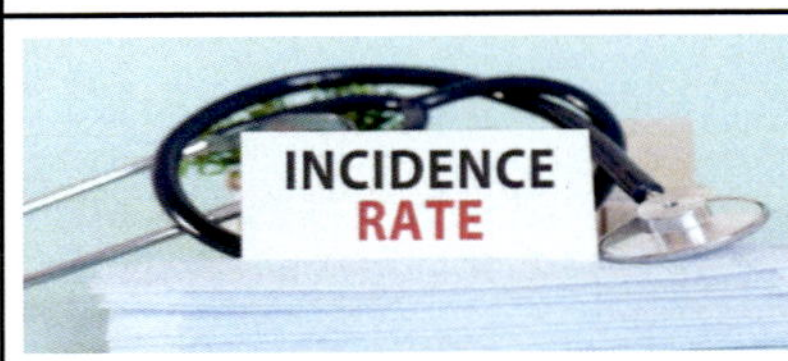
Population health	Population health is the health status and outcomes of a group of people, rather than the health of each individual.	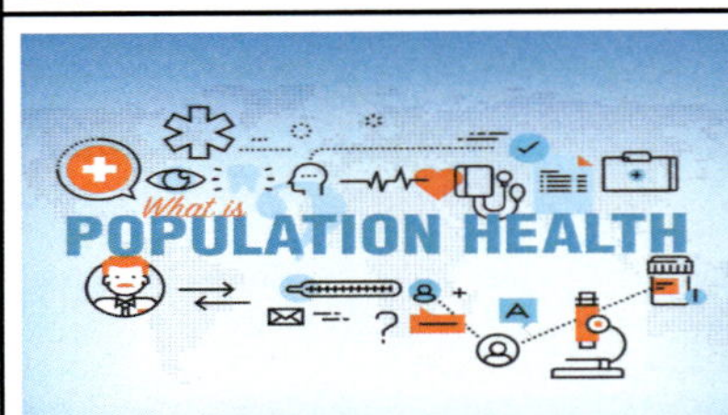
Years Lived with Disability (YLDs)	A measure of morbidity, which is the loss of healthy life years due to living in a less-than-perfect health state. YLDs are calculated by multiplying the number of incident cases by the duration and disability weight of the health state.	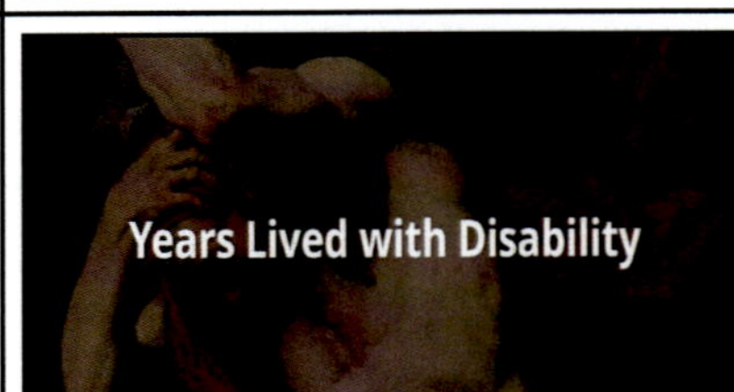

2.1. Absence of Disease and Infirmity

One of the factors that determine health is the existence or absence of illness or infirmity, which affects health. It's interesting to note that to be deemed completely healthy or well-being, one must not have disease or infirmity, which are included in this definition of health. "A condition of the living animal or plant body or of one of its parts that impairs normal functioning and is typically manifested by distinguishing signs and symptoms" is the definition of "disease" according to the Western biomedical perspective. The prefixes dis- (lack of) and ease (freedom from pain) were hyphenated to form the word disease in the fourteenth century. Disease, in the Oxford English Dictionary, meant discomfort or not feeling well. The word "disease" was used in the 16th century to describe particular ailments or diseases.

Similarly, "the quality or state of being of poor or deteriorated vitality" is what the word "infirmity" refers to. The 14th century is when it first appeared as well. These days, the condition is the more accepted term for infirmity, and we will stick with it for the duration of this textbook. It should be noted that according to these definitions, infirmity or condition suggests a broader focus with less distinct or obvious characteristics, whereas disease suggests a more narrow and identifiable focus through signs, symptoms, and pathology that can be observed. As we proceed with our quest to define and quantify the burden of disease, this distinction will become increasingly evident and significant.

2.1.1. The Biomedical Paradigm in Global Health and Disease

It is crucial to recognize that the majority of current global health work is dominated by and uses Western biomedical understandings of disease and infirmity. The WHO's influence in the years following World War II, when "the focus was on improving the health of people within individual nations by strengthening their biomedical prevention and treatment capacities," is largely to blame for this. We do, however, know that there is a human dimension to health that includes cultural beliefs and behavior, so it is imperative to alter the prevalent perceptions of illness and infirmity as limited medical technical issues. To "see beyond dominant assumptions to assess the actual role of local conditions and social experiences in the making of health and sickness—disease understanding develops at the local level, as do social responses to limit adverse health outcomes through social and cultural adjustments" is something we can keep learning from non-Western perspectives. These viewpoints take into account the opinions, voices, and cultural customs of underrepresented groups. For instance, sickness is viewed from an indigenous viewpoint as the result of an imbalance between the four basic dimensions of the spiritual, intellectual, physical, and emotional realms. This viewpoint makes it possible to implement more comprehensive, locally driven health promotion and equity initiatives.

2.1.2. Disease (and Condition) Causation

After discussing the definition of disease, let's look at its causes. The epidemiologic triangle, also known as the triad, is one of the most basic models of disease causation. This concept is frequently applied to the study of infectious diseases. An external agent, a vulnerable host, and the environment that unites the host and agent make up the triad. According to this model, illness arises from an agent's interaction with a susceptible host in a setting that facilitates the agent's transfer from a source to that host. Figure 2.1. illustrates this model in two different ways.

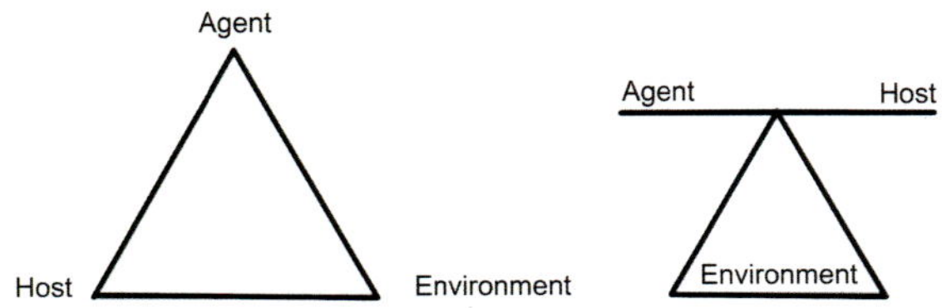

Figure 2.1. *Epidemiologic Triad Model. One model shows the agent, host, and environment as having equal influence. The other model shows agent and host as variables dependent on each other and the environment.*

Source: https://pubh110.digital.uic.edu/section-1-2-defining-measuring-the-burden-of-disease-part-i/.

To cause disease, agent, host, and environmental variables interact in several intricate ways. These three elements must interact and balance differently to treat different diseases. Evaluation of all three elements and their interactions is typically necessary to develop appropriate, workable, and efficient public health interventions to control or prevent disease.

2.1.2.1. Agent

An infectious microorganism or pathogen, such as a virus, bacteria, parasite, or other microbe, was originally referred to as an agent. In general, the agent must exist for disease to manifest; however, the agent's presence by itself does not always result in disease. The pathogenicity—the capacity of an organism to cause disease—and the dose of the organism are two important factors that determine whether exposure to it will cause illness.

The definition of an agent has evolved to encompass both physical and chemical causes of illness or injury. These include physical forces (like the repetitive mechanical forces linked to carpal tunnel syndrome) and chemical contaminants (like the L-tryptophan contaminant that causes eosinophilia-myalgia syndrome).

2.1.2.2. Host

A host is a person who has the potential to contract an illness. Numerous host-specific characteristics also referred to as risk factors, can affect a person's exposure to, susceptibility to, or reaction to a causative agent. In addition to age and sex, behavior like personal hygiene, sexual practices, and other choices frequently impact opportunities for exposure. A person's genetic make-up, nutritional and immunological status, anatomical structure, presence of disease or medication, and psychological make-up can all affect their susceptibility to an agent and how they respond to it.

2.1.2.3. Environment

The term "environment" describes external elements influencing the agent and exposure opportunity. Environmental factors encompass physical elements like climate and geology, biological elements like insects that spread the agent, and socioeconomic elements like population density, hygienic conditions, and access to healthcare.

The Epidemiologic Triad model can be used to understand the causes of conditions or infirmities, although it is most commonly used to understand the causation of diseases. A condition requires the presence of a host, an agent (which need not always be a microorganism), and the environment in which the host and agent interact.

2.2. Common Diseases and Conditions

The top 20 common diseases and conditions in the world as of 2019 that are causing serious concern in the field of global health are briefly reviewed here. While many of them might be well-known to you, some might need a brief refresher. (Bautista et al., 2020) (Bilcke et al., 2008) (see Table 2.1).

Table 2.1. *Top 20 Global Health Diseases 2019*

1. Ischaemic Heart Disease	The most common form of heart disease, in which narrowed or blocked coronary arteries have difficulty supplying sections of the heart muscle with the blood they need (ischemia).
2. Stroke	Blockage or rupture of a blood vessel supplying the brain; often leads to impaired brain function or death.
3. Chronic Obstructive Pulmonary Disease	(COPD) is the name for a group of lung conditions that cause breathing difficulties. It includes emphysema which is damage to the air sacs in the lungs and chronic bronchitis which is long-term inflammation of the airways.
4. Lower Respiratory Infections	A lower respiratory tract infection (RTI) occurs when there is an infection of the lungs, specifically in the lower airways. This infection is usually caused by a virus, but it can also be caused by bacteria or other less common organisms and pneumonia is an example.
5. Neonatal Conditions	Neonatal conditions are defined as conditions occurring during the first month after birth (0- 28 days). Among many neonatal conditions are premature birth, neonatal infections and birth asphyxia which is a lack of oxygen and blood flow to the brain.
6. Trachea, Bronchus, Lung Cancers	Cancer is a disease in which cells in the body grow out of control. When cancer starts in the trachea, it is called trachea cancer. When it starts in the mucous glands and ducts of the lung airways (bronchi) it is called bronchial cancer and when it starts in the lungs, it is called lung cancer.
7. Alzheimer's Disease and other Dementias	Alzheimer's disease is a brain disorder that slowly destroys memory and thinking skills and, eventually, the ability to carry out the simplest tasks. Dementia is the loss of cognitive functioning — thinking, remembering, and reasoning — to such an extent that it interferes with a person's daily life and activities.
8. Diarrheal Diseases	Diarrheal diseases are usually associated with infections in the intestinal tract, which can be caused by a variety of bacterial, viral and parasitic organisms. Infection is spread through contaminated food or drinking-water which results in cholera or from person-to-person as a result of poor hygiene causing rotavirus.
9. Diabetes Mellitus	A disease in which the body does not properly produce or use insulin, resulting in abnormally high levels of sugar (glucose) in the blood.
10. Kidney Diseases	Chronic kidney diseases (CKD) can affect your body's ability to clean your blood, filter extra water out of your blood, and help control your blood pressure. Main cause of death is lack of dialysis or kidney transplant treatments.
11. Cirrhosis of the Liver	A chronic disease of the liver that progressively destroys the liver's ability to aid in digestion and detoxification.
12. Road Injury	Road injuries or death due to traffic crashes that result from speeding, impaired/distracted driving, unsafe road quality, non-use of vehicle restraints or helmets, unsafe vehicles or lack of enforcement of traffic laws.
13. Tuberculosis	Tuberculosis (TB) is caused by bacteria (Mycobacterium tuberculosis) that most often affect the lungs and spread from person to person through the air.

14. Hypertensive Heart Disease	A group of heart diseases caused by high blood pressure. Hypertension is a major risk factor for stroke, especially haemorrhagic and lacunar strokes, because it puts excess stress on the walls of blood vessels and damages their delicate inner lining.
15. Colon and Rectum Cancers	Colon cancer is a type of cancer that begins in the large intestine (colon). Rectal cancer is a type of cancer that begins in the rectum. In both cases it usually begins as small, noncancerous (benign) clumps of cells called polyps that form on the inside of the colon or rectum.
16. Stomach Cancer	Stomach cancer, also called gastric cancer, begins when cells in the stomach start to grow out of control.
17. Self-Harm	Deliberate non-suicidal injury to one's own body tissue, as cutting or burning the skin, or pulling out hair, in a physical manifestation of emotional distress.
18. Falls	Advertently coming to rest on the ground, floor or other lower level, excluding intentional change in position to rest in furniture, wall or other objects.
19. HIV/AIDS	Abbreviation for human immunodeficiency virus, the virus that leads to acquired immunodeficiency syndrome (AIDS). HIV damages immune cells so that they are no longer able to fight off other infections.
20. Breast Cancer	Breast cancer is a disease in which cells in the breast grow out of control. There are different kinds of breast cancer. The kind of breast cancer depends on which cells in the breast turn into cancer.

Source: https://pubh110.digital.uic.edu/section-1-2-defining-measuring-the-burden-of-disease-part-i/.

2.3. Classification of Diseases and Conditions

On the other hand, there is a specific vocabulary used in public and global health when discussing disease classification schemes and categories. This will be particularly crucial when the topic of the Global Burden of Disease comes up. There are, in fact, numerous classifications and vocabulary used in the field of global health; some examples are "diseases of poverty," "diseases of wealth," "emerging infectious diseases," "re-emerging infectious diseases," and neglected tropical diseases.

The most common way the field of global health classifies and talks about diseases is by putting diseases into three groups as follows:

- ***Group I: Communicable Diseases***: Communicable Diseases are also referred to as infectious diseases. As we noted above, the disease agent is a micro-organism which results in an infection of the host in their environment.
- ***Group II: Non-communicable Diseases***: Non-communicable diseases (NCDs) are also referred to as chronic diseases. In this case, the host is exposed to several non-infectious agents such physical or behavioural factors (i.e., exercise, diet) in their environment.
- ***Group III: Injuries***: Injuries do not fit neatly into the classic notion of disease. However, they are an important contributor to how we conceptualize and measure the burden of disease because they can result in the development of a disease (accidental exposure to chemicals resulting in skin or respiratory diseases). Similar to NCDs, the host is exposed to non-infectious agents in their environment (often the workplace).

2.3.1. A Comment on Mental Health/Neurological Diseases and Conditions

While neurological and mental health disorders are frequently classified as non-communicable or chronic diseases, they can also be classified as a fourth group that consists of three subcategories:

1. Substance use disorders like alcohol or opioid use;
2. Neurological diseases like Parkinson's and Alzheimer's disease;
3. Mental health disorders like depression and bipolar disorder.

In Table 2.2, you will see a summary of Disease Classifications and some examples.

Table 2.2. *Global Health Disease Classifications and Some Examples*

Disease Type	**Disease Group Number**	**Examples**
Communicable or Infectious Disease	I	Lower Respiratory Infections (pneumonia), Diarrhoeal diseases (e.g. Cholera), Tuberculosis, HIV/AIDS, Ebola, Measles, Syphillis
Non-Communicable Diseases (NCDs) or Chronic Diseases	II	Heart Disease, Stroke, COPD, Cancers, Diabetes, Alzheimer's Disease and Related Dementias, Chronic Kidney Disease, Liver Cirrhosis, Hypertensive Heart Disease
Injuries	III	Road Injuries, Self-Harm, Falls

Source: https://pubh110.digital.uic.edu/section-1-2-defining-measuring-the-burden-of-disease-part-i/.

2.4. Epidemiology

The Greek terms epi, which means on or upon, demos, which means people, and logos, which means the study of, are the origin of the word epidemiology. Epidemiology is the study of how health conditions and events are distributed among populations, how they are caused, and how to use this knowledge to control health issues. The words in bold are highlighted for the following reasons.

- **Study** – Epidemiology is a scientific discipline with sound methods of scientific inquiry at its foundation
- **Distribution** – is concerned with the **frequency** and **pattern** of health events in a population

The term "**frequency**" describes the quantity of health events within a population, such as the number of cases of diabetes or COVID-19. A **pattern** is the frequency of health-related events by person, place, and time. Time patterns can be annual, seasonal, weekly, daily, hourly, or any other type of time breakdown that could affect the likelihood of an illness or injury. Geographic variance, distinctions between urban and rural areas, and the placement of workplaces or educational institutions are examples of place patterns. Personal characteristics encompass a person's age, sex, marital status, socioeconomic status, behavior, and environmental exposures, all of which may be linked to an increased risk of disease, injury, or disability.

The causes of disease and other events related to health are known as **determinants**, along with other relevant factors. They evaluate whether the demographics, immunologic or genetic makeup, behavior, exposure to the environment, and other so-called potential risk factors of groups with varying disease rates differ. Ideally, the results offer enough proof to guide timely and efficient public health prevention and control actions.

2.4.1. Health-Related States or Events

Anything that has an impact on a population's health can be considered a health-related state or event. This can include illnesses, trauma, congenital abnormalities, workplace health, maternal-child health, and environmental health. They may also include genetics and actions linked to health and well-being, such as the quantity of exercise and the use of seat belts.

2.4.2. Specified Populations

An epidemiologist is interested in the overall health of a population or community. Stated differently, the community serves as the epidemiologist's "patient.." As a result, when dealing with an ill individual, the roles of the epidemiologist and the clinician differ. For instance, both parties are interested in determining the accurate diagnosis when a patient with diarrheal disease appears. However, the epidemiologist concentrates on determining the exposure or source that caused the illness, the number of other people who may have been similarly exposed, the possibility of further spread in the community, and interventions to prevent additional cases or recurrences. In contrast, the clinician typically focuses on treating and caring for the individual.

2.4.3. Application

Epidemiology is more than just "the study of" health in a population; it also entails utilizing the insights gleaned from research to inform community-based interventions. Epidemiology is a science and an art in practice. The epidemiologist "diagnoses" the health of a community and suggests appropriate, workable, and acceptable public health interventions to control and prevent disease in the community using the scientific methods of descriptive and analytical epidemiology as well as experience, epidemiologic judgment, and knowledge of local conditions.

2.4.4. Uses and Functions of Epidemiology

Numerous applications have been made of epidemiology and the data gathered from epidemiologic research. The following describes two typical uses.

2.4.4.1. Assessing the Community's Health

Epidemiologic data is used by public health officials in charge of developing, implementing, and assessing policies as a factual basis for their decisions. Finding and analyzing pertinent data sources by person, place, and time is necessary to evaluate the health of a community or population (descriptive epidemiology).

- What are the actual and potential health problems in the community?
- Where are they occurring?

- Which populations are at increased risk?
- Which problems have declined over time?
- Which ones are increasing or have the potential to increase?
- How do these patterns relate to the level and distribution of public health services available?

Hippocrates, the father of medicine, was also a public health-oriented person and maybe even an early epidemiologist. Notice how in his famous piece 'On Airs, Waters and Places' he recognizes that time (seasons), place (particular locality, wind, and waters) and person (lifestyle behaviours) are important to investigating disease.

2.4.4.2. Searching for Causes

The goal of much epidemiologic research is to identify the causative variables that affect an individual's risk of illness. Finding the cause will ideally allow for the implementation of the necessary public health measures. Epidemiology frequently offers sufficient data to enable sensible action. One well known example involves the removal of the handle from the Broad St pump following John Snow's investigation of cholera in the Golden Square area of London in 1854. Snow charted the cholera cases that were happening in the neighbourhood. The hand pump's locations are indicated by the X's. As you can see, the majority of the incidents happened close to the Broad Street pump. After Snow's pump handle was removed, there were a lot fewer cholera case. He reasoned that the excess of cholera cases could be attributed to the water coming from the pump.

2.4.5. Public Health Surveillance

The process of continuously gathering, analyzing, interpreting, and disseminating health data to inform public health policy and decision-making is known as public health surveillance. The same goes for surveillance: keeping an eye on the community's pulse.

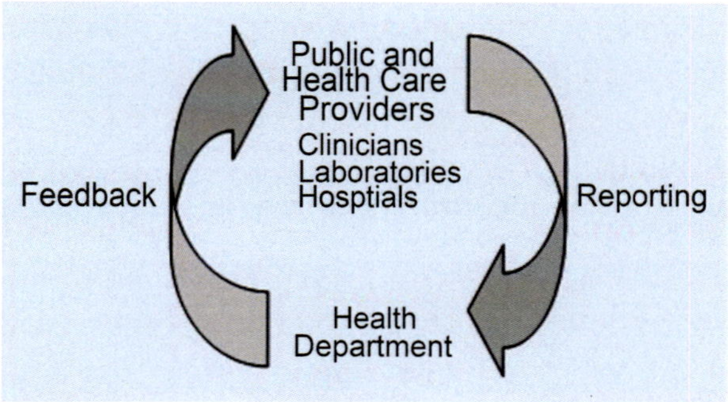

Figure 2.2: *Surveillance information flows from public and health care providers such as clinicians, laboratories, hospitals, and health departments. Feedback flows from health departments back to public and health care providers.*

Source: *https://pubh110.digital.uic.edu/section-1-2-defining-measuring-the-burden-of-disease-part-i/.*

Understanding the continuing patterns of disease occurrence and potential is the goal of public health surveillance, also known as "information for action," to facilitate the efficient and effective application of investigation, control, and preventive measures. This is achieved by methodically gathering, assessing, and disseminating pertinent health data to individuals engaged in disease prevention and public health decision-making, along with providing an interpretation of the data (see **Figure 2.2**).

2.4.6. Types of Epidemiology

There are two subfields within epidemiology, known as descriptive epidemiology and analytical epidemiology. The goal of descriptive epidemiology is to compile and arrange information about the individuals impacted (e.g., the traits of the sick individuals), time (e.g., when they get sick), and location (e.g., where the illness's potential source may have been encountered). The goal of analytical epidemiology is to identify the type of health issue and its cause. Analytic epidemiology quantifies associations between exposures and outcomes and tests hypotheses regarding the source of the issue by using comparison groups to provide baseline or expected values. Shortly put, the 5 W's (Who, When, Where, What, Why) are frequently asked by epidemiologists.

Person, time, and place are all covered by descriptive epidemiology.

As with all scientific endeavours, the practice of epidemiology relies on a systematic approach. In very simple terms, the epidemiologist:

- **Counts** cases or health events, and describes them in terms of time, place, and person;
- **Divides** the number of cases by an appropriate denominator to calculate rates; and
- **Compares** these rates over time or for different groups of people.

Before counting cases, however, the epidemiologist must decide what a case is. This is done by developing a case definition.

2.4.6.1. Defining a Case

A case definition is a set of accepted standards used to determine if an individual is afflicted with a specific disease, syndrome, or other medical condition. To ensure comparability, some case definitions—particularly those used for global health surveillance—have been created and accepted as international standards. Every case is equal when a standard case definition is used, regardless of who identified it, when it happened, or where. Moreover, it is possible to compare the quantity or rate of disease cases found in one location or time with that from another.

Global public health officials can, for instance, compare the number of COVID-19 cases that occurred in Senegal in March 2000 with the number that occurred there in March 1999 using a standard case definition. Alternatively, they could assess the difference between the 2000 global rate and the COVID-19 Senegal rate. If a difference is noticed between groups using the same standard case definition, it is more likely to be the result of actual differences in the cases' classifications. Whether describing an influenza pandemic or a local rise in all-terrain vehicle crashes, epidemiologists aim for a similar level of comprehensiveness.

The five W's mentioned above—case definition (What), person (Who), time (When), place (Where), and causes/risk factors/modes of transmission (Why)—are, nevertheless, frequently substituted by synonyms by epidemiologists.

Compiling and analyzing data by who, time, and place is desirable for several reasons.

- First, by looking at the data carefully, the epidemiologist becomes very familiar with the data. He or she can see what the data can or cannot reveal based on the variables available, its limitations (for example, the number of records with missing information for each important variable), and its eccentricities (for example, all cases range in age from 2 months to 6 years, plus one 17-year-old.).
- Second, the epidemiologist learns the extent and pattern of the public health problem being investigated — which months, which neighbourhood, and which groups of people have the most and least cases.
- Third, the epidemiologist creates a detailed description of the health of a population that can be easily communicated with tables, graphs, and maps.
- Fourth, the epidemiologist can identify areas or groups within the population that have high rates of disease.

This information in turn provides important clues to the causes of the disease, and the clues can be turned into testable hypotheses. Let's take a more in-depth look at Person, Time, and Place characteristics.

2.4.6.2. Person

Age, sex, race/ethnicity, and socioeconomic status are examples of "person" attributes.

Organization and analysis of data by "person" may make use of intrinsic characteristics of people (e.g., age, sex, race), biological characteristics (e.g., immune status), acquired characteristics (e.g., marital status), activities (e.g., occupation, leisure activities, use of medications, tobacco, or drugs), or environmental factors (e.g., socioeconomic status, access to medical care) because personal characteristics may influence illness. The two most often examined "person" characteristics are age and sex, which are included in practically all data sets. However, analyses of other personal variables are typically required, depending on the disease and the available data. Typically, epidemiologists start by examining each variable independently when analyzing personal data. It is sometimes possible to look at two factors a, like age and sex. Tables and graphs are typically used to display personal data.

1. Age

   Given that nearly all health-related events vary with age is likely the most significant "person" attribute. Age-related variations in several factors also occur, such as susceptibility, exposure opportunity, latency or incubation period of the disease, and physiologic response (which influences the development of the disease among other things).

2. Sex

   For many diseases, men are more likely than women to become ill and die. The sex-related differences in certain diseases can be attributed to genetic, hormonal, anatomical, or other innate differences between the sexes. These innate variations have an impact on physiological reactions or susceptibility.

3. Ethnic and Racial Groups

   Epidemiologists may find it interesting to examine individual data according to biological, cultural, or social categories, such as race, nationality, religion, or social groups like tribes and other socially or geographically marginalized groups. Variations in racial, ethnic, or other group variables could be due to variations in exposure or susceptibility, or variations in other factors like socioeconomic status and access to healthcare that affect the risk of disease.

4. Socioeconomic Status

   Measuring socioeconomic status is a challenging task. It is composed of numerous factors, including social standing, living conditions, family income, educational attainment, and census track. The easiest-to-measure variables might not fully capture the idea as a whole. Even so, epidemiologists frequently use factors like occupation, family income, and educational attainment, although they are aware that these are not exact indicators of socioeconomic status.

2.4.6.3. Time

Diseases appear and disappear over time. Certain changes happen regularly, while others happen unpredictably. Influenza (winter) and West Nile virus infection (August–September) are two illnesses that happen in the same season every year. Conversely, illnesses like salmonellosis and hepatitis B can strike at any time. Health officials can plan for seasonal diseases and apply preventative and control measures, like mosquito repellent or influenza vaccination campaigns, to minimize their incidence. Researchers can study the causes and modes of transmission of diseases that occur infrequently before creating tailored interventions to manage or stop the disease from spreading. In either case, tracking disease occurrence in the community and determining the effectiveness of public health interventions depend on the ability to visualize disease occurrence patterns over time.

1. Secular (Long-Term) Trends

Long-term or secular trends in the occurrence of the disease can be seen by graphing the annual cases or rate of the disease over several years. These graphs are used by health officials to determine whether disease incidence is trending upward, downward, or nearly flat, to evaluate programs or make policy decisions, to infer the cause of a disease's increase or decrease in occurrence (especially if the graph shows the dates of related events), and to use historical trends as a predictor of future disease incidence.

2. Seasonality

To display any seasonal patterns in the occurrence of diseases, they can be plotted by week or month over one year or longer. Certain illnesses, like influenza, are known to exhibit distinct seasonal patterns of occurrence. Seasonal variations may lead to theories regarding the mode of infection transmission, behavioural traits associated with increased risk, and additional potential causes of the illness.

2.4.6.4. Place

Understanding the geographic scope and variation of the issue can be gained by characterizing the incidence of disease by location. A place's place of residence as well as any other geographic location connected to the occurrence of the disease are included in the description by place. These sites could be the hospital unit, school district, birthplace, place of employment, diagnosis or report location, or recent travel destinations. The unit could be a street address, a hospital wing, or an operating room, or it could be as big as a continent or a nation. Place can sometimes refer to a place category rather than a specific place, such as urban or rural, domestic or foreign, institutional or non-institutional.

Communities at higher risk of illness can be identified through location-based data analysis. Even though the data does not explain why these individuals are more likely to get sick, it can help produce theories that can be investigated in follow-up research. For instance, is a community more vulnerable because of the genetic susceptibility, lack of immunity, risky behaviours, exposure to contaminated food or local toxins? Is the increased risk, especially in the case of a communicable disease, due to features of the agent causing the illness, such as a particularly virulent strain, friendly breeding sites, or the presence of the vector that spreads the organism to humans? Or is the increased risk due to the environment that brings the agent and the host together, such as population density in urban areas, which raises the risk of disease transmission between individuals? (Lopez et al., 2006) (Murray et al., 2000).

2.5. Disability-Adjusted Life Years

The World Bank's 1993 World Health Report, Investing in Health, was the source of the DALY concept. The World Bank needed a metric that allowed health outcomes to be compared between nations in order to estimate the global burden of disease. Therefore, equity concerns played a key role in the creation of the DALYs.

The number of potentially healthy life years lost as a result of morbidity, disability, and death is known as the disability-adjusted life years or DALYs. This measure quantifies the health gap from a life lived in perfect health. Therefore, a disease burden of 100 DALYs per 1000 people annually would indicate a loss of 100 years of healthy life for every 1000 people. Thus, diseases or risk factors that cause a greater number of DALYs have a greater impact on public health. Both a morbidity and a mortality component make up the DALY. Years Lived with Disability (YLDs), which measure the number of years of healthy life lost as a result of having subpar health, are used to quantify morbidity. The number of incident cases multiplied by the health state's duration and disability weight yields the YLDs for a given condition. Introduced in the GDB 2010 study, an alternative prevalence-based version of the YLD is calculated by multiplying the number of prevalent cases by the disability weight. The disability weight, which represents the relative reduction in HRQoL on a scale from zero (perfect health) to one (worst possible health state), is an important component in both versions. Years of Life Lost (YLLs), or the number of years of healthy life lost due to passing away before a set life expectancy, are used to measure mortality. The residual life expectancy at the age of death multiplied by the number of deaths yields the YLLs. One way to extend the standard DALY formulas is to apply time discounting or age weighting. Yet, not all writers agree with these so-called social weighting functions. As a result, even in the most recent GBD updates, the use of age weighting and time discounting is decreasing.

2.5.1. Data Needs

It is clear that the caliber of the input data directly affects the caliber of the DALY estimate. Therefore, accurate incidence (or prevalence) and mortality data are essential to get the most accurate DALY estimate. The ideal source of data would be a nationally representative system that, using a precise set of diagnostic criteria, continuously tracks the occurrence of all disorders in the population. Since there is no such registration, one must make use of what is already in place. There are numerous sizable and significant data generation systems in operation in Belgium.

- The national health surveys (performed in 1997, 2001, 2004, 2008 and 2013)
- The National Cancer Registry
- The 40 national reference centers and 16 national reference laboratories for human microbiology
- The network of sentinel GPs and sentinel microbiology laboratories

The mandatory reporting of specific agents.

These data sources can offer important insights into the prevalence of the diseases and risk factors included, even with the degree of under-reporting and under-ascertainment taken into consideration.

Because of the strict privacy regulations in place, it is challenging to use healthcare providers' data directly in Belgium. Nonetheless, some information is provided as Minimal Clinical, Hospital, Nursing, and Psychiatric Information. These data sources offer useful information for estimating the direct costs associated with health care because they are limited to the financial impact of diseases. Given that non-aggregated data are made available, the announced intention to update the disease classification system to ICD-10-BE (International Classification of Disease, 10th Revision – Belgian Modification) in the Medical Data of the Minimal Hospital Data may prove valuable for health impact assessment studies.

There are several regional data collection methods in addition to the national data collection systems. Due to the disparities in databases and data collection practices among the various Belgian regions, it may be difficult to consistently use these data sources to produce burden estimates pertinent to the country. Furthermore, the diseases that are being reported vary by region, which results in partial availability of routine data for a portion of the nation.

One may turn to international databases or data from nearby nations when local data are not accessible. But Vanthomme et al. report indicating that the inability to use three major health databases (i.e., WHO-HFA, OECD, and EUROSTAT) promptly can be a significant impediment. Furthermore, when extrapolating data from nearby nations, it is assumed that the state of health in Belgium is comparable to that of its neighbours.

The absence of a distinct national system for collecting health data is the primary cause of the lack of data harmonization in the Belgian system. Public and private institutions have launched several separate initiatives, but there is a lack of communication between these various players. There are multiple registries for the same illness (e.g., diabetes registry), however, there are situations when it's unclear at what point a patient is added to a particular registry. Furthermore, it is impossible to combine registries due to differences in the codes used to define the disease, identify patients, and specify the follow-up period. One reason for this inconsistent system of health data collection is the division of health responsibilities among the federal, state, regional, and local levels.

Lastly, many diseases, particularly those brought on by chemicals, are not adequately reported in Belgium, including foodborne diseases (FBD). Due to the lack of priority given to these diseases in Belgium and the difficulty in assessing the impact of FBD on public health, there is a dearth of information.

2.5.2. DALY as a Summary Measure of Population Health

To express a population's health as a single numerical index, summary measures of population health (SMPH) integrate data on mortality with that on a wide range of non-fatal health outcomes. A wide range of potential uses for these summary measures include comparing the health of two populations, tracking changes in a population's health over time, identifying and measuring health disparities within a population, giving appropriate and balanced attention to the effects of non-fatal health outcomes on population health overall, setting priorities for the delivery of health services and planning, guiding research and development initiatives, and evaluating the advantages of health interventions to facilitate cost-effectiveness analyses.

Health expectancies and health gaps are the two main categories into which the vast array of summary measures that have been developed in the past fall. Time is a suitable metric that is used in both classes to assess the influence of both mortality and non-fatal health outcomes. Health expectancies are useful for communicating to a general audience and summarizing the average health attainment of a population. They estimate the average time that a person could expect to live in a defined state of health. Health gaps are used to measure the discrepancy between a population's actual and ideal states of health. They expand on the concept of mortality gaps by including time spent in states other than ideal health. While health gap measures allow for the categorical attribution of fatal and nonfatal injuries and BoDs to a comprehensive and mutually exclusive set of disease and injury causes, health expectancy measures do not naturally lend themselves to disaggregation by categorically defined causes. A health gap measure was selected for the GBD project and a new SMPH, the DALY, was developed because one of the primary objectives in selecting an SMPH for quantifying the GBD is to enable identification of the relative magnitude of various health problems, including diseases, injuries, and risk factors. The DALY is now the most popular composite health gap measure and the most widely used SMPH, thanks to the significant GBD projects.

2.5.3. Years of Life Lost (YLL), Years Lived with Disability (YLD), and Their Sum, the DALY

The DALY offers a distinctive viewpoint that unifies fatal and non-fatal outcomes while still permitting each to be investigated independently. It does this by combining data on mortality and morbidity into a single figure expressed in units of healthy life lost. One year of healthy life lost is equal to one DALY. Years of life lost (YLLs), which account for the age at which death occurs, are used to quantify mortality to facilitate the aggregation and comparison of the burdens of various illnesses and injuries. The number of deaths at each age is multiplied by the average life expectancy for that age to determine the YLL. The conversion of morbidity to years lived with disability (YLDs) is used. The term "YLD" stands for "lost years of full health." The degree of disability that each condition imposes on disease-affected individuals is measured using disability weights, which range from 0 (perfect health) to 1 (equivalent to death). The number of incident cases multiplied by the disease's expected mean duration and disability weight yields the YLD. The reference life expectancy, disability weights, time discounting, and age weights are among the social value decisions that must be made during the planning phase and are included in these metrics, as they are in all other SMPHs, either explicitly or implicitly. These value decisions have been hotly contested since the 1990 GBD study. In GBD 2010, the Institute for Health Metrics and Evaluation (IHME) unveiled a more straightforward version of DALYs. In that study, age weights and time discounting were eliminated, and prevalence YLD was utilized instead of incidence YLD. This led to a YLD computation procedure where the disability weight associated with a sequela is multiplied by the prevalence of the sequela. Non-fatal health outcomes can be measured using incidence- or prevalence-based metrics, although the YLL calculation is intrinsically based on an incidence-based viewpoint.

2.6. Prevalence

Prevalence is the percentage of individuals who have a certain risk factor or disease at a specific time. The starting point of a study is called the baseline time. For example, in a cohort study, each participant receives a full physical examination at the baseline. During this examination, we identify if each individual has a history of cardiovascular disease (CVD). The prevalence of CVD is calculated by dividing the number of existing cases of CVD by the total number of participants examined. This measurement is known as the point prevalence (PP) of CVD, indicating the level of disease at a particular time (i.e., at baseline).

$$\text{Point prevalence} = \frac{\text{Number of persons with disease}}{\text{Number of persons examined at baseline}}$$

Example 2.1

The fifth examination of the offspring in the Framingham Heart Study was conducted between 1991 and 1995. A total of n = 3799 participants participated in the fifth examination. Table 2.3 shows the numbers of men and women with diagnosed CVD at the fifth examination. The point prevalence of CVD among all participants attending the fifth examination of the Framingham Offspring Study is 379 / 3799 = 0.0998 or 9.98%. The point prevalence of CVD among men is 244 / 1792 = 0.1362, or 13.62%, and the point prevalence of CVD among women is 135 / 2007 = 0.0673, or 6.73%.

Table 2.3. *Men and Women with Diagnosed CVD*

	Free of CVD	History of CVD	Total
Men	1548	244	1792
Women	1872	135	2007
Total	3420	379	3799

Source: Lisa M. Sullivan. Essentials of Biostatistics in Public Health, Third Edition. Jones & Bartlett Learning.

Data on the prevalence of CVD among participants who were and were not smokers at the time of the Framingham Offspring Study's fifth examination are shown in Table 2.4. About 20 percent (744 / 3799) of the participants in the Framingham Offspring Study's fifth exam admitted to smoking at the time of the test. The point prevalence of CVD in current smokers is 81 / 744 = 0.1089 or 10.89 percent, and in non-smokers, it is 298 / 3055 = 0.0975 or 9.75 percent. (Pinheiro et al., 2011) (Scully et al., 2004).

Table 2.4. *Smoking and Diagnosed CVD*

	Free of CVD	History of CVD	Total
Nonsmoker	2757	298	3055
Current smoker	663	81	744
Total	3420	379	3799

Source: Lisa M. Sullivan. Essentials of Biostatistics in Public Health, Third Edition. Jones & Bartlett Learning.

2.7. Incidence

In epidemiological research, our main focus is frequently on predicting the chances of developing a disease rather than the percentage of people who currently have the disease. Prevalence represents the latter, while incidence indicates the likelihood of contracting a disease among individuals who do not currently have it and are at risk of developing it during a specified period. To include only individuals who are free of CVD, we eliminate participants from our fixed cohort at baseline who have a history of CVD (i.e., individuals who are actually "at risk" of contracting a disease). We keep track of these participants prospectively for ten years, noting whether or not each person develops CVD during that time. We can directly calculate the likelihood or risk of developing CVD over ten years if we can track each person for ten years and determine whether or not they develop the disease. To be more precise, we take the ratio of newly diagnosed CVD cases to all participants who were initially free of the disease. This is referred to as cumulative incidence (CI):

$$\text{Cumulative incidence} = \frac{\text{Number of persons who develop a disease during a specified period}}{\text{Number of persons at risk (at baseline)}}$$

The percentage of participants who contract an illness throughout a given observation period is represented by cumulative incidence. The total number of individuals at risk and the total number of disease-free individuals included at baseline are the same. The calculation of cumulative incidence is predicated on the assumption that each of these people is monitored for the full observation duration. In certain situations, such as an acute disease outbreak with a brief period of observation or follow-up, this might be feasible. However, in longer studies, it may be challenging to monitor each participant for the onset of disease since some participants may move, refuse to communicate with researchers, or pass away during the study's follow-up period. It is challenging to follow every participant in this example due to the older cohort (as is the case in most studies of cardiovascular disease and other diseases that are more common in older people) and the lengthy follow-up period (10 years). Later, the problems that occur and the solutions for inadequate follow-up are discussed.

2.7.1. Problems Estimating the Cumulative Incidence

Estimating the cumulative incidence of disease can be challenging due to a variety of issues. Since incidence studies are by nature longitudinal (e.g., five or ten years of follow-up), some research participants might disappear during that time. Some study participants can withdraw, for others to move, and for still others to pass away during the follow-up period. Additionally, various study designs might permit participants to arrive at various times (i.e., there is a rolling or extended enrolment period; participants are not all enrolled at baseline). Participants are often followed for varying periods for these and other reasons. We could limit our focus to individuals who finish the entire follow-up, but doing so would mean missing out on important data.

2.7.2. Person-Time Data

Once more, the general goal of epidemiological research is to determine the likelihood of contracting an illness (incidence) over a specific amount of time (e.g., ten years). The cumulative incidence is predicated on the assumption that every member of the population is informed of their disease status and that the entire population at risk is monitored for the duration of the observation period. By taking advantage of the different amounts of time that each participant contributes to the study, the unit of analysis is changed from the person or study participant to one that is explicitly defined: person-time. One can use months or years as the time unit (e.g., person-years or person-months). Assume, for instance, that a person enrols in a study in 1990 and is monitored until 2000, at which time it is concluded they are free of disease. A second participant joined the study in 1995 and became ill with the research disease in 2000. While the second person contributes five years of disease-free follow-up time before getting the disease, the first person contributes ten years of disease-free follow-up time. Using all of this data, we would like to calculate the disease's incidence. These two individuals provide a combined 15 years of disease-free time.

2.7.3. Incidence Rate

By dividing the total follow-up time (i.e., the sum of all disease-free person-time) by the number of new cases, the incidence rate is calculated using all available data. Rates are estimations that show the possibility or risk of an individual changing their disease status (e.g., developing a disease) in a given amount of time, and they aim to address the issue of differing follow-up times. The total amount of the disease-free follow-up period—that is, the period of time during which participants are thought to be at risk of contracting the disease—is the denominator. Rates are expressed as an integer value per multiple of participants over a specified period (e.g., the incidence of the disease is 12 per 1000 person-years) and are based on a specific period (e.g., 5 years, 10 years).

The ratio of newly diagnosed cases to total person-time units is used to calculate the incidence rate (IR), also known as the incidence density (ID). These person-time units can be person-months (e.g., 360 months, 60 months) or person-years (e.g., one person may contribute 10 years of follow-up, whereas another may contribute 5 years of follow-up). The total amount of time that each participant was at risk—that is, their time without illness—is the denominator. A rate with a particular time interval (e.g., 5 per 1000 person-years) is reported for the IR or ID. The incidence rate is given as follows:

$$\text{Incidence rate} = \text{IR} = \frac{\text{Number of persons who develop disease during a specified period}}{\text{Sum of the lengths of time during which persons are disease-free}}$$

The incidence rate is typically multiplied by a multiple of 10 (e.g., 100, 1000, or 10,000) for presentation purposes to obtain an integer value (see Example 2.2).

Example 2.2

Take a second look at the fifth assessment of the children in the Framingham Heart Study. A total of n = 3799 participants attended the fifth examination, and 379 of them had a history of CVD, as shown in Example 2.1. As a result, at the fifth examination, n = 3420 participants were free of CVD. Let's say we track each participant's progression of CVD for the ensuing ten years. The percentage of men and women who develop CVD over a 10-year follow-up period is displayed in **Table 2.5**.

Table 2.5. *Men and Women who Develop CVD*

	No CVD	Develop CVD	Total
Men	1358	190	1548
Women	1753	119	1872
Total	3111	309	3420

Source: Lisa M. Sullivan. Essentials of Biostatistics in Public Health, Third Edition. Jones & Bartlett Learning.

Because not every participant is followed for the full 10-year period, with the mean follow-up time being 7 years, we are unable to accurately estimate cumulative incidence based on previous data. The assumption that each of the 3111 individuals free of CVD would be followed for 10 years is incorrect. Instead, we should add up all available follow-up times and calculate an incidence rate. **Table 2.6** presents the disease-free follow-up times for men and women, as well as the corresponding incidence rates. These rates are reported as 190 per 10,000 person-years for men and 98 per 10,000 person-years for women, which can also be interpreted as 19 per 1000 men per 10 years and 9.8 per 1000 women per 10 years.

Table 2.6. *Total Disease-Free Time in Men and Women*

	Develop CVD	Total Follow-Up Time (years)	IR
Men	190	9984	0.01903
Women	119	12,153	0.00979
Total	309	22,137	0.01396

Source: Lisa M. Sullivan. Essentials of Biostatistics in Public Health, Third Edition. Jones & Bartlett Learning.

Person-time is the unit of analysis, and the denominator of the incidence rate is the total amount of time observed without illness (e.g., an individual's years in Example 2.2). Comparatively, the person serves as the unit of analysis and the denominator of the cumulative incidence is determined at the start of the study (baseline). It is important to remember that rates have a dimension—the quantity of new cases per person-time unit—and are frequently misinterpreted for proportions, also known as probabilities, or percentages, which have no dimensions and range from 0 to 1, 0% to 100%. The distinction between the prevalence, cumulative incidence, and incidence rate is shown in Example 2.3. It is noteworthy that, in contrast to the cumulative incidence, where the time component is only part of the interpretation, the time component is an integral part of the denominator of the incidence rate.

Example 2.3

Let us consider a six-person prospective cohort study. Every subject is enrolled at baseline, and the study's objective is to track every subject for ten years. Some participants develop CVD, some discontinue the study, and some pass away during the follow-up period. The follow-up experiences for every participant are shown in **Figure 2.3**. In this case, the following occurs: Participant 1 develops CVD six years into the study; Participant 2 passes away nine years into the study but is free of CVD; Participant 3 survives the entire follow-up period without developing any disease; Participant 4 develops CVD two years into the study and passes away after eight years; Participant 5 withdraws from the study after seven years without developing any disease; and Participant 6 develops CVD five years into the study.

We now calculate prevalence, cumulative incidence, and incidence rate using the information from Example 2.3.

- Prevalence of CVD at baseline = 0 /6 = 0, or 0%
- Prevalence of CVD at 5 years = 2 / 6 = 0.333, or 33%
- Prevalence of CVD at 10 years = 2 / 3 = 0.666, or 67%

- (Note that we can only assess disease status at 10 years in Participants 1, 3, and 6.)
- Cumulative incidence of CVD at 5 years = 2 / 6 = 0.333, or 33%

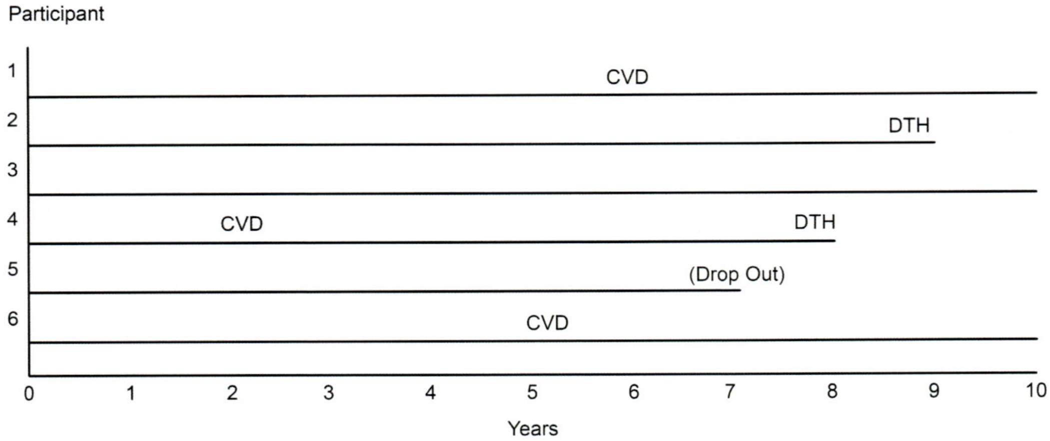

Figure 2.3. *Course of follow-up for six participants.*

Source: Lisa M. Sullivan. Essentials of Biostatistics in Public Health, Third Edition. Jones & Bartlett Learning.

We are unable to estimate the cumulative incidence of CVD at ten years because we do not have complete follow-up data for Participants 2, 4, or 5. We calculate the incidence rate to utilize all of the data that is available.

- The incidence rate of CVD = 3 / (6 + 9 + 10 + 2 + 7 + 5) = 3 / 39 = 0.0769
- We can report this as an incidence rate of CVD of 7.7 per 100 person-years.
- The incidence rate of death per person-year = 2 / (10 + 9 + 10 + 8 + 7 + 10) = 2 / 54 = 0.037
- We can report this as an incidence rate of death of 3.7 per 100 person-years.

It can be observed that the incidence rates are reported as the number of events per person-time, while the prevalence and cumulative incidence are expressed as percentages (they can also be expressed as proportions or probabilities).

2.8. Comparing the Extent of Disease Between Groups

Comparing groups in terms of the severity of the disease or the chance of contracting the disease is frequently interesting. One way to characterize these groups could be through exposure to potentially harmful agents (e.g., whether exposed or not), by a specific sociodemographic trait (e.g., men or women), or by a specific risk factor (e.g., whether they smoke now or not). Ratios or difference measures are the general categories for popular comparative measures. Ratio measures are used to compare things relative to one another, while difference measures are used to compare things absolute. To compare prevalence or incidence measures between comparison groups, one can create differences or ratios.

2.8.1. Difference Measures: Risk Difference and Population Attributable Risk

The absolute impact of the exposure or the absolute impact of the relevant risk factor on prevalence or incidence is measured by the risk difference (RD), also known as excess risk. The difference in point prevalence, cumulative incidence, or incidence rates between groups is known as the risk difference and can be calculated as follows:

$$\text{Risk difference} = RD = PP_{\text{exposed}} - PP_{\text{unexposed}}$$

$$RD = CI_{\text{exposed}} - CI_{\text{unexposed}}$$

$$RD = IR_{\text{exposed}} - IR_{\text{unexposed}}$$

We calculated the point prevalence of CVD in smokers and non-smokers in Example 2.1. Those who reported smoking during the fifth Framingham Offspring Study examination are considered exposed. By deducting the point prevalence for non-smokers from the point prevalence for smokers, the risk (prevalence) difference in CVD for smokers compared to non-smokers is calculated using data from Example 2.1. The absolute risk (prevalence) of CVD is 0.0114 higher in smokers than in non-smokers, according to the risk difference of 0.1089 – 0.0975 = 0.0114. The excess risk connected with exposure to the risk factor is represented by the risk difference, which can also be calculated by taking the difference in cumulative incidences or incidence rates between comparison groups. We calculated the incidence rates of CVD in men and women in Example 2.2. Here, the comparison groups are determined by sex rather than whether or not a risk factor was exposed. Therefore, we can calculate the risk difference by deducting the incidence rate for men from the incidence rate for women, or the other way around. The method used will determine how the results are interpreted. Using data from Example 2.2, the incidence rate difference between men and women is 190/10,000 person-years for men and 98/10,000 person-years for women, or 92/10,000 person-years. This suggests that men experience 92 more CVD events per 10,000 person-years than women do.

The risk difference in point prevalence or cumulative incidence can have values between –1 and 1. The risk difference in incidence rates can have values between ∞ and ∞ events per person-time. When the risk for those exposed is higher than the risk for those unexposed, the risk difference is positive. When the risk for those who are exposed is lower than the risk for those who are not, there is a negative risk difference. The risk difference is zero if exposure to the risk factor has no bearing on the likelihood of contracting the illness. The null or no-difference value of the risk difference is equal to zero.

An additional measure of difference that quantifies the relationship between a risk factor and the incidence or prevalence of disease is the population-attributable risk (PAR). This is how the population-attributable risk is calculated:

$$Population\ attributable\ risk = PAR = \frac{PP_{overall} - PP_{unexposed}}{PP_{overall}}$$

$$PAR = \frac{CI_{overall} - CI_{unexposed}}{CI_{overall}}$$

$$PAR = \frac{IR_{overall} - IR_{unexposed}}{IR_{overall}}$$

The difference between the total risk (exposed and unexposed individuals combined) and the risk of the unexposed is first evaluated in order to calculate the population attributable risk. This difference is typically displayed as a percentage after being divided by the total risk. Utilizing the information provided in Example 2.1, which contrasts the prevalence of CVD in smokers and non-smokers, the point prevalence of CVD for every participant present at the Framingham Offspring Study's fifth examination is 379 / 3799 = 0.0998. As a result, 2.3 percent of the common cases of CVD could be prevented if smoking exposure were to end. This is indicated by the population-attributable risk, which is calculated as (0.0998 – 0.0975) / 0.0998 = 0.023 or 2.3 percent. The range of 0 percent to 100 percent is commonly used to express the population-attributable risk. One way to interpret the magnitude of population-attributable risk is as the proportion of risk (prevalence or incidence) linked to the risk factor. The population-attributable risk is 0% if exposure to the risk factor has no bearing on the likelihood of contracting a disease (i.e., none of the risks is associated with exposure to the risk factor). The population-attributable risk is defined as the percentage of risk (prevalence or incidence) that could be eliminated if the exposure or risk factor were removed. It also presumes a causal relationship between the risk factor and disease.

2.8.2. Ratios: Relative Risk, Odds Ratio, and Rate Ratio

A useful metric for comparing the incidence or prevalence of disease between two groups is the relative risk (RR), sometimes known as the risk ratio. The calculation involves calculating the ratio of the corresponding cumulative incidences or prevalence. In general, the group of reference (e.g., individuals who are not exposed, do not have the risk factor, or are enrolled in the control group during a clinical trial) is taken into account in the denominator:

$$Relative\ risk = RR = \frac{PP_{exposed}}{PP_{unexposed}}$$

$$RR = \frac{CI_{exposed}}{CI_{unexposed}}$$

The rate ratio, also known as the incidence density ratio, is the ratio of incidence rates between two groups. The rate ratio of incident CVD in men compared to women, using the data from Example 2.2, is (190/10,000 person-years)/(98/10,000 person-years) = 1.94. Consequently, men have a 1.94 times higher incidence of CVD per person-year than women do.

Since the relative risk is based on a baseline (or comparative) level, it is frequently thought to be a more accurate indicator of the magnitude of the effect than the risk difference (or attributable risk). Based on the information in Example 2.1, smokers have a relative risk of CVD of 0.1089 / 0.0975 = 1.12, meaning that smokers have a 1.12 higher prevalence of CVD than nonsmokers. The relative risk and the rate ratio will both be 1 if exposure to the risk factor has no bearing on the likelihood of contracting an illness. The relative risk ranges from 0 to ∞. The null or no-effect value of the relative risk or the rate ratio is defined as 1.

It is not possible to calculate a relative risk under some study designs. Rather, the effect is measured by computing an odds ratio. Let's say we wish to evaluate the association between a specific risk factor's exposure and the presence of a disease in case-control research. In a case-control study, participants are chosen based on their results; some are considered cases, meaning they meet the condition of interest, while others are considered controls.

Example 2.4

The association between common cardiovascular disease and common hypertension at the offspring's fifth examination in the Framingham Heart Study is displayed in Table 2.7. The ratio of people with hypertension to those with CVD is 181 / 840 = 0.215. The percentage of people with CVD who do not have hypertension is 188 / 2942 = 0.064. In contrast to probabilities, which are based on the number of events to the number of non-events, odds are calculated using the number of events divided by the total sample size. A person with hypertension has 181 / 659 = 0.275 odds of having CVD. A person without hypertension has 188 / 2754 = 0.068 odds of having CVD.

People with hypertension are 3.36 times more likely to have prevalent CVD than people without hypertension, according to the relative risk of CVD for those with and without hypertension, which is 0.215 / 0.064 = 3.36. Although it is based on the ratio of odds, the computation of the odds ratio is similar. The odds ratio, which is 0.275 / 0.068 = 4.04, can be understood as follows: Compared to those without hypertension, those with hypertension have 4.04 times the risk of developing CVD.

Table 2.7. *Prevalent Hypertension and Prevalent CVD*

	No CVD	CVD	Total
No hypertension	2754	188	2942
Hypertension	659	181	840
Total	3413	369	3782

Source: Lisa M. Sullivan. Essentials of Biostatistics in Public Health, Third Edition. Jones & Bartlett Learning.

An odds ratio's invariance property is arguably its most crucial feature. The odds that a person with CVD has hypertension are 181 / 188 = 0.963, based on the information in Table 2.7. It is 659/2754 = 0.239 odds that a person without CVD has hypertension. For hypertension, the odds ratio is thus 0.963 / 0.239 = 4.04. Compared to those without CVD, those with CVD have 4.04 times higher odds of having hypertension. A relative risk does not hold this property. For instance, 181 / 369 = 0.491 represents the percentage of people with CVD who have hypertension. The ratio of people without cardiovascular disease (CVD) with hypertension is 659 / 3413, or 0.193. For hypertension, the relative risk is 0.491 / 0.193 = 2.54.

The odds ratio's invariance property makes it a perfect measure of association for a case-control study. For instance, if we were to conduct a case-control study on the potential connection between cigarette smoking and a rare form of cancer (e.g., a cancer believed to affect less than 1% of the general population), using individuals with the rare cancer as cases and similar cancer-free individuals as controls. Participants are asked if they have ever smoked or currently smoke cigarettes. In this study, both former and current smokers are classified as smokers. The data can be found in Table 2.8.

Table 2.8. *Smoking and Cancer*

	Cancer (Case)	No Cancer (Control)	Total
Smoker	40	29	69
Nonsmoker	10	21	31
Total	50	50	100

Source: Lisa M. Sullivan. Essentials of Biostatistics in Public Health, Third Edition. Jones & Bartlett Learning.

Due to the method used to gather the data, we are unable to determine the cancer incidence in the entire sample or smokers or non-smokers using these data. This sample shows that 10 / 31 = 0.32, or 32 percent of non-smokers, and 40 / 69 = 0.58, or 58 percent of smokers, have cancer, but this is an uncommon form of the disease. Because the sample was specifically created to include an equal number of cases and controls, these estimates do not accurately reflect the situation. If we had used a cohort study design and randomly selected participants from the general population, we might have needed to sample a larger number of people—perhaps over 10,00 to obtain enough cases for analysis. We can use the odds ratio from this case-control study to estimate the relationship between smoking and cancer. Smokers have 40 / 29 = 1.379 odds of developing cancer, while non-smokers have 10 / 21 = 0.476 odds. According to the odds ratio of 1.379 / 0.476 = 2.90, smokers are 2.9 more likely to develop cancer than non-smokers. Observe that this corresponds to the probability ratio of smoking among cancer cases relative to controls, i.e., that is, (40 / 10) / (29 / 21) = 4 / 1.38 = 2.90.

One helpful and significant feature of a case-control study is the ability to estimate an odds ratio. The odds ratio calculated in a research project with a prospective sampling plan (i.e., selecting representative groups of smokers and non-smokers and tracking the incidence of cancer) is comparable to the odds ratio determined by a method of retrospective sampling (i.e., collecting data on smoking status, and selecting representative groups of cancer patients and cancer-free patients).

The odds ratio can be calculated by comparing the point prevalence (PP) or cumulative incidence (CI) of a disease to its complementary proportion (1 – PP) or (1 – CI), respectively. It represents the odds of developing the disease for individuals who were exposed versus those who were not exposed. When using cumulative incidences, the odds ratio is defined as:

$$\text{Odds ratio} = \frac{CI_{exposed} / (1 - CI_{exposed})}{CI_{unexposed} / (1 - CI_{unexposed})}$$

When the disease under investigation is rare—typically defined as having a prevalence or cumulative incidence of less than 10 percent—the odds ratio will roughly represent the relative risk. Because of this, when the prevalence or cumulative incidence is low, it is common to interpret an odds ratio in the same way as a relative risk.

2.8.3. Issues with Person-Time Data

One of the unique features of person-time data that requires consideration is censoring. When the noteworthy event (e.g., not every person has their disease status) is noted, typically because of time constraints (e.g., the study's follow-up period expires, participants leave the study early, or they opt-out). Right, censoring is the most prevalent kind of censoring that takes place in epidemiological studies. Assume that we carry out a long-term research project and track participants' potential development of CVD over time. The time to event for participants who develop CVD is known; for the remaining subjects, we only know that the event did not develop during the study observation period. These individuals have a longer time-to-event, also known as their survival time, than the observation period. These periods, which are censored for analytical purposes, are known as Type I censored or right-censored periods. Strategies to manage survival time, which is also known as time-to-event data. (Snow et al., 1936) (Walter et al., 2016)

A Closer Look

Relationships between Prevalence and Incidence

The prevalence (proportion of the population with the disease at a point in time) of a disease depends on the incidence (risk of developing disease within a specified time) of the disease as well as the duration of the disease. If the incidence is high but the duration is short, the prevalence (at a point in time) will be low by comparison. In contrast, if the incidence is low but the duration of the disease is long, the prevalence will be high. When the prevalence of the disease is low (less than 1%), the prevalence is approximately equal to the product of the incidence and the mean duration of the disease (assuming that there have not been major changes in the course of the disease or its treatment). Hypertension is an example of a disease with a relatively high prevalence and low incidence (due to its long duration). Influenza is an example of a condition with low prevalence and high incidence (due to its short duration).

The incidence rate is interpreted as the instantaneous potential to change the disease status (i.e., from non-diseased to diseased, also called the hazard) per unit of time. An assumption that is implicit in the computation of the IR or ID is that the risk of disease is constant over time. This is not a valid assumption for many diseases because the risk of disease can vary over time and among certain subgroups (e.g. persons of different ages have different risks of disease). It is also very important that only persons who are at risk of developing the disease of interest are included in the denominator of the estimate of incidence. For example, if a disease is known to affect only people over 65 years of age, then including disease-free follow-up time measured on study participants less than 65 years of age will underestimate the true incidence. Person-times measured in these participants should not be included in the denominator as these participants are not truly at risk of developing the disease before age 65.

Prevalence and incidence measures are important measures that quantify the extent of disease and the rate of development of disease in study populations. Understanding the difference between prevalence and incidence is critical. Prevalence refers to the extent of a disease at a point in time, whereas incidence refers to the development of disease over a specified time. Because it can be difficult to ascertain disease status in every participant in longitudinal studies—particularly when the follow-up period is long—measures that take into account all available data are needed. Incidence rates that account for varying follow-up times are useful measures in epidemiological analysis.

The formulas to estimate and compare prevalence and incidence are summarized in Table 2.9.

Table 2.9. *Summary of Key Formulas*

Measure	Formula
Point prevalence (PP)*	$\frac{\text{Number of persons with disease}}{\text{Number of persons examined at baseline}}$
Cumulative incidence (CI)*	$\frac{\text{Number of persons who develop disease during a specified period}}{\text{Number of persons at risk (at baseline)}}$
Incidence rate (IR)	$\frac{\text{Number of persons who develop disease during a specified period}}{\text{Sum of the lengths of time during which persons are disease-free}}$
Risk difference (RD)	$PP_{exposed} - PP_{unexposed}, CI_{exposed} - CI_{unexposed}, IR_{exposed} - IR_{unexposed}$
Population attributable risk (PAR)	$\frac{PP_{overall} - PP_{unexposed}}{PP_{overall}}, \frac{CI_{overall} - CI_{unexposed}}{CI_{overall}}, \frac{IR_{overall} - IR_{unexposed}}{IR_{overall}}$
Relative risk (RR)	$\frac{PP_{exposed}}{PP_{unexposed}}, \frac{CI_{exposed}}{CI_{unexposed}}$
Odds ratio (OR)	$\frac{PP_{exposed}/(1-PP_{exposed})}{PP_{unexposed}/(1-PP_{unexposed})}, \frac{CI_{exposed}/(1-CI_{exposed})}{CI_{unexposed}/(1-CI_{unexposed})}$

* Can also be expressed as a percentage.

Source: *Lisa M. Sullivan. Essentials of Biostatistics in Public Health, Third Edition. Jones & Bartlett Learning.*

Summary

- In the Western biomedical perspective, the term disease is defined as 'a condition of the living animal or plant body or of one of its parts that impairs normal functioning and is typically manifested by distinguishing signs and symptoms.
- The word infirmity refers to 'the quality or state of being of poor or deteriorated vitality.
- Agent originally referred to an infectious microorganism or pathogen: a virus, bacterium, parasite, or other microbe.
- Host refers to the human who can get the disease. A variety of factors intrinsic to the host, sometimes called risk factors, can influence an individual's exposure, susceptibility, or response to a causative agent.
- Environment refers to extrinsic factors that affect the agent and the opportunity for exposure. Environmental factors include physical factors such as geology and climate, biologic factors such as insects that transmit the agent, and socioeconomic factors such as crowding, sanitation, and the availability of health services.
- Epidemiology is the study (scientific, systematic, data-driven) of the distribution (frequency, pattern) and determinants (causes, risk factors) of health-related states and events (not just diseases) in specified populations (patient is a community, individuals viewed collectively), and the application of (since epidemiology is a discipline within public health) this study to the control of health problems.
- Prevalence refers to the proportion of participants with a risk factor or disease at a particular point in time.
- Cumulative incidence reflects the proportion of participants who become diseased during a specified observation period. The total number of persons at risk is the same as the total number of persons included at baseline who are disease-free.
- The incidence rate (IR), also called the incidence density (ID), is computed by taking the ratio of the number of new cases of disease to the total number of person-time units available. These person-time units may be person-years (e.g., one individual may contribute 10 years of follow-up, whereas another may contribute 5 years of follow-up) or person months (e.g., 360 months, 60 months). The denominator is the sum of all of the participants' time at risk (i.e., disease-free time).
- The risk difference (RD), also called excess risk, measures the absolute effect of the exposure or the absolute effect of the risk factor of interest on prevalence or incidence.
- The relative risk (RR), also called the risk ratio, a useful measure to compare the prevalence or incidence of disease between two groups. It is computed by taking the ratio of the respective prevalence or cumulative incidences

References

1. Bautista-Valarezo, E., Duque, V., Verdugo Sánchez, A. E., et al. (2020). Towards an indigenous definition of health: An explorative study to understand the indigenous Ecuadorian people's health and illness concepts. *International Journal for Equity in Health, 19*, 101. https://doi.org/10.1186/s12939-020-1142-8

2. Bilcke, J., Van Damme, P., De Smet, F., Hanquet, G., Van Ranst, M., & Beutels, P. (2008). The health and economic burden of rotavirus disease in Belgium. *European Journal of Pediatrics, 167*, 1409–1419. https://doi.org/10.1007/s00431-008-0684-3
3. Lopez, A. D., Mathers, C. D., Ezzati, M., Jamison, D. T., & Murray, C. J. L. (Eds.). (2006). *Global Burden of Disease and Risk Factors*. Washington, D.C.: World Bank.
4. Lopez, A., Mathers, C., Ezzati, M., Jamison, D., & Murray, C. (2006). *Global Burden of Disease and Risk Factors*. New York: Oxford University Press.
5. Murray, C. J. L., Salomon, J. A., & Mathers, C. D. (2000). A critical examination of summary measures of population health. *Bulletin of the World Health Organization, 78*, 981–994.
6. Murray, C. J. L., Salomon, J. A., Mathers, C. D., & Lopez, A. D. (Eds.). (2002). *Summary Measures of Population Health: Concepts, Ethics, Measurement and Applications*. Geneva: World Health Organization.
7. Pinheiro, P., Plaß, D., & Krämer, A. (2011). The burden of disease approach for measuring population health. In A. Krämer, M. M. Khan, & F. Kraas (Eds.), *Health in Megacities and Urban Areas* (pp. 21–38). Heidelberg: Physica-Verlag.
8. Scully, J. L. (2004). What is a disease? *EMBO Reports, 5*(7), 650–653. https://doi.org/10.1038/sj.embor.7400195
9. Singer, M., & Erickson, P. I. (2013). *Global Health: An Anthropological Perspective*. Waveland Press.
10. Snow, J. (1936). *Snow on Cholera*. London: Humphrey Milford: Oxford University Press.
11. Walter, M., & Andersen, C. (2016). *Indigenous Statistics: A Quantitative Research Methodology*. Routledge.

Chapter 3

SUMMARIZING DATA COLLECTED IN THE SAMPLE

Contents

Introduction 64
3.1. Data Collection Methods 66
3.2. Why Select a Sample? 83
3.3. Types of Variables 87
Summary 97
References 97

Introduction

Concisely describing the data at hand is the first step in analyzing it. Listing each data point can be used to complete this step in smaller studies. However, this process is usually time-consuming or unfeasible, and even if it were feasible, it would not provide a comprehensive view of the data. This is how the fundamental issue in statistics can be put: Take a look at sample data X_1, X_n, where the first sample point is represented by X_1 and the nth sample point by X_n. What conclusions or inferences about population P, assuming that the sample is taken from it, can be drawn from the sample?

Before this question can be answered, the data must be summarized as succinctly (concisely, briefly) as possible, since the number of sample points is frequently large and it is easy to lose track of the overall picture by looking at all the data at once. One type of measure useful for summarizing data defines the center, or middle, of the sample. This type of measure is a measure of central tendency (location).

Before attempting the measures of central tendency and dispersion, let's see some of the notations that are used frequently. Notations: $\sum$ is read as Sigma (the Greek Capital letter for S) means the sum of

Suppose n values of a variable are denoted as x_1, x_2, x_3...., x_n then $\sum x_i = x_1, + x_2, + x_3 + ... x_n$ where the subscript i range from 1 up to n

Example: Let $x_1=2$, $x_2 = 5$, $x_3=1$, $x_4 =4$, $x_5=10$, $x_6= -5$, $x_7 = 8$

Since there are 7 observations, i range from 1 up to 7

i. $\sum x_i = 2+5+1+4+10-5+8 = 25$

ii. $(\sum x_I)^2 = (25)^2 = 625$

iii. $\sum x_I^2 = 4 + 25 + 1 + 16 + 100 + 25 + 64 = 235$

- ***Rules for Working with Summation***

1. $\sum (x_i + y_i) = \sum x_i + \sum y_i$, where the number of x values = the number of y values.
2. $\sum K x_i = k \times \sum x_i$, where K is a constant.
3. $\sum K = n \times K$, where K is a constant.

Orientation and Directional Terms

<table>
<tr><th>Term</th><th>Definition</th><th>Illustration</th></tr>
<tr><td>Frequency distribution</td><td>Frequency distribution is a representation, either in a graphical or tabular format, that displays the number of observations within a given interval. The frequency is how often a value occurs in an interval while the distribution is the pattern of frequency of the variable.</td><td>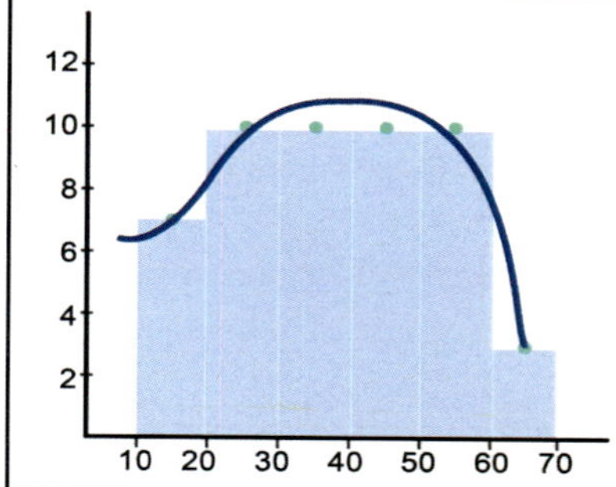
</td></tr>
<tr><td>Bar chart</td><td>Bar chart is a chart or graph that presents categorical data with rectangular bars with heights or lengths proportional to the values that they represent. The bars can be plotted vertically or horizontally. A vertical bar chart is sometimes called a column chart.</td><td>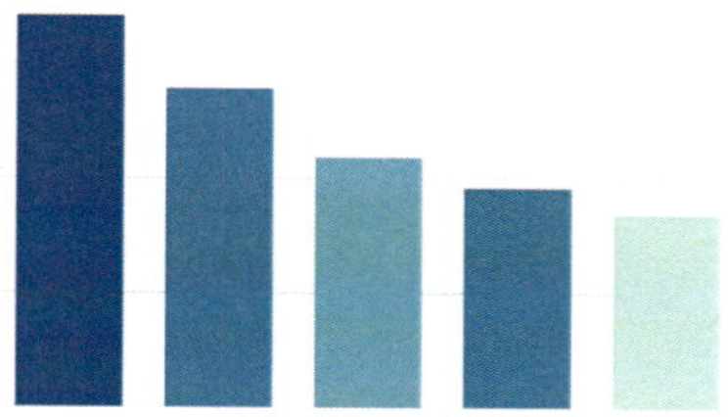</td></tr>
<tr><td>Histogram</td><td>Histogram is a bar graph-like representation of data that buckets a range of classes into columns along the horizontal x-axis. The vertical y-axis represents the number count or percentage of occurrences in the data for each column.</td><td>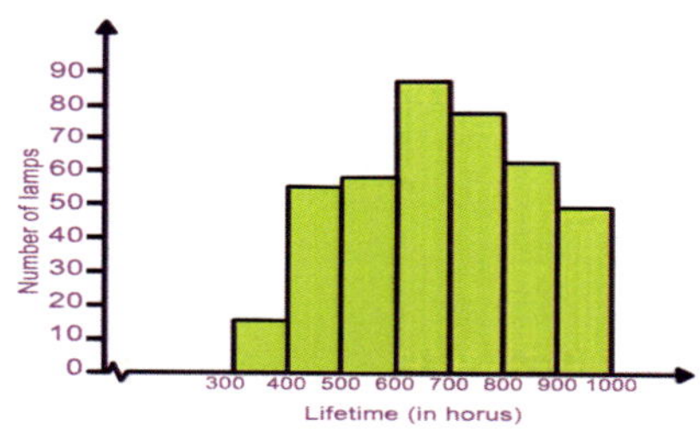
</td></tr>
<tr><td>Simple Random Sampling</td><td>Simple random sampling is a type of probability sampling in which the researcher randomly selects a subset of participants from a population. Each member of the population has an equal chance of being selected. Data is then collected from as large a percentage as possible of this random subset.</td><td>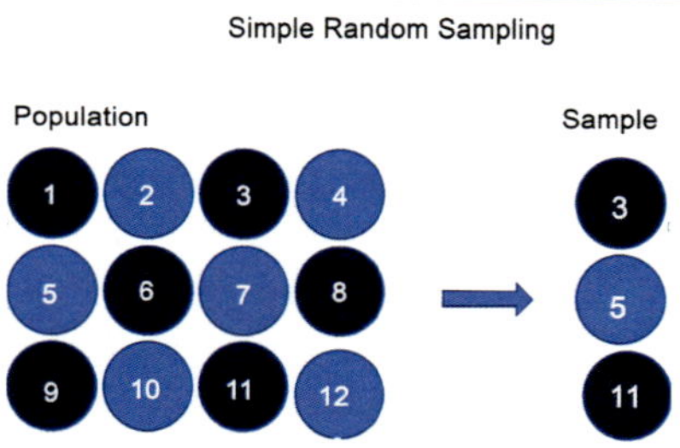
</td></tr>
<tr><td>Systematic sampling</td><td>Systematic sampling is a probability sampling method where researchers select members of the population at a regular interval – for example, by selecting every 15th person on a list of the population. If the population is in a random order, this can imitate the benefits of simple random sampling.</td><td>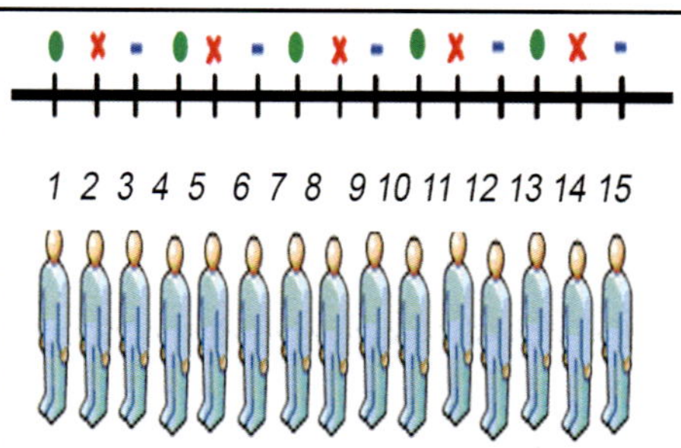
</td></tr>
</table>

3.1. Data Collection Methods

Through the use of data collection techniques, we are able to gather information about people, things, and phenomena as well as the environments in which they occur in a methodical manner. We must be methodical in the way we gather data. It will be challenging to provide a comprehensive response to our research questions if data are gathered randomly.

Various data collection techniques can be used such as:

- Observation
- Face-to-face and self-administered interviews
- Postal or mail method and telephone interviews
- Using available information
- Focus group discussions (FGD)
- Other data collection techniques – Rapid appraisal techniques, 3L technique, Nominal group techniques, Delphi techniques, life histories, case studies, etc.

1. ***Observation***: The method of observation entails methodically choosing, observing, and recoding human behavior as well as those of other phenomena and elements of their environment in order to obtain (gain) specific information. It covers every approach, from straightforward visual observations to the application of advanced machinery and measurements, as well as sophisticated facilities and equipment like X-ray, radiography, biochemistry, microscopes, clinical exams, and microbiological examinations. Before any data is actually collected, lay out the guidelines for the observations.
2. ***Advantages***: Gives relatively more accurate data on behavior and activities.
3. ***Disadvantages***: Investigators or observer's own biases, prejudice, desires, and etc. and needs more resources and skilled human power during the use of high level machines.
4. ***Interviews and self-administered questionnaire***: The two methods for gathering research data that are most frequently used are probably interviews and self-administered questionnaires. Thus, creating effective "questioning tools" is a crucial and time-consuming step in the creation of the majority of research proposals.

Once the decision has been made to use these techniques, the following questions should be considered before designing our tools:

- What exactly do we want to know, according to the objectives and variables we identified earlier? Is questioning the right technique to obtain all answers, or do we need additional techniques, such as observations or analysis of records?
- Of whom will we ask questions and what techniques will we use? Do we understand the topic sufficiently to design a questionnaire, or do we need some loosely structured interviews with key informants or a focus group discussion first to orient ourselves?
- Are our informants mainly literate or illiterate? If illiterate, the use of self-administered questionnaires is not an option.
- How large is the sample that will be interviewed? Studies with many respondents often use shorter, highly structured questionnaires, whereas smaller studies allow more flexibility and may use questionnaires with several open-ended questions.

Interviews can be less or more structured depending on the decision that has been made.

Unstructured interviews are adaptable; the questions' content and sequence change from one interview to the next. The investigators do not predetermine the precise questions to be asked or the sequence in which they will be asked; they simply know what they hope to find out. In other circumstances, a more uniform approach might be employed, with the questions' phrasing and sequence determined beforehand. This could be a self-administered questionnaire where the respondent reads the questions and fills in the answers on his own (sometimes with the help of an interviewer who "stands by" to help if needed), or it could be a highly structured interview where the questions are asked systematically.

In community medicine research, standardized approaches to questioning are typically preferred because they increase the likelihood of reproducible data. Less structured interviews might be helpful in intensive studies of perceptions, attitudes, motivation, and affective reactions, as well as in preliminary surveys where the goal is information to aid in the planning of a study later on rather than factors for analysis. One of the hallmarks of qualitative (as opposed to quantitative) research is unstructured interviews.

The use of self-administered questionnaires is simpler and cheaper; such questionnaires can be administered to many persons simultaneously (e.g., to a class of students), and unlike interviews, can be sent by post. On the other hand, they demand a certain level of education and skill on the part of the respondents; people of a low socio-economic status are less likely to respond to a mailed questionnaire.

When conducting a questionnaire-based interview, the investigator selects agents referred to as enumerators, who visit the respondents in person, hand them the questionnaire, ask them the questions it contains, and note their responses. These may be conducted over the phone or in person.

1. ***Face-to-face and telephone interviews***: An effective interviewer can pique and sustain the respondent's interest and foster a rapport (understanding, harmony) and environment that facilitates question-answering. The interviewer can calm any anxiety that may have arisen. If a question is unclear, the interviewer may ask it again and, if required (and in compliance with predetermined guidelines), offer an explanation or alternative wording. It is difficult to include optional follow-up or probing questions in self-administered questionnaires that should only be asked if previous responses are contradictory or inconclusive. Additionally, observations can be made during in-person interviews. With the crucial caveat that they are carried out by qualified interviewers, interviews are generally preferable to self-administered questionnaires, aside from their costs.
2. ***Mailed Questionnaire Method***: With this approach, a questionnaire with several questions about the area of study is created by the investigator. The questionnaires are mailed to the informants along with a kind cover letter outlining the details, the purposes and goals of gathering the data, and a request for cooperation on the part of the respondents to provide accurate responses and return the completed questionnaire. Usually, the investigator covers the cost of return postage to guarantee a prompt response. The primary issues with postal questionnaires are that they may underrepresent subjects with lower levels of literacy and that response rates are typically rather low.
3. ***Use of documentary sources***: Clinical and other personal records, death certificates, published mortality statistics, census publications, etc. Examples include:

- Official publications of the Central Statistical Authority
- Publication of Ministry of Health and Other Ministries
- News Papers and Journals.
- International Publications like Publications by WHO, World Bank, UNICEF
- Records of hospitals or any Health Institutions.

Even though using data from documents can save time and money, it is still important to ensure that the data is accurate and comprehensive. The primary author of the data and the user may have different goals in mind.

1. ***Problems in Gathering Data***: It is important to recognize some of the main problems that may be faced when collecting data so that they can be addressed in the selection of appropriate collection methods and the training of the staff involved.

   Common problems might include:

- Language barriers
- Lack of adequate time
- Expense
- Inadequately trained and experienced staff
- Invasion of privacy
- Suspicion
- Bias (spatial, project, person, season, diplomatic, professional)
- Cultural norms (e.g., which may preclude men from interviewing women)

3.1.1. Choosing a Method of Data Collection

Information that is timely, accurate, relevant, and useful is essential for decision-makers. These data are expensive to collect, process, and analyze. Finding methods that produce information that is timely, relevant, affordable, and essential for immediate use is the difficult part. Certain approaches prioritize cost-effectiveness and timeliness. Others focus on methodological rigor and accuracy when employing scientific approaches. Two categories could apply to the statistical data, depending on the sources.

3.1.1.1. Primary Data

Primary data are those that are gathered directly from the source by the researcher to support a particular investigation or study. These are unique data that are primarily produced by surveys that are carried out by individuals or academic institutions. As the investigator can extract accurate information by dispelling any doubts the respondents may have had about specific questions, first-hand information gathered by the investigator is more trustworthy and accurate. Since the responses to a variety of questions are obtained instantly, high response rates may be attained. It enables questions about complex subjects to be explained.

3.1.1.2. Secondary Data

Secondary data are those that are used by investigators that have previously gathered data. For the organization that collected the data, these are primary data; however, when someone else uses them for their own gain, they become secondary data. Journals, reports, government publications, professional publications, and research organization publications are good sources of secondary data. It costs less money and effort to gather secondary data. These data can also be used more effectively, and occasionally their quality may even be higher because they were gathered by individuals who received specialized training for that very purpose. However, these data must be used extremely carefully because they may contain many errors. After all, the primary agency's motivation for gathering the data may have been different from the user's. Second, it's important to carefully examine the validity of the secondary data because it's possible that bias was introduced, the sample size was insufficient, or there were definitional or arithmetic errors.

Generally speaking, the accuracy of the information that a method of data collection yields plays a major role in the method choice. In this sense, "accuracy" refers to both the relevance of the information as well as its correspondence with objective reality, though this is undoubtedly a component of the concept. The degree to which the approach will yield an accurate measurement of the variable the researcher wants to examine is this issue.

The selection of the method of data collection is also based on practical considerations, such as:

1. The need for personnel, skills, equipment, etc. about what is available and the urgency with which results are needed.
2. The acceptability of the procedures to the subjects – the absence of inconvenience, unpleasantness, or untoward consequences.
3. The probability that the method will provide good coverage, i.e., will supply the required information about all or almost all members of the population or sample. If many people will not know the answer to the question, then the question is not an appropriate one.

A legitimate factor to take into account could be the investigator's experience with a study technique. That a scientist formulates problems in a way that calls for the application of specific techniques unique to him to solve them should not come as a significant surprise.

3.1.2. Types of Questions

We must first go over the different kinds of questions that are included in questionnaires before looking at the steps involved in creating one. Open-ended and closed questions are the two main categories of questions based on how they are posed and documented.

3.1.2.1. Open-Ended Questions

Free-form answers to open-ended questions should be noted using the respondent's own words. There are no options available for the respondent to select from.

Such questions are useful to obtain information on:

- Facts with which the researcher is not very familiar,
- Opinions, attitudes, and suggestions of informants, or
- Sensitive issues.

For example

- Can you describe exactly what the traditional birth attendant did when your labour started?
- What do you think are the reasons for a high drop-out rate of village health committee members?
- What would you do if you noticed that your daughter (schoolgirl) had a relationship with a teacher?

3.1.2.2. Closed Questions

Closed questions offer a list of possible options or answers from which the respondents must choose. When designing closed questions one should try to:

- Offer a list of options that are exhaustive and mutually exclusive
- Keep the number of options as few as possible.

Closed questions are useful if the range of possible responses is known.

For example

What is your marital status?

1. Single
2. Married/living together
3. Separated/divorced/widowed

Have your every gone to the local village health worker for treatment?

1. Yes
2. No

Closed questions may also be used if one is only interested in certain aspects of an issue and does not want to waste the time of the respondent and interviewer by obtaining more information than one needs.

3.1.2.3. Requirements of Questions

Face validity is a requirement, meaning the question we create must provide an accurate and pertinent measurement for the variable. For instance, it might seem obvious that birth weight data recorded in an obstetrics ward is more reliable than data gathered from mothers who are questioned.

- ***Must be unambiguous*** – how questions are worded can 'make or break' a questionnaire. Questions must be unambiguous. They must be phrased in language that it is believed the respondent will understand and that all respondents will understand in the same way. To ensure clarity, each question should contain only one idea; 'double-barrelled' questions like 'Do you take your child to a doctor when he has a cold or has diarrhea?' are difficult to answer, and the answers are difficult to interpret.
- ***Must not be offensive*** – whenever possible it is wise to avoid questions that may offend the respondent, for example those that deal with intimate matters, those which may seem to expose the respondent's ignorance, and those requiring him to give a socially unacceptable answer.
- ***The questions should be fair*** – They should not be phrased in a way that suggests a specific answer and should not be loaded. Short questions are generally regarded as preferable to long ones.
- ***Sensitive questions*** – It may not be possible to avoid asking 'sensitive' questions that may offend respondents, e.g., those that seem to expose the respondent's ignorance. In such situations, the interviewer (questioner) should do it very carefully and wisely.

3.1.3. Steps in Designing a Questionnaire

A quality questionnaire requires multiple drafts to design. We should focus on the content of the first draft. In the second, we ought to examine the questions' phrasing and order closely. Next, we ought to carefully examine the questionnaire's format. To ensure that the questionnaire provides us with the information we need and that both the respondents and we are comfortable with it, we should conduct a test run. Before we can use the questionnaire to actually collect data, it usually needs to be further adjusted.

3.1.3.1. Step 1: Content

1. ***Take your objectives and variables as your starting point.***

   Select the questions that will help you define and measure your variables and accomplish your goals. You should review the variables you selected when creating the questionnaire and, if necessary, add, remove, or modify some of them. You might even decide at this point to modify some of your goals.

3.1.3.2. Step 2: Formulating Questions

1. ***Formulate one or more questions that will provide the information needed for each variable.***

   Make sure your questions are sufficiently clear and specific to prevent varying responses from different respondents. For instance, it would be inappropriate to ask a general question like "Where do community members typically seek treatment when they are sick?" as each respondent may have a different response in mind.

- One informant may think of measles with complications and say he goes to the hospital, another of cough and say goes to the private pharmacy;
- Even if both think of the same disease, they may have different degrees of seriousness in mind and thus answer differently;
- In all cases, self-care may be overlooked.
- The question, therefore, as a rule has to be broken up into different parts and made so specific that all informants focus on the same thing. For example, one could:
- Concentrate on an illness that has occurred in the family over the past 14 days and ask what has been done to treat it from the onset; or
- Concentrate on several diseases, ask whether they have occurred in the family over the past X months (chronic or serious diseases have a longer recall period than minor ailments), and what has been done to treat each of them from the onset.

2. ***Check whether each question measures one thing at a time.***

   The question, "How large an interval would you and your husband prefer between two successive births?" for instance would be better off being split into two sections because the husband and wife may disagree on the ideal interval.

3. ***Avoid leading questions.***

   If a question implies a particular response, it is leading. For instance, there isn't much space for a "no" response or other options when asked, "Do you agree that the district health team should visit each health center monthly?" A more appropriate question might be, "Do you think that district health teams should visit each health center? If yes, how often?" There are situations when a question is leading because it assumes something. For instance, asking "What did you do when your child had diarrhoea the last time?" assumes that the child has already experienced diarrhoea. The following would be a better series of questions: "Has your child had diarrhoea? If so, when was the last time? Did you treat it? If so, how?

3.1.3.3. Step 3: Sequencing of Questions

1. ***Design your interview schedule or questionnaire to be "consumer friendly."***

- The sequence of questions must be logical for the respondent and allow as much as possible for a "natural" discussion, even in more structured interviews.

- At the beginning of the interview, keep questions concerning "background variables" (e.g., age, religion, education, marital status, or occupation) to a minimum. If possible, pose most or all of these questions later in the interview. (Respondents may be reluctant to provide "personal" information early in an interview)
- Start with an interesting but non-controversial question (preferably open) that is directly related to the subject of the study. This type of beginning should help to raise the informants' interest and lessen suspicions concerning the purpose of the interview (e.g., that it will be used to provide information to use in levying taxes).
- Pose more sensitive questions as late as possible in the interview (e.g., questions about income, sexual behavior, or diseases with the stigma attached to them, etc.
- Use simple everyday language.

Make the questionnaire as short as possible. Interview two parts if the nature of the topic requires a long questionnaire (more than 1 hour).

3.1.3.4. Step 4: Formatting the Questionnaire

When you finalize your questionnaire, be sure that:

- Each questionnaire has a heading and space to insert the number, data and location of the interview, and, if required the name of the informant. You may add the name of the interviewer to facilitate quality control.
- Layout is such that questions belonging together appear together visually. If the questionnaire is long, you may use subheadings for groups of questions.
- Sufficient space is provided for answers to open-ended questions.
- Boxes for pre-categorized answers are placed in a consistent manner half of the page.

3.1.3.5. Step 5: Translation

To standardize the questions asked, the questionnaire must be translated if the interview will be conducted in one or more local languages. It should be translated again into the original language after being translated. After that, you can assess any discrepancies between the two versions and decide how to finally phrase complex ideas.

3.1.4. Methods of Data Organization and Presentation

Raw data is the information gathered from surveys. Most of the time, the abundance of unsorted data does not immediately reveal any meaningful information. The way collected data are arranged must be such that the information they hold is condensed and can display patterns of variation. Only when the properties of the data are known can specific methods of analysis be chosen. Several methods of data organization and presentation, including order arrays, tables, and diagrams, are employed for this project's main goal.

3.1.4.1. Frequency Distributions

Data can be better understood and compared quickly by organizing it into tables or various types of graphs. When dealing with large amounts of data, such as from a health center's records, tables are helpful for condensing information. Creating a frequency distribution is often done to present data in a meaningful way and detect any patterns that may not be apparent in the raw data.

1. ***Array (ordered array):*** The information is organized into a sequential list of numbers, either in an increasing or decreasing sequence. This allows us to understand the range of values and the overall distribution of the data. An ordered array is the most suitable format when dealing with small data sets (typically less than 20). For example, in a study where 400 individuals were surveyed about the number of full-length movies watched on television in the past week, the following distribution of the data was obtained.

Table 3.1. *Distribution of the Data Collected*

Number of movies	Number of persons	Relative frequency (%)
0	72	18.0
1	106	26.5
2	153	38.3
3	40	10.0
4	18	4.5
5	7	1.8
6	3	0.8
7	0	0.0
8	1	0.3
Total	400	100.0

Source: https://www.cartercenter.org/resources/pdfs/health/ephti/library/lecture-notes/env-health-science-students/ln-biostat-hss-final.pdf.

In the distribution above, the variable under consideration is represented by the number of movies, the frequency by the number of people, and the entire distribution is referred to as a frequency distribution, specifically a simple frequency distribution.

2. ***A categorical distribution***: Non-numerical information can also be represented in a frequency distribution. Seniors of a high school were interviewed on their plan after completing high school. The following data give plans of 548 seniors of a high school.

Seniors' Plan	Number of Senior
Plan to attend college	240
May attend college	146
Plan to or may attend a vocational school	57
Will not attend any school	105
Total	548

Suppose a social scientist wishes to investigate the age distribution of people arrested in a nation. When dealing with extensive datasets, it is frequently possible to present a clear and comprehensive picture while retaining enough information by organizing the data into multiple class intervals, as illustrated below.

Age (years)	Number of persons
Under 18	1,748
18 – 24	3,325
25 – 34	3,149
35 – 44	1,323
45 – 54	512
55 and over	335
Total	10,392

This kind of frequency distribution is called grouped frequency distribution.

Although frequency distributions offer a clear and concise representation of the data, they are not always sufficient for all purposes. In most cases, certain information can only be ascertained using the original data. For example, it is impossible to determine how many of the arrested individuals are over 62 or how many are 19 years old based on the grouped frequency distribution above.

The construction of grouped frequency distribution consists essentially of four steps:

1. Choosing the classes,
2. sorting (or tallying) of the data into these classes,
3. counting the number of items in each class, and
4. displaying the results in the form of a chart or table

Determining the number of classes and the range of values that each class should cover—that is, from where each class should go—are key components of selecting an appropriate classification scheme. Both of these decisions are somewhat subjective, but they also rely on the type of data, how accurate it is, and what the distribution is meant to accomplish.

- Less than 6 or more than 20 classes are rarely used; fifteen is usually a good number; the precise number we use in a given scenario primarily depends on how many measurements or observations we have to group.

A guide on the determination of the number of classes (k) can be the Sturge's Formula, given by:

$K = 1 + 3.322 \times \log(n)$, where n is the number of observations

And the length or width of the class interval (w) can be calculated by:

$W = (\text{Maximum value} - \text{Minimum value})/K = \text{Range}/K$

- Every measurement or observation is always assigned to a single class; that is, classes must be mutually exclusive. To achieve this, we must ensure that the greatest and smallest values are included in the classification, that no value can fall into a potential gap between classes, and that classes do not overlap—that is, that classes do not share any values.

  Note that the Sturges rule should not be regarded as final, but should be considered as a guide only. The number of classes specified by the rule should be increased or decreased for convenient or clear presentation.

- Establishing class limits: (i) Class limits have to be precise and unambiguous. Stated differently, open-end classes should be avoided because they make it challenging, if not impossible, to calculate some potentially interesting further descriptions. These include classes greater than 65, less than 10, and so forth. (ii) The initial position, i. e. the first class's lower limit should be set so that each class's frequency is concentrated close to the middle of the class interval. This is required because the midpoint of each class is assumed to represent the value of all items included in the frequency of that class when interpreting a frequency table and performing calculations based on it.

It is important to watch whether they are given to the nearest inch or the nearest tenth of an inch, whether they are given to the nearest ounce or the nearest hundredth of an ounce, and so forth. For instance, to group the weights of certain animals, we could use the first of the following three classifications if the weights are given to the nearest kilogram, the second if the weights are given to the nearest tenth of a kilogram, and the third if the weights are given to the nearest hundredth of a kilogram:

Weight (kg)	**Weight (kg)**	**Weight (kg)**
10 - 14	10.0 - 14.9	10.00 - 14.99
15 - 19	15.0 - 19.9	15.00 - 19.99
20 - 24	20.0 - 24.9	20.00 - 24.99
25 - 29	25.0 - 29.9	25.00 - 29.99
30 - 34	30.0 - 34.9	30.00 - 34.99

3. ***Cumulative and Relative Frequencies***: Cumulative frequencies are total frequencies that result from adding the frequencies of two or more classes. Finding the total number of items whose values are less than or greater than a given value is made easier by these frequencies. Conversely, relative frequencies indicate each values or class's frequency as a percentage of the overall frequency.

   Note. When constructing a cumulative frequency distribution, the resulting frequency distribution is referred to as "less than cumulative frequency distribution" if the accumulation is started from the lowest size of the variable to the largest size, and "more than cumulative frequency distribution" if the accumulation is started from the highest value to the lowest value. Less than cumulative frequencies are the most prevalent cumulative frequencies.

4. ***Mid-Point of a class interval and the determination of Class Boundaries:*** The value of an interval that falls halfway between a class's upper true limit (UTL) and lower true limit (LTL) is known as the interval's mid-point, or class mark (X_c). It is calculated as:

$$X_c = \frac{\text{Upper Class Limit} + \text{Lower Class Limit}}{2}$$

The limits that are mathematically determined to make an interval of a continuous variable continuous in both directions and to have no gaps between classes are known as true limits, also sometimes referred to as class boundaries. If one could measure precisely, the tabulated limits would match the true limits.

3.1.4.2. Statistical Tables

Numerical data is presented in rows and columns in a systematic and orderly manner in a statistical table. Stubs are arranged horizontally in rows, and captions are arranged vertically in columns. Counting the frequency (number of occurrences) for each category of the variables and grouping the data into mutually exclusive categories are the steps involved in using tables to organize data. For qualitative variables, these mutually exclusive categories are naturally-occurring groupings. For example, Sex (Male, Female), Marital status (single, Married, divorced, widowed, etc.), Blood group (A, B, AB, O), Method of Delivery (Normal, forceps, Cesarean section, etc.), etc. are some qualitative variables with exclusive categories. In the case of large size quantitative variables like weight, height, etc. measurements, the groups are formed by amalgamating continuous values into classes of intervals. There are, however, variables which have frequently used standard classes. One of such variables, which have wider applications in demographic surveys, is age. The age distribution of a population is described based on the following intervals:

< 1	20-24	45-49
1-4	25-29	50-54
5-9	30-34	55-59
10-14	35-39	60-64
15-19	40-44	65+

Based on the purpose for which the table is designed and the complexity of the relationship, a table could be either of simple frequency table or cross tabulation. When individual observations only pertain to one variable, a simple frequency table is utilized; in contrast, a cross tabulation is used to determine the frequency distribution of one variable by a subset of another variable. A clear illustration of the data distribution pattern is provided by the relative frequency, in addition to frequency counts. The frequency counts are displayed as percentages. When dealing with basic frequency distributions (such as those found in Table 3.2), the total of all observed frequencies, or 210, serves as the denominator for the percentages.

In contrast, the choice of the denominator in cross-tabulated frequency distributions with row and column totals is determined by the variable of interest that needs to be compared over the other variable's subset. For instance, Table 3.4 compares the immunization status of mothers in various marital status groups, which is of interest. Hence, the denominators for the computation of proportion of mothers under each marital status group will be the total number of mothers in each marital status category, i.e., row total.

3.1.4.2.1. Construction of Tables

Although there are no hard and fast rules to follow, the following general principles should be addressed in constructing tables.

1. Tables should be as simple as possible.
2. Tables should be self-explanatory. For that purpose
   - o Title should be clear and to the point (a good title answers: what? when? where? How classified? and it be placed above the table.
   - o Each row and column should be labelled.
   - o Numerical entities of zero should be explicitly written rather than indicated by a dash. Dashed are reserved for missing or unobserved data.
   - o Totals should be shown either in the top row and the first column or in the last row and last column.
3. If data are not original, their source should be given in a footnote.

- *Examples*
- ***Simple or one-way table***: While cross-tabulation is used to determine the frequency distribution of one variable

by the subset of another variable, a simple frequency table is utilized when individual observations only pertain to one variable. Apart from frequency counts, the relative frequency is employed to distinctly illustrate the data distribution pattern. It displays the proportions of a specified frequency count.

Table 3.2. *Overall Immunization Status of Children*

Immunization status	Number	Percent
Not immunized	75	35.7
Partially immunized	57	27.1
Fully immunized	78	37.2
Total	210	100.0

Source: https://www.cartercenter.org/resources/pdfs/health/ephti/library/lecture-notes/env-health-science-students/ln-biostat-hss-final.pdf.

- ***Two-way table***: This table, which is created when the stub or the caption is split into two or more sections, has two features. The choice of the denominator in cross-tabulated frequency distributions with row and column totals is made in light of the variable of interest that has to be compared over the other variable's subset. Table 3.3, for instance, compares the immunization status of mothers in various marital status groups.

Hence, the denominators for the computation of the proportion of mothers under each marital status group will be the total numbers of mothers in each marital status category, i.e., row total.

Table 3.3. *TT Immunization by Marital Status of the Women of Childbearing Age*

Marital Status	Immunization Status				Total
	Immunized		Non Immunized		
	No.	%	No.	%	
Single	58	24.7	177	75.3	235
Married	156	34.7	294	65.3	450
Divorced	10	35.7	18	64.3	28
Widowed	7	50.0	7	50.0	14
Total	231	31.8	496	68.2	727

Source: https://www.cartercenter.org/resources/pdfs/health/ephti/library/lecture-notes/env-health-science-students/ln-biostat-hss-final.pdf.

- ***Higher Order Table***: When it's preferred to have a single table that represents three or more characteristics. Therefore, the table would take the form as indicated in table 3.4 below and would be referred to as a higher order table if it were desired to represent the profession, "sex," and "residence" of the study participants.
- *Example*

  A study on the level of job satisfaction among physicians and nurses in urban and rural settings was conducted. The sex and place of residence (rural versus urban) of the physicians and nurses questioned were included in a cross-tabulation that was created to characterize the sample (see Table 3.4).

Table 3.4. *Distribution of Health Professionals by Sex and Residence*

		Residence		
Profession/Sex		Urban	Rural	Total
Doctors	Male	8 (10.0)	35 (21.0)	43 (17.7)
	Female	2 (3.0)	16 (10.0)	18 (7.4)
Nurses	Male	46 (58.0)	36 (22.0)	82 (33.7)
	Female	23 (29.0)	77 (47.0)	100 (41.2)
Total		79 (100.0)	164 (100.0)	243 (100.0)

Source: https://www.cartercenter.org/resources/pdfs/health/ephti/library/lecture-notes/env-health-science-students/ln-biostat-hss-final.pdf.

3.1.4.3. Diagrammatic Representation of Data

A well-drawn graph enables readers to quickly get a general understanding of the data being presented. A graph often makes it easier and faster to see the relationship between numbers of different magnitudes than a table does. It is not always the case that figures are interesting, and as they get bigger and more numerous, they become so confusing and uninteresting that nobody would want to study them unless they had a special interest. Their research is more cognitively taxing without producing, for the most part, any scientific findings. One of the goals of statistical methods is to make statistical data more easily comprehensible by reducing their size. To achieve this goal, tabulation, averages, percentages, and classification techniques are typically applied. However, the diagrammatic representation method (visual aids) is probably a more straightforward and comprehensible approach. It entails the presentation of statistical data as lines, curves, maps, and geometric figures.

3.1.4.3.1. Importance of Diagrammatic Representation

1. They have greater attraction than mere figures. They give delight to the eye and add a spark of interest.
2. They help in deriving the required information in less time and without any mental strain.
3. They facilitate comparison.
4. They may reveal unsuspected patterns in a complex set of data and may suggest directions in which changes are occurring. This warns us to take immediate action.
5. They have greater memorizing value than mere figures. This is so because the impression left by the diagram is lasting.

3.1.4.3.2. Limitations of Diagrammatic Representation

1. The technique of diagrammatic representation is made use only for purposes of comparison. It is not to be used when comparison is either not possible or is not necessary.
2. Diagrammatic representation is not an alternative to tabulation. It only strengthens the textual exposition of a subject, and cannot serve as a complete substitute for statistical data.
3. It can give only an approximate idea and as such where greater accuracy is needed diagrams will not be suitable.
4. They fail to bring to light small differences

3.1.4.3.3. Construction of Graphs

The choice of the particular form among the different possibilities will depend on personal choices and/or the type of the data.

- Bar charts and pie chart are commonly used for qualitative or quantitative discrete data.
- Histograms, frequency polygons are used for quantitative continuous data.

There are, however, general rules that are commonly accepted about construction of graphs.

1. Every graph should be self-explanatory and as simple as possible.

2. Titles are usually placed below the graph and it should again question what? Where? When? How classified?
3. Legends or keys should be used to differentiate variables if more than one is shown.
4. The axes label should be placed to read from the left side and from the bottom.
5. The units in to which the scale is divided should be clearly indicated.
6. The numerical scale representing frequency must start at zero or a break in the line should be shown.

3.1.4.3.4. Examples of Diagrams

1. Bar Chart

   The frequency distribution of discrete variables and attributes, or categorical series, can be represented and compared using bar diagrams. All of the bars in a bar diagram must have the same width and spacing between them in order to represent data.

There are different types of bar diagrams, the most important ones are:

- ***Simple bar chart***: The bar in this one-dimensional diagram represents the entire magnitude. The size (frequency) of the figure represented is indicated by the height or length of each bar (see **Figure 3.1**).

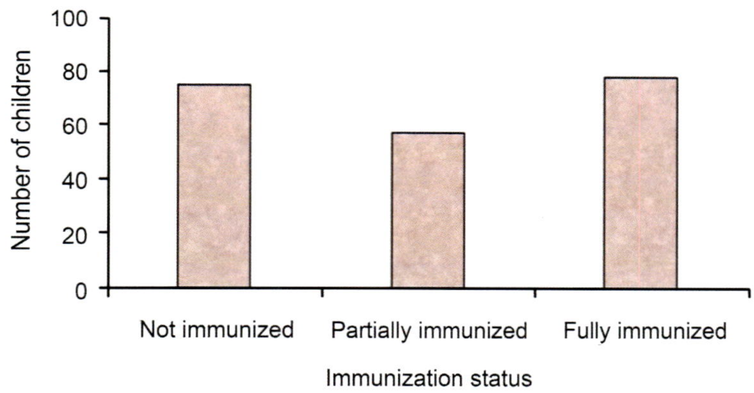

Figure 3.1. *Immunization status of children (Simple Bar Chart).*

Source: https://www.cartercenter.org/resources/pdfs/health/ephti/library/lecture-notes/env-health-science-students/ln-biostat-hss-final.pdf.

- ***Multiple bar chart***: The component figures in this kind of chart are displayed as distinct bars that are next to one another. The true value of each component figure is represented by the height of the bar. It shows the pattern of distribution for multiple variables (see **Figure 3.2**).

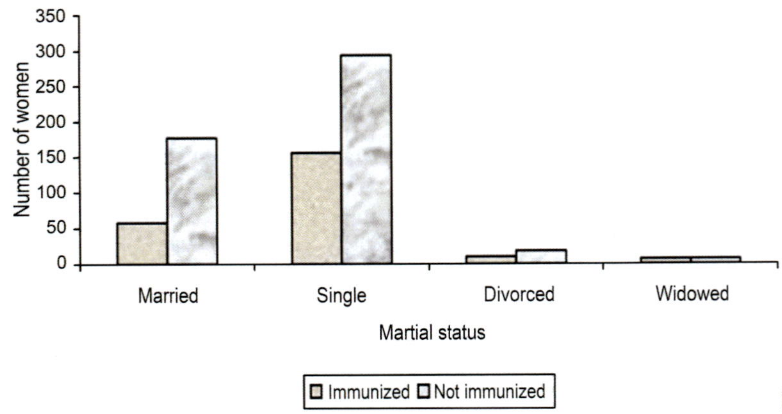

Figure 3.2. *TT Immunization status by marital status of women 15-49 years (Multiple Bar Chart).*

Source: https://www.cartercenter.org/resources/pdfs/health/ephti/library/lecture-notes/env-health-science-students/ln-biostat-hss-final.pdf.

- ***Component (or sub-divided) Bar Diagram***: Bars are separated into the figure's component elements. When each total is built up from two or more component figures, these kinds of diagrams are created. They can be of two kind:

i. ***Actual Component Bar Diagrams***: When the individual component lengths and the bars' overall height accurately depict actual figures (see **Figure 3.3**).

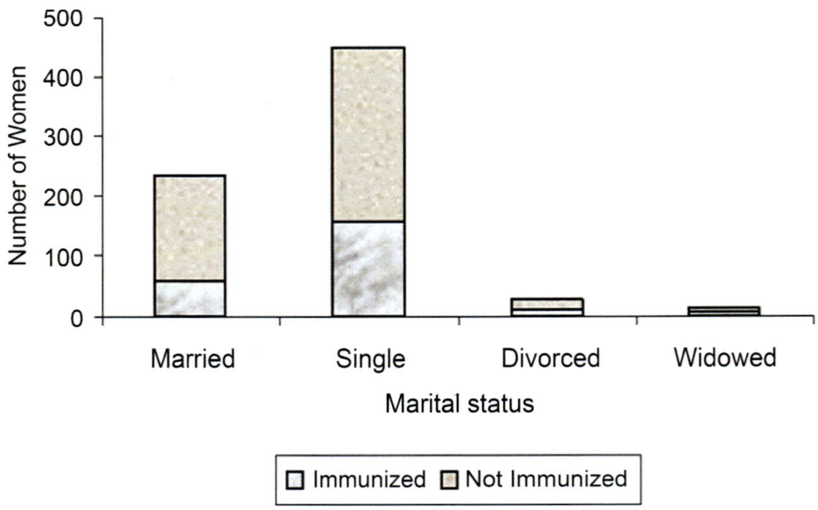

Figure 3.3. *TT Immunization status by marital status of women 15-49 years (Actual Component Bar Diagram).*

Source: https://www.cartercenter.org/resources/pdfs/health/ephti/library/lecture-notes/env-health-science-students/ln-biostat-hss-final.pdf.

ii. ***Percentage Component Bar Diagram***: Where the lengths of each individual component indicate the proportion that each component makes up of the overall total. Note that a series of such bars will all be the same total height, i.e., 100 percent (see **Figure 3.4**).

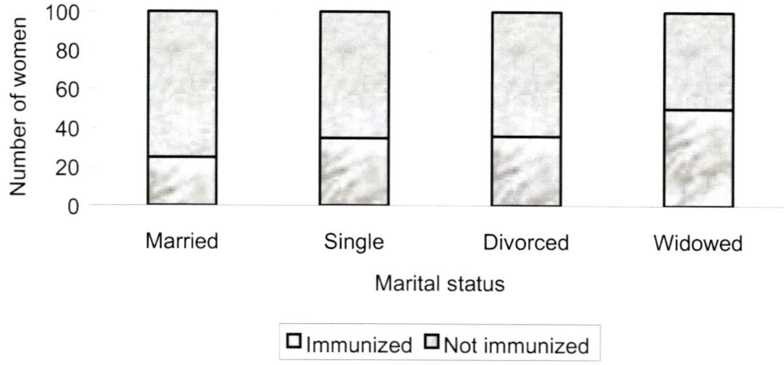

Figure 3.4. *TT Immunization status by marital status of women 15-49 years (Percentage Component Bar Diagram).*

Source: https://www.cartercenter.org/resources/pdfs/health/ephti/library/lecture-notes/env-health-science-students/ln-biostat-hss-final.pdf.

2. Pie-chart (qualitative or quantitative discrete data)

   It is a circle with sectors proportionate to the frequencies in which it is divided (see **Figure 3.5**).

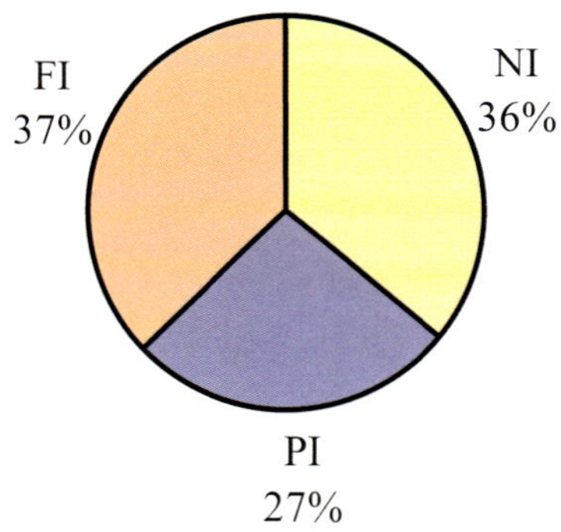

Figure 3.5. *Immunization status of children (Pie Chart).*

Source: https://www.cartercenter.org/resources/pdfs/health/ephti/library/lecture-notes/env-health-science-students/ln-biostat-hss-final.pdf.

3. Histograms (quantitative continuous data)

   The graph of a continuous measurement variable's frequency distribution is called a histogram. It is constructed on the basis of the following principles:

   The horizontal axis is a continuous scale that extends from the distribution's extreme ends to its middle. The variable name and the measurement units must be written on it.

A vertical rectangle is drawn for each class in the distribution, with (i) its base on the horizontal axis that extends from the class boundary to the other class boundary. The histogram rectangles are never separated by a gap. (ii) The width of the class intervals will establish the bases of each rectangle. Adjusting for different class interval magnitudes is required when presenting a distribution with an unequal class-interval using a histogram.

Example: Consider the data on time (in hours) that 80 college students devoted to leisure activities during a typical school week: (see Figure 3.6).

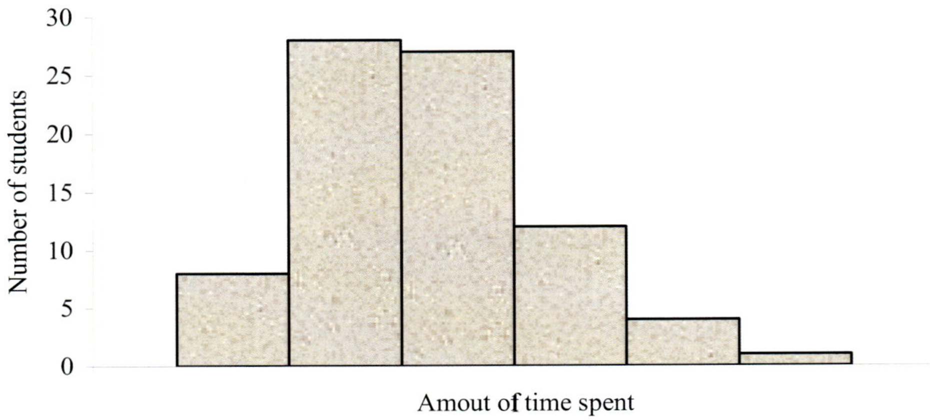

Figure 3.6. *Histogram for the amount of time college students devoted to leisure activities.*

Source: https://www.cartercenter.org/resources/pdfs/health/ephti/library/lecture-notes/env-health-science-students/ln-biostat-hss-final.pdf.

3.1.4.4. Frequency Polygon

A frequency polygon is created by joining the midpoints of the tops of the neighbouring rectangles on the histogram with line segments. The total area under the polygon and the total area under the histogram are equal when the polygon is extended to the X-axis slightly outside the range of the lengths.

Note that it is not essential to draw a histogram to obtain a frequency polygon. It can be drawn without erecting rectangles of histogram as follows: (see Figure 3.7).

1. The scale should be marked in the numerical values of the midpoints of intervals.
2. Erect ordinates on the midpoints of the interval – the length or altitude of an ordinate representing the frequency of the class on whose mid-point it is erected.
3. Join the tops of the ordinates and extend the connecting lines to the scale of sizes.
4. Example: Consider the above data on time spent on leisure activities

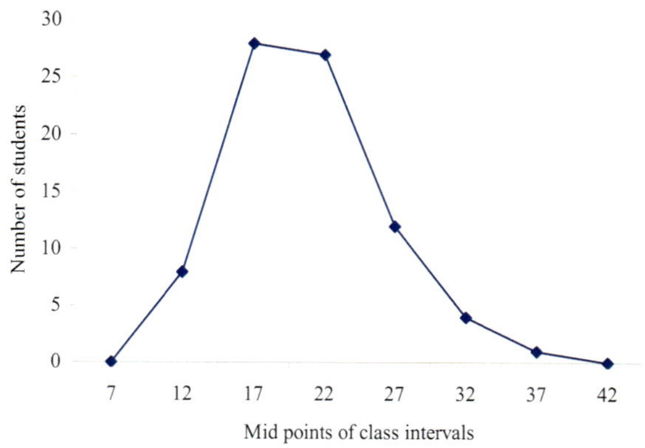

Figure 3.7. *Frequency polygon curve on time spent for leisure activities by students.*

Source: https://www.cartercenter.org/resources/pdfs/health/ephti/library/lecture-notes/env-health-science-students/ln-biostat-hss-final.pdf.

3.2. Why Select a Sample?

Frequently, it is either too costly or not feasible to gather information on an entire population. By using carefully selected samples, accurate statistical estimates of population parameters can still be obtained. Even in cases where a complete count of the population is necessary, such as in a U.S. decennial census, sampling can be utilized to enhance estimates for key subpopulations (such as states, counties, cities, or precincts). In a recent national election, it was revealed that the result of a presidential election in a single state (Florida) was uncertain due to various counting errors or exclusion rules. This highlights the fact that even when every vote is thought to be tallied accurately, there may still be inaccuracies; surprisingly, a sample estimate might be more precise than a complete count. To provide an example of the use of sampling in government agencies, the Internal Revenue Service (IRS) is mentioned. The IRS does not have the resources to scrutinize each tax return for errors or fraud; instead, they select a sample of returns for review. By employing statistical techniques, the IRS aims to increase the likelihood of identifying returns that may contain errors or fraud within the sample. Another instance involves reliability studies, which may involve destructive testing methods. For instance, a medical device company often tests the peel strength of its packaging material to ensure that it maintains sterility for medical products like catheters. These catheters will be utilized in delicate procedures involving patients' hearts, making the maintenance of sterility crucial to prevent infections. When conducting reliability tests, it is possible to sample only a small proportion of the packages to avoid wasting good packaging. However, accurate statistical inferences necessitate selecting adequately large samples.

Choosing a sample effectively and appropriately is one of the main challenges in statistics; sample selection aims to be as accurate as possible to derive meaningful conclusions about the characteristics of the population from the sample's results. You might not be aware of how crucial the sample drawing technique is at this point. But as history has shown us, it is very simple to draw the wrong conclusions when samples are selected incorrectly. Inappropriate sampling is frequently evident in the outcomes of radio and television surveys. We refer to this subtle issue as a selection bias. Although we have a larger target audience in mind, the poll only includes people who chose to participate in the survey after listening to a specific TV or radio program. The audience may lean more Republican than the intended demographic, for example, if the program features a Republican commentator on a political topic. As such, the survey's results won't accurately represent the intended audience. In this instance, we're presuming that the response rate was high enough to ensure that, in the case of a random sample, the results would be trustworthy. This kind of sampling error is also known as response bias by statisticians. When volunteers are asked to participate in a survey, bias like this frequently arises. The people who answer the poll might not be representative of the target population, even though viewers or listeners of a certain radio or TV show are. Because of this, credible polling companies like Harris and Gallup employ proven statistical techniques to guarantee that the sample is representative of the general population.

3.2.1. Simple Random Sampling

Taking a basic random sample is one of the simplest and most practical ways for statisticians to draw trustworthy conclusions about a population. Unbiased estimates of population parameters are guaranteed by random sampling. When a sample estimate is considered unbiased, it indicates that the population parameter is equal to the average of all possible samples. A basic random sample can be used to mathematically demonstrate biasedness, a statistical property derived from probability theory. Choosing a sample of size n from a population of size N is the idea behind simple random sampling. We will use combinatorial mathematics later in this text to demonstrate the total number of ways (let's say Z) to choose a sample of size n from a population of size N. A method known as simple random sampling offers an equal chance 1/Z of choosing any one of these Z samples. According to this statement, every member of the population has an equal chance of being chosen for the sample.

A random sample selection technique based on random number tables. Let's say we wish to use the mean of a sample (a statistic) to estimate the population mean (a parameter). Keep in mind that we are not claiming that the population parameter will be equal to the estimate from each individual sample. We would get the population parameter by averaging all possible means if we were to choose every sample of a fixed size (n) from the parent population. The central limit theorem specifies a conceptual problem regarding the relationship between the population parameter and the mean of all possible sample means. For the time being, it suffices to state that we do not produce every possible sample of size n in the majority of applications. In reality, we only use one sample to get the parameter estimate. Even the accuracy (i.e., proximity to the parameter value) of individual estimates is not guaranteed by the unbiasedness property of sample means.

3.2.2. Convenience Sampling

As the name implies, convenience sampling involves selecting patients or samples randomly and in an easy-to-manage manner. These kinds of samples are known as "grab bag" samples by certain researchers. Being representative of the population—that is, reflecting the fundamental traits of the population from which the samples were drawn—is a desirable quality in samples. Convenience sample representativeness is unfortunately not guaranteed, so estimates derived from these samples are probably biased. Convenience samples, however, have been employed in situations where drawing a random sample is extremely challenging or impossible. Convenience sample-based study results are descriptive and can be used to guide future investigations, but they shouldn't be interpreted as generalizations about the population being studied. Finally, we would like to point out that although random sampling yields objective estimates of population parameters, it does not ensure balance in any given sample that is chosen at random. All samples of size n from a population of size N are equally possible in random sampling. Although a large number of these samples exhibit demographic balance, some do not. The sample with the n smallest values for the population parameter and the sample with the n largest values are two extreme examples of non-representative samples. These samples are not balanced, so they can both produce inaccurate estimates. As an illustration (concerning point 2), let's say that a catheter ablation procedure has a 95% success rate. In other words, for a sample size of 20, we should only anticipate roughly one failure. Though it is unlikely, it is still possible that we will choose a random sample of 20 people and find that every single one of them has had an ablation procedure fail.

3.2.3. Systematic Sampling

When a sampling frame, or an exhaustive list of all the individuals or items that make up the population, is available, systematic sampling is frequently employed. The process is to start at an arbitrary but predetermined initial point in the table, or go to the top of the list and choose the first person. The initial point that is selected doesn't matter; it just initiates the process and needs to be specified for it to be repeated. Next, we choose the n + 2 person on the list, skipping the next n names. After n people are skipped, we keep skipping people and choose the next one.

As an illustration of systematic sampling, consider the following scenario: a researcher needs to choose 30 patients from a list of 5000 names (the list, which conveniently defines the population from which we are sampling, is called the sampling frame). The procedure would be as follows: the researcher would choose the first patient on the list, skip to the thirty-second name on the list, choose that name, skip the next thirty names and choose the next name after that, and so on until a total of thirty names were chosen. The sampling interval, or the total number of cases skipped, is 30 in this instance.

We first determined the sampling interval in the previous process. We wouldn't finish the list because we would only go through about 800 of the 5000 names. Alternatively, we could decide on a specific proportion of patients, say 1 percent. That means that for a list of 5000, the sample size would be 50. Suppose we skip 100 names from the list; the first patient will be 1, the second 102, the third 203, the fourth 304, the fifth 405 and so on until we reach the last one, the fiftieth number, 4950. The decision of how many names to skip is subjective. Here, we almost reach the end of the list, and each sample is chosen at random from the list.

As you can see, having such a comprehensive list makes systematic sampling simple and convenient. It is a perfectly valid sampling technique if there is no correlation between the characteristics we are measuring and the order in which the individuals are on the list. We might be able to persuade ourselves that this circumstance is real in some applications. Nonetheless, there are instances where systematic sampling can be extremely harmful. Let's say, for instance, that age is one of the population traits we are interested in. Let's now assume that 50 communities in Southern California make up the population. Every community has one hundred residents. To create our sample frame, we first sort each member of each community by age, going from the youngest to the oldest, and then we arrange the communities in a certain order, like alphabetical order by community name. We want n = 50 here, where N = 5,000. Selecting the first person from each community would be one method of selecting a systematic sample. By choosing the first person on the list and ignoring the other 99, we could have gotten the sample. However, doing so would force us to choose the youngest person in each community, which would result in a highly skewed estimate of the population's average age that is closer to the low end. Comparably, we would be biased toward the high side because we would only choose the oldest person in each community if we decided to ignore the first 99 people and always take the hundredth. When the variable of interest is periodic (with period n) in the sampling frame's sequence order, systematic sampling may cause problems. When groups of elements occur in a list in a cyclical pattern rather than evenly distributed throughout, the situation is referred to as periodic. The parts of the list where these elements are concentrated are referred to as peaks, and the sections where they are absent are referred to as troughs. We will only choose the peak values if we begin at a peak value and skip n people in the sequence. Troughs would have the same outcome. Our estimate will be skewed to the high side for the scenario where we choose the peaks and to the low side for the scenario where we choose the trough.

Here is an example of the foregoing source of sampling error, called a periodic or list effect. If we used a very long list such as a telephone directory for our sampling frame and needed to sample only a few names using a short sampling interval, it is possible that we could select by accident a sample from a portion of the list in which a certain ethnic group is concentrated. The resulting sample would not be very representative of the population. If the characteristics of interest to us varied considerably by ethnic group, our estimate of the population parameter could be very biased.

3.2.4. Stratified Random Sampling

An appropriate proportion or representation of each stratum (subgroup) in the sample is ensured by using stratified random sampling, which is a modification of simple random sampling. When it is known that there is variation in data variability amongst the subgroups, stratified random sampling can also be utilized to increase sample estimate accuracy. The method of stratified random sampling is very simple. We define m subgroups or strata. For the ith subgroup, we select a simple random sample of size n_i. We follow this procedure for each subgroup. The total sample size of n is then $\sum_{i=1}^{n} n_i$.

The notation Σ stands for the summation of the individual n_i's. For example, if there are three groups, then $\sum_{i=1}^{3} n_i = n_1 + n_2 + n_3$. Generally, we have a total sample size "n" in mind.

In many cases, stratified random sampling yields a more accurate and unbiased estimate of the population mean than simple random sampling with the same total sample size n, as shown by statistical theory. When we select large values of ni for the subgroups with the highest variability and small values for the subgroups with the lowest variability, the estimate's precision increases.

3.2.5. Cluster Sampling

Statistical analysts occasionally choose cluster samples as an alternative to the previously mentioned sampling techniques. Cluster sampling is a sampling technique where the element chosen is a group, known as a cluster, as opposed to an individual. The clusters might be city blocks, for instance. Frequently, the U.S. Cluster sampling is a practical method of sampling, according to the Bureau of the Census. The Bureau may choose city blocks at random from a list of city blocks in a specific city in order to conduct a survey. Every head of household in each chosen city block would be interviewed by the Bureau. In many cases, this approach will be more cost-effective than alternative sampling strategies, especially if the Census Bureau needs to dispatch staff members to the communities to carry out the in-person interviews. Cluster sampling is frequently quite effective. Since the clusters are chosen at random, the samples may be representative of the population, allowing for the objective estimation of the population's size or the mean value for a given parameter. There may occasionally be a decrease in estimate precision when compared to simple random sampling, but this drawback may be made up for by the savings on data collection expenses. Although clusters can have equal or unequal sizes, equal-size clusters have an easier mathematical solution. The theory for equal cluster sizes is developed in the three texts mentioned above, followed by a discussion of the more complex case of unequal cluster sizes.

3.2.6. Bootstrap Sampling

We will cover both parametric and nonparametric statistical inference techniques in this text. Bootstrap is one such nonparametric statistical method that allows conclusions to be drawn without depending on parametric models of the population distribution. Without making parametric assumptions about the distribution being sampled, nonparametric techniques offer a way to get sample estimates or test hypotheses. Let's go over sampling with replacement and sampling without replacement before delving deeper into the bootstrap. Assume that we are choosing items from our population in a specific order. Sampling with replacement is used when we choose the first item from our population and then let it stay on the list of things that can be chosen again, and we keep choosing in this manner. In contrast to sampling with replacement, simple random sampling involves eliminating every item from the pool of potential subsequent selections. Thus, there is no repetition of observations in simple random sampling. Sampling without replacement is used in simple random sampling. One way to approximate the bootstrap process is through the use of Monte Carlo (random sampling) techniques. The bootstrap becomes a useful procedure despite requiring a lot of computational power thanks to this approximation. Using a replacement from the original sample, a random sample is taken as part of the bootstrap sampling process. In other words, we resample or take samples from a sample. A method for creating a basic random sample (sampling from the population without replacement). Because basic random sampling and bootstrap sampling are so similar. First, a bootstrap sample is created by sampling from a sample rather than a population. Secondly, replacement is used during the sampling process as opposed to non-replacement. These are the main distinctions between bootstrap sampling and simple random sampling. (Chernick et al., 1999) (Cochran et al., 1977).

3.3. Types of Variables

Depending on the kind of data (or variables) that are available, different procedures are used for data summarization and further analysis. Therefore, it's critical to comprehend the classification process for variables.

There are three general classifications of variables:

- ***Discrete Variables***: variables that assume only a finite number of values, for example, race categorized as non-Hispanic white, Hispanic, black, Asian, other. Discrete variables may be further subdivided into:
- ***Dichotomous variables***: Discrete variables with only two options, e.g., yes or no, lived or died, male or female. Exposure to a particular risk factor (e.g., current smoking) could be a dichotomous variable (yes or no). Prevalent disease status is another example of a dichotomous variable, e.g., classifying each individual as having or not having the disease of interest at a point in time.
- ***Categorical variables (or nominal variables)***: Categorical variables, sometimes called nominal variables, are similar to ordinal variables except that the responses are unordered. Race/ethnicity is an example of a categorical variable, for which response options might be white, black, Hispanic, American Indian or Alaskan Native, Asian or Pacific Islander, or other. Another example

of a categorical variable is blood type with response options A, B, AB, and O.

- ***Ordinal variables***: Discrete variables that have ordered values such as self-reported health status with response options "Excellent, Very Good, Good, Fair, Poor." While the response options are ordered, they are not necessarily equally spaced.
- ***Continuous Variables***: These are sometimes called quantitative or measurement variables; they can take on any value within a range of plausible values. For example, total serum cholesterol level, height, weight, and systolic blood pressure are example of continuous variables.
- ***Time to Event Variables***: these reflect the time of a particular event such as a heart attack, cancer remission, or death.

3.3.1. Frequency Distribution Tables for Dichotomous Variables

A comprehensive physical examination was part of the 7th examination, which 3,539 participants in the Framingham Heart Study offspring cohort finished between 1998 and 2001. A frequency distribution table summarizing the variables recorded includes sex (see Table 3.5).

Table 3.5. *Frequency Distribution Table for Sex*

Sex	Frequency	Relative Frequency, %
Male	1,625	45.9
Female	1,914	54.1
Total	**3,539**	**100.0**

Source:https://sphweb.bumc.bu.edu/otlt/mph-modules/bs/bs704_summarizingdata/BS704_SummarizingData3.html.

The relative frequencies, which are calculated by dividing the frequency in each response category by the sample size (e.g., 1,625/3,539 = 0.459), are displayed in the third column. Relative frequencies of dichotomous variables are frequently expressed as percentages (by multiplying by 100).

The investigators also recorded whether or not the subjects were being treated with antihypertensive medication, as shown below (see Table 3.6).

Table 3.6. *Frequency Distribution Table for Treatment with Antihypertensive Medication*

Treatment	Frequency	Relative Frequency (%)
No	2,313	65.5
Yes	1,219	34.5
Total	**3,532**	**100.0**

Source: https://sphweb.bumc.bu.edu/otlt/mph-modules/bs/bs704_summarizingdata/BS704_SummarizingData3.html.

3.3.1.1. Missing Data

Despite having a sample size of 3,539, the table above shows that there are only 3,532 valid responses. This suggests that for this specific question, seven people had missing data.

Table 3.7. *Treatment with Antihypertensive Medication in Men and Women*

Sex	Number on Treatment / n	Relative Frequency, %
Male	611/1,622	37.7
Female	608/1,910	31.8
Total	**1,219/3,532**	**34.5**

Source: *https://sphweb.bumc.bu.edu/otlt/mph-modules/bs/bs704_summarizingdata/BS704_SummarizingData3.html.*

Studies may contain missing data for a number of reasons. The analysis's findings could be skewed if there is a large amount of missing data or if there is a consistent pattern of missing answers. Comparing two or more groups based on a dichotomous outcome variable can occasionally be interesting. For example, suppose we wish to compare the extent of treatment with antihypertensive medication in men and women, as summarized in the table below (see Table 3.7).

In this case, there are two dichotomous variables: sex and treatment status. The relative frequency of treatment for each sex must be determined by dividing the number of treatments by the sample size for that sex due to the unequal numbers of men and women. Although the frequencies of men and women receiving treatment are nearly equal, the relative frequencies show that men receive treatment at a higher rate than women. Also take note of the fact that the rightmost column's sum, which represents the relative frequency of treatment among all participants (men and women combined), is not 100 percent as it was in earlier examples.

3.3.2. Frequency Distribution Tables for Categorical Variables

Remember that categorical variables are unranked variables that have two or more distinct responses. The Framingham Heart Study measures a variety of categorical variables, such as smoking status, handedness (left or right), and marital status. The summary table's response or category order can be altered because the responses are not sorted; for instance, the categories could be shown alphabetically or even from most frequent to least frequent.

Table 3.8 below summarizes data on marital status from the Framingham Heart Study. The mutually exclusive and exhaustive categories are shown in the first column of the table. The frequencies, or numbers of participants in each response category, are shown in the middle column and the relative frequencies, as percentages, are shown in the rightmost column.

Table 3.8. *Frequency Distribution Table for Marital Status*

Marital Status	Frequency	Relative Frequency, %
Single	203	5.8
Married	2,580	73.1
Widowed	334	9.5
Divorced	367	10.4
Separated	46	1.3
Total	**3,530**	**100.0**

Source: https://sphweb.bumc.bu.edu/otlt/mph-modules/bs/bs704_summarizingdata/BS704_SummarizingData3.html.

The question about marital status elicited n = 3,530 valid answers (9 participants did not provide data on marital status). The sample's marital status is 73.1%, with only 10% of participants having a divorce. Ten percent more are widowed, 6% are single, and 1% are not together.

3.3.3. Frequency Distribution Tables for Ordinal Variables

Certain discrete variables are ordinal by nature. Apart from naturally occurring ordered categories (e.g., excellent, very good, good, fair, and poor), researchers will occasionally gather data on continuously distributed measures before classifying them to facilitate clinical decision making.

Heart Association use the following classification of blood pressure:

- **Normal:** systolic blood pressure <120 and diastolic blood pressure <80
- **Pre-hypertension:** systolic blood pressure between 120-139 or diastolic blood pressure between 80-89
- **Stage I hypertension:** systolic blood pressure between 140-159 or diastolic blood pressure between 90-99

- **Stage II hypertension:** systolic blood pressure of 160 or more or diastolic blood pressure of 100 or more

The American Heart Association uses the following classification for total cholesterol levels:

- **Desirable:** total cholesterol <200 mg/dL,
- **Borderline high risk:** total cholesterol between 200–239 mg/dL and
- **High risk:** total cholesterol of 240 mg/dL or greater

Body mass index (BMI) is computed as the ratio of weight in kilograms to height in meters squared and the following categories are often used:

- **Underweight:** BMI <18.5
- **Normal weight:** BMI between 18.5-24.9
- **Overweight:** BMI between 25-29.9
- **Obese:** BMI of 30 or greater

All of these are instances of typical continuous measures that have been classified into ordinal variables. The frequency distribution table for the ordinal blood pressure variable is shown in the table below. The first column of the table displays the categories, which are mutually exclusive and comprehensive. The middle column displays the frequencies, or the total number of participants in each response category, while the rightmost columns display the relative frequencies as percentages. Relative frequencies and cumulative relative frequencies are the two main summary statistics for ordinal variables (see Table 3.9).

Table 3.9. *Frequency Distribution for Blood Pressure Category*

Blood Pressure	Frequency	Relative Frequency (%)	Cumulative Frequency	Cumulative Relative Frequency, %
Normal	1,206	34.1	1,206	34.1
Pre-Hypertension	1,452	41.1	2,658	75.2
Stage I Hypertension	653	18.5	3,311	93.7
Stage II Hypertension	222	6.3	3,533	100.0
Total	**3,533**	**100.0**		

Source: https://sphweb.bumc.bu.edu/otlt/mph-modules/bs/bs704_summarizingdata/BS704_SummarizingData3.html.

That the cumulative frequencies show how many patients have a given blood pressure level or lower. For instance, 2,658 individuals have pre-hypertension or normal blood pressure 3,311 patients have Stage I hypertension, normal, or prehypertension conditions. When summarizing ordinal variables, the cumulative relative frequencies come in very handy as they show the percentage (between 0 and 100 percent) or proportion (between 0 and 1) of patients who are at a given level or below 75.2% of the patients in this instance are either pre-hypertensive or have normal blood pressure, meaning they are not considered hypertensive. Observe that the cumulative frequency for the last (highest) blood pressure category equals the sample size (n = 3,533), and the cumulative relative frequency is 100%, signifying that every patient falls within or reaches the highest level.

3.3.4. Descriptive Statistics for Continuous Variables

We chose a small subset (n = 10) of Framingham Heart Study participants to give a detailed description of the computations used for numerical and graphical summaries of continuous variables. The table below displays the data values for these ten participants. The body mass index (BMI), is derived from the height and weight measurements, is shown in the rightmost column.

Table 3.10. *Data Values for a Small Sample*

Participant ID	Systolic Blood Pressure	Diastolic Blood Pressure	Total Serum Cholesterol	Weight	Height	**Body Mass Index**
1	141	76	199	138	63.00	24.4
2	119	64	150	183	69.75	26.4
3	122	62	227	153	65.75	24.9
4	127	81	227	178	70.00	25.5
5	125	70	163	161	70.50	22.8
6	123	72	210	206	70.00	29.6
7	105	81	205	235	72.00	31.9
8	113	63	275	151	60.75	28.8
9	106	67	208	213	69.00	31.5
10	131	77	159	142	61.00	26.8

Source: https://sphweb.bumc.bu.edu/otlt/mph-modules/bs/bs704_summarizingdata/BS704_SummarizingData5.html.

The sample size (n=10 in this example) is the first summary statistic that should be reported for a continuous variable, as well as for any discrete variable. Greater precision and weight are obtained from larger sample sizes. There is a limit, though, beyond which expanding the sample size will not significantly improve the analysis's precision. We'll go into more detail about sample size calculations in a later module.

Because this sample is small (n=10), it is easy to summarize the sample by inspecting the observed values, for example, by listing the diastolic blood pressures in ascending order:

62 63 64 67 70 72 76 77 81 81

The last two blood pressure readings barely surpass the upper limit, which is deemed normal when it is less than 80 mm Hg. Nevertheless, summary statistics are required for large samples since examining each data value alone cannot produce a meaningful summary.

The two key components of a useful summary for a continuous variable are:

1. a description of the center or 'average' of the data (i.e., what is a typical value?) and

2. an indication of the variability in the data.

3.3.4.1. Sample Mean

The word "average" in biostatistics is very broad and can be used to describe a variety of statistics. The most commonly known is the sample mean, which is calculated by taking the total of all the values and dividing it by the size of the sample.

For the sample of diastolic blood pressure in the table above, the sample mean is computed as follows:

Sample mean = (62+63+64+67+70+72+76+77+81+81) /10 = 71.3

To simplify the formulas for sample statistics (and for population parameters), we usually denote the variable of interest as "X." X is simply a placeholder for the variable being analyzed. Here X=diastolic blood pressure.

The general formula for the sample mean is:

$$\bar{X} = \frac{\Sigma X}{n}$$

The X with the bar over it represents the sample mean, and it is read as "X bar." The Σ indicates summation (i.e., the sum of the X's or sum of the diastolic blood pressures in this example).

It is customary to report one extra decimal place in summary statistics for continuous variables rather than the number of decimal places measured. Because weight, total serum cholesterol, and diastolic blood pressure were measured to the closest integer, the summary statistics are given to the tenth place. Since height was measured to the nearest hundredths of an inch, the summary statistics are presented to the thousandths of an inch. The body mass index was calculated to the tenth of a percent, and summary statistics are presented to the hundredth of a percent.

3.3.4.2. Median

A second measure of the "average" value is the sample median, which is the middle value in the ordered data set, or the value that separates the top 50% of the values from the bottom 50%. The value in the ordered data set with an odd number of observations is the median; that is, the value with an equal number of values above and below it. The median, in an ordered data set with an even number of observations (n = 10), is defined as the mean of the two middle values. The median is (70+72)/2 = 71 in the sample of n = 10 diastolic blood pressures because the two middle values are 70 and 72. Diastolic blood pressures range from 71 to 71 in half of the cases. The sample mean and sample median are extremely similar in this instance. The mean and median provide different information about the average value of a continuous variable. Suppose the sample of 10 diastolic blood pressures looked like the following:

62 63 64 67 70 72 76 77 81 140

The sample's diastolic blood pressures are below 77.2, so while the sample mean (x "bar") in this instance is 772/10 = 77.2, we do not believe this to be a typical value. The calculation of the mean is impacted by the extreme value of 140. The median for the same sample is 71. Extreme or outlying values have no bearing on the median. Because of this, in situations where there are extreme values (i.e., very small or very large values in comparison to the others), the median is preferred over the mean. The mean is the preferred measure of a typical value when there are no extreme values; this is partly because the mean is computed taking into account each observation. A sample's mean and median will have similar values if it contains no extreme values. A more formal approach to identifying extreme values and when the median should be applied is given below.

Table 3.11 displays the sample means and medians for each of the continuous measures for the sample of n=10 in Table 3.10.

Table 3.11. *Means and Medians of Variables in Subsample of Size n=10*

Variable	Mean	Median
Diastolic Blood Pressure	71.3	71
Systolic Blood Pressure	121.2	122.5
Total Serum Cholesterol	202.3	206.5
Weight	176.0	169.5
Height	67.175	69.375
Body Mass Index	27.26	26.60

Source:https://sphweb.bumc.bu.edu/otlt/mph-modules/bs/bs704_summarizingdata/BS704_SummarizingData5.html.

For each continuous variable measured in the subsample of n=10 participants, the means and medians are not identical but are relatively close in value suggesting that the mean is the most appropriate summary of a typical value for each of these variables. (If the mean and median are very different, it suggests that there are outliers affecting the mean.)

3.3.4.3. Mode

The mode, or most frequent value, is a third way to measure a typical value for a continuous variable. Table 3.10 above shows that the diastolic blood pressure mode is 81, the total cholesterol level mode is 227, and the height mode is 70.00. This is because each of these values occurs twice while the other values only appear once. There are ten different values for each of the other continuous variables, so there isn't a mode because no value occurs more frequently than any other. Suppose the diastolic blood pressures had been:

62 63 64 64 70 72 76 77 81 81

In this sample there are two modes: 64 and 81. The mode is a useful summary statistic for a continuous variable. It is not presented instead of either the mean or the median, but rather in addition to the mean or median.

3.3.4.4. Range

The variability in the sample is the second component of a continuous variable that needs to be summed up. The sample range is a somewhat imprecise but significant indicator of a sample's variability. The sample range is computed as follows:

Sample Range = Maximum – Minimum Value

Table 3.12 displays the sample ranges for each of the continuous measures in the subsample of n=10 observations.

Table 3.12. *Ranges of Variables in Subsample of Size n=10*

Variable	Minimum	Maximum	Range
Diastolic Blood Pressure	62	81	19
Systolic Blood Pressure	105	141	36
Total Serum Cholesterol	150	275	125
Weight	138	235	97
Height	60.75	72.00	11.25
Body Mass Index	22.8	31.9	9.1

A variable's range is determined by its measurement scale. Blood pressure is expressed in millimetres of mercury, weight in pounds, total cholesterol in milligrams per decilitre, and so forth. Total serum cholesterol has a wide range; in the sample of size n=10, the minimum and maximum varied by 125 units. On the other hand, the participants' heights, which range from 11.25 inches, are more uniform. The range, which is dependent on just two values in the data set, is a crucial descriptive statistic for a continuous variable. The sample range should be interpreted cautiously because, similar to the mean, it can be impacted by extreme values. As seen below, the standard deviation is the most commonly used way to quantify variability for a continuous variable. (Dunn et al., 1977) (Kuzma et al., 2001)

A Closer Look

Bootstrapping Method

Bootstrapping is a resampling technique that is used in statistics to stimulate samples from a data set by using the replacement technique. Bootstrapping is a technique that makes it possible to determine standard errors, infer population data, and guarantee effective testing of the data. The Bootstrapping Method is a resampling statistical technique used in statistics and machine learning that tests a dataset by substituting the sample, thereby evaluating the statistics of a given population. Using random replacement, a dataset is sampled repeatedly in this technique. A statistical test that belongs to the class of resampling techniques, this method makes the greatest effort to guarantee the accuracy and objectivity of the statistics examined. The Bootstrapping method, in contrast to other sampling distribution techniques, repeatedly uses study samples to apply the replacement technique and guarantee that the stimulated samples produce an accurate evaluation. To assess a sample statistic's accuracy, the bootstrapping method is known to create new samples or resamples from the samples that already exist. The procedure generates new fictitious samples via the replacement technique, which aids in the testing of an estimated value.

Here are 3 quick steps that are involved in the Bootstrapping method -

- Randomly choose a sample size.
- Pick an observation from the training dataset in random order.
- Combine this observation with the sample chosen earlier.

The term "bootstrapped samples" or "bootstrap sample size" refers to the samples that are selected in the representative sample size. The samples that are not selected, on the other hand, are known as the "Out-of-the-bag" samples, and they form the testing dataset. Using the bootstrapping method, a machine learning model is trained on the training dataset, or bootstrapped samples, and then tested on a fresh dataset, the Out-of-the-bag samples.

The method's goal is to give the model the ability to forecast outcomes for the out-of-the-bag samples, which typically produce a Gaussian or normal distribution. In order to improve results, the replacement technique is applied, repeating the above steps for a minimum of twenty-five times. It should be noted that in order to test the model's accuracy more effectively, a small sample size must be selected, and the procedure must be repeated several times. An incredibly insightful resampling process, the bootstrapping method is used to quantify a model's uncertain loopholes.

Bootstrap sampling is applied in health science:

- ***Parameter Estimation***: Bootstrap sampling allows researchers to estimate parameters of interest, such as means, proportions, or regression coefficients, along with their associated uncertainty. By resampling from the original dataset with replacement, multiple bootstrap samples are generated. From these samples, statistics of interest are computed, providing estimates of parameters along with confidence intervals.

- ***Hypothesis Testing***: Bootstrap methods can be employed for hypothesis testing in health science research. Instead of relying on theoretical distributions, bootstrap resampling generates empirical distributions of test statistics under the null hypothesis. This approach is particularly useful when traditional parametric assumptions are violated or when the data distribution is unknown.
- ***Model Validation***: In health science, researchers often develop predictive models for various purposes, such as disease prognosis or treatment outcome prediction. Bootstrap techniques can be utilized for internal validation of these models. By repeatedly resampling from the dataset, researchers can assess the stability and performance of the model, estimating measures like prediction error or model accuracy.
- ***Assessment of Uncertainty***: Uncertainty quantification is crucial in health science research, especially when making decisions based on limited data. Bootstrap sampling provides a robust way to estimate uncertainty by generating multiple bootstrap samples and computing statistics of interest from each sample. This allows researchers to obtain confidence intervals or quantiles for parameters or model predictions, aiding in informed decision-making.
- ***Non-parametric Analysi***s: Many health science datasets may have non-normal or complex distributions. Bootstrap techniques offer a non-parametric approach to analyzing such data, as they do not rely on specific assumptions about the underlying distribution. This flexibility makes bootstrap sampling particularly valuable when dealing with real-world health data, which often exhibit heterogeneity and variability.

Summary

- Primary Data are those data, which are collected by the investigator himself for the purpose of a specific inquiry or study. Such data are original in character and are mostly generated by surveys conducted by individuals or research institutions.
- The concept of simple random sampling involves the selection of a sample of size n from a population of size N. Later in this text, we will show, through combinatorial mathematics, the total number of possible ways (say Z) to select a sample of size n out of a population of size N.
- Stratified random sampling is a modification of simple random sampling that is used when we want to ensure that each stratum (subgroup) constitutes an appropriate proportion or representation in the sample.
- As an alternative to the foregoing sampling methods, statisticians sometimes select cluster samples. Cluster sampling refers to a method of sampling in which the element selected is a group (as distinguished from an individual), called a cluster. For example, the clusters could be city blocks.
- Bootstrap Sampling is a method that involves drawing of sample data repeatedly with replacement from a data source to estimate a population parameter.
- A bootstrapping approach is an extremely useful alternative to the traditional method of hypothesis testing, as it's fairly simple and it mitigates some of the pitfalls encountered within the traditional approach.
- In biostatistics, the term 'average' is a very general term that can be addressed by several statistics. The one that is most familiar is the sample mean, which is computed by summing all of the values and dividing by the sample size.

References

1. American Heart Association. (n.d.). Retrieved from http://www.americanheart.org
2. Chernick, M. R. (1999). *Bootstrap Methods: A Practitioner's Guide*. New York: Wiley.
3. Cochran, W. G. (1977). *Sampling Techniques* (3rd ed.). New York: Wiley.
4. Davison, A. C., & Hinkley, D. V. (1997). *Bootstrap Methods and Their Applications*. Cambridge, England: Cambridge University Press.
5. Dunn, O. J. (1977). *Basic Statistics: A Primer for the Biomedical Sciences* (2nd ed.). New York: Wiley.
6. Hoaglin, D. C. (2003). John W. Tukey and data analysis. *Statistical Science, 18*(3), 311–318.
7. Kuzma, J. W., & Bohnenblust, S. E. (2001). *Basic Statistics for the Health Sciences* (4th ed.). Mountain View, CA: Mayfield.
8. Little, R. J. A., & Rubin, D. B. (1987). *Statistical Analysis with Missing Data*. New York: John Wiley & Sons.
9. MacCallum, R. C., Zhang, S., Preacher, K. J., & Rucker, D. D. (2002). On the practice of dichotomization of quantitative variables. *Psychological Methods, 7*, 19–40.

10. Mooney, C. Z., & Duval, R. D. (1993). *Bootstrapping: A Nonparametric Approach to Statistical Inference*. Newbury Park, CA: Sage.

11. Scheaffer, R. L., Mendenhall, W., & Ott, L. (1979). *Elementary Survey Sampling* (2nd ed.). Boston: Duxbury Press.

12. The Expert Panel. (1993). Expert panel on detection, evaluation and treatment of high blood cholesterol in adults: Summary of the second report of the NCEP expert panel (Adult Treatment Panel II). *Journal of the American Medical Association, 269*, 3015–3023.

Chapter

BASIC PROBABILITY

4

Contents

Introduction 99
4.1. Elementary Sets as Events and their Complements 103
4.2. Independent and Disjoint Events 103
4.3. Probability Rules 105
4.4. Permutations and Combinations 107
4.5. Probability Distribution 109
4.6. The Binomial Distribution 114
4.7. The Monty Hall Problem 115
4.8. A Quality Assurance Problem 117
4.9. Improved Diagnostic Accuracy Through Probability-Based Diagnosis 119
Summary 124
References 124

Introduction

A mathematical construct called probability is used to calculate the chance of occurrence for events that are subject to chance. An event is said to be subject to change when there are at least two possible outcomes and the outcome is uncertain.

The roots of probability are found in gambling. Games of chance offer useful illustrations of potential outcomes. For instance, we might be interested in finding the likelihood that two dice will yield the number 11, the likelihood that a ball will land on red in a roulette wheel, the likelihood that the Yankees will win today's baseball game, or the likelihood of drawing a full house in a hand of poker.

Within the field of health science, we might be curious about the likelihood that a sick patient will live for five years or longer after receiving a new medical treatment. Making decisions, like whether or not to treat a sick patient, is made easier when we are aware of the likelihood of certain outcomes.

Certain probabilities are taken for granted. Most people believe that there is a 0.5 chance that a pregnant woman will give birth to a boy instead of a girl. We may believe this because the population of the world appears to be almost evenly divided. In actuality, vital statistics indicate that the likelihood of having a boy at birth is 0.514.

Given that girls typically live longer than boys, perhaps this is how nature keeps things in balance. Therefore, even though 51.4% of babies are boys, the proportion of men over 50 may actually be lower than 50% of the total population over 50. Therefore, even though over 51% of children born worldwide are boys, the average sex distribution across all age groups may be closer to 50%. The uncertainty of many life events serves as another example of probability. We have no idea when the next earthquake will occur or if it will rain tomorrow. A formal method for calculating the likelihood of these erratic occurrences is probability. In probability, the mechanism generating uncertain or random outcomes is described by a mathematical model based on mathematical axioms and theorems. Our probability model will allocate a number between 0 and 1 to each event. Events with a value of 1 are certain to occur, and those with a value of 0 are impossible.

An event's assigned probability value, such as 0.6, which ranges from 0 to 1, has a frequency interpretation. Typically, when we assign a probability, we are addressing a singular event. Probabilities are frequently used to describe potential future occurrences.

Consider an event's occurrence as the result of an experiment. Assume that we have unlimited opportunities to repeat this experiment. If we were to assert a probability of 0.6 for the event, this would imply that, following numerous runs of the experiment, we would find that the proportion of times the event transpired would be nearly 60% of the possible results. Consequently, the event would not occur in about 40% of the experiments. These probability concepts related to frequency are significant because we will revisit them in the context of statistical inference.

By first defining the set of all possible elementary events, assigning a probability to each elementary event, and then adding up all of the elementary event probabilities that imply the occurrence of A, one can calculate the probability of an event A. The terms "mutually exclusive" refer to the distinct nature of the elementary events.

When we refer to elementary events A_1 and A_2 as "mutually exclusive," we mean that if A1 occurs, then A_2 cannot occur, and vice versa. As we will see later, this property is required to sum probabilities. Let's say we have an event A such that both A1 and A_2 imply the occurrence of A, and that if A_1 occurs, A_2 cannot occur, or if A_2 occurs, A_1 cannot occur (i.e., A_1 and A_2 are mutually exclusive elementary events). The probability that an event will occur, P (A), is defined as follows: $P(A) = P(A_1) + P(A_2)$.

If each elementary event has the same probability of happening, we can simplify this equation even further. Then, we declare the events to be equally likely. Every elementary event has a probability of 1/k if there are k different elementary events and they are all equally likely. Let us assume that m, the number of favorable outcomes, is made up of m elementary events. Assume furthermore that any event A will transpire when any of these m advantageous elementary events take place, with $m < k$. According to the previous assertion, there are m favorable events out of k equally likely, distinct, elementary events. As a result, the probability that any one of the m elementary events connected to A will occur is equal to the sum of the probabilities that A will occur. This likelihood is only m/k. Since m represents the distinct ways that A can occur and k represents the total possible outcomes, a common description of probability in this simple model is:

$$P(A) = \frac{m}{k} = \frac{\{\text{number of favorable outcomes}\}}{\{\text{number of possible outcomes}\}}$$

- ***Example 4.1. Tossing a Coin Twice***

Let's say the coin is fair—that is, it doesn't favor heads or tails—and let's write H for heads and T for tails.

According to the fairness assumption, there is a P(H) = 1/2 chance of heads and a P(T) = 1/2 chance of tails on each trial. Furthermore, we make the assumption that each trial is statistically independent, which means that the results of any one trial are unrelated to each other. We will define statistical independence mathematically in a moment, but for the time being, just consider it to mean that the trials are independent of one another.

There are four equally likely elementary outcomes to our coin toss experiment. These results, which are {H, H}, {H, T}, {T, H}, and {T, T}, are indicated as ordered pairs. For instance, the pair {H, T} indicates a tail on the second trial and a head on the first. The independence assumption gives each of the four elementary events a 1/4 chance of occurring.

Let's say we wish to determine the likelihood that event A = {one head and one tail} will occur. If {H, T} or {T, H} occurs, then A happens. P(A) thus equals 1/4 + 1/4 = 1/2.

Take event B = {at least one head occurs} as an example now. If any of the elementary events {H, H}, {H, T}, or {T, H} take place, then B may also happen. Thus, 1/4 + 1/4 + 1/4 = 3/4 is P(B).

- ***Example 4.2. Role Two Dice one Time***

It is assumed that there is no correlation between the two dice. We are interested in the faces that sum up to 7, 11, or 2. Sum the two faces. Ascertain the likelihood of rolling a total of 2, 7, 11, or 11.

There are six faces on each die, each numbered from one to six dots. It is assumed that there is an equal 1/6 chance of each face landing up. For a pair of dice in this scenario, there are 36 equally likely elementary outcomes. Pairs represent these basic results; for example, {3, 5} indicates a roll of three on one die and five on the other.

The 36 elementary outcomes are:

{1, 1}, {1, 2}, {1, 3}, {1, 4}, {1, 5}, {1, 6}, {2, 1}, {2, 2}, {2, 3}, {2, 4}, {2, 5}, {2, 6}, {3, 1}, {3, 2}, {3, 3}, {3, 4}, {3, 5}, {3, 6}, {4, 1}, {4, 2}, {4, 3}, {4, 4}, {4, 5}, {4, 6}, {5, 1}, {5, 2}, {5, 3}, {5, 4}, {5, 5}, {5, 6}, {6, 1}, {6, 2}, {6, 3}, {6, 4}, {6, 5}, and {6, 6}.

Assign the sums of 7 to A, 11 to B, and 2 to C. To get to 7, 11, and 2, all we need to do is find and count every elementary outcome. Dividing each sum by 36 then gives us the answers:

We can get a sum of seven with {1, 6}, {2, 5}, {3, 4}, {4, 3}, {5, 2}, or {6, 1}, which has a probability of 1/6 ≈ 0.167. To get a sum of eleven, we need {5, 6} or {6, 5}, with a probability of 1/18 ≈ 0.056. To roll a 2 (snake eyes), we need {1, 1}, giving us a probability of 1/36 ≈ 0.028.

Orientation and Directional Terms

Term	Definition	Illustration
Statistical inference	Statistical inference is the process of using data analysis to infer properties of an underlying distribution of probability. Inferential statistical analysis infers properties of a population, for example by testing hypotheses and deriving estimates. It is assumed that the observed data set is sampled from a larger population.	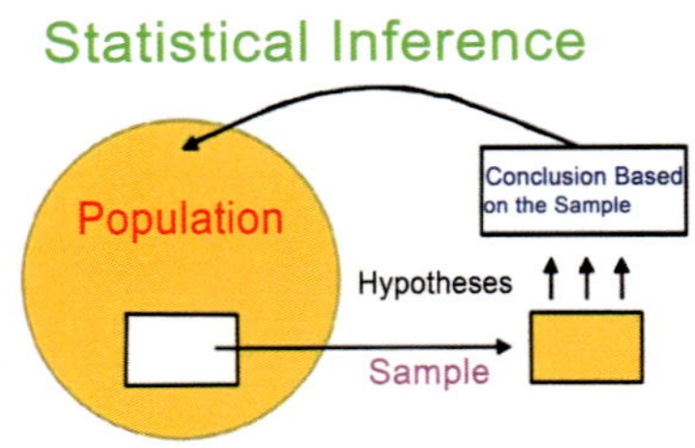
Mutually exclusive events	Mutually exclusive events are those events that do not occur at the same time. For example, when a coin is tossed then the result will be either head or tail, but we cannot get both the results. Such events are also called disjoint events since they do not happen simultaneously.	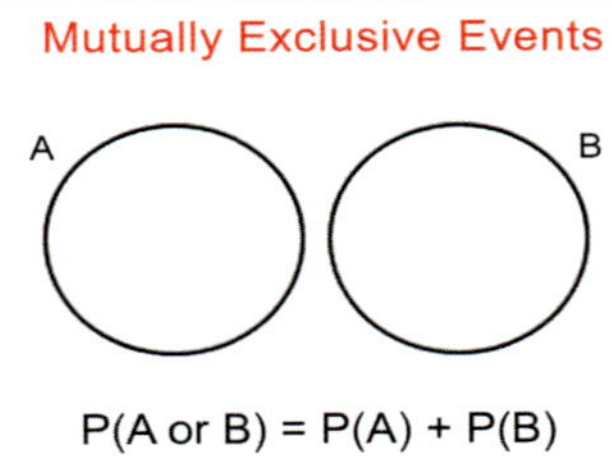
Disjoint events	Disjoint events are disjointed, or not connected. Another way of looking at disjoint events are that they have no outcomes in common. This definition can be easier to wrap your head around if you think of the opposite: overlapping events have one or more outcomes in common.	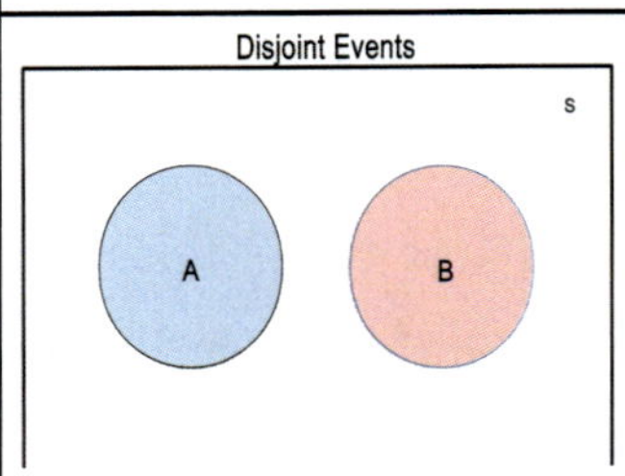
Venn diagrams	Venn diagrams are the diagrams that are used to represent the sets, relation between the sets and operation performed on them, in a pictorial way.	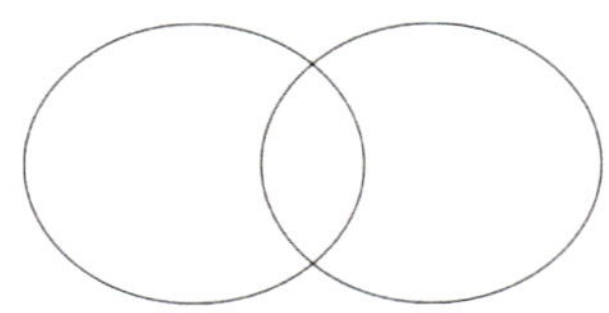

4.1. Elementary Sets as Events and their Complements

The basic elements of a probability model are the elementary events, which are indivisible and form the foundation of the model. These events cannot be broken down any further into smaller components and together make up the entire set of elementary events. The set of elementary events is just the collection of all the elementary events. In example 2, the event {1, 1} "snake eyes" is an elementary event. The set [{1, 1}, {1, 2}, {1, 3}, {1, 4}, {1, 5}, {1, 6}, {2, 1}, {2, 2}, {2, 3}, {2, 4}, {2, 5}, {2, 6}, {3, 1}, {3, 2}, {3, 3}, {3, 4}, {3, 5}, {3, 6}, {4, 1}, {4, 2}, {4, 3}, {4, 4}, {4, 5}, {4, 6}, {5, 1}, {5, 2}, {5, 3}, {5, 4}, {5, 5}, {5, 6}, {6, 1}, {6, 2}, {6, 3}, {6, 4}, {6, 5}, and {6, 6}] is the set of elementary events.

The set containing all of the elementary events is commonly represented by the Greek letter omega, Ω. Another name for this set is the universal set. We have P(Ω) = 1 for Ω. The null set, also known as the empty set, is the set that is denoted by Ø and contains no events. P(Ø) = 0 is the result for the empty set Ø.

For any set A, A^c denotes the complement of A. The complement of set A is just the set of all elementary events not contained in A. From Example 2, if A = {sum of the faces on the two dice is seven}, then A = [{1, 6}, {2, 5}, {3, 4}, {4, 3}, {5, 2}, {6, 1}] and the set Ac is the set [{1, 1}, {1, 2}, {1, 3}, {1, 4}, {1, 5}, {2, 1}, {2, 2}, {2, 3}, {2, 4}, {2, 6}, {3, 1}, {3, 2}, {3, 3}, {3, 5}, {3, 6}, {4, 1}, {4, 2}, {4, 4}, {4, 5}, {4, 6}, {5, 1}, {5, 3}, {5, 4}, {5, 5}, {5, 6}, {6, 2}, {6, 3}, {6, 4}, {6, 5}, and {6, 6}] .

We can calculate the probability of event Ω by simply counting the elementary events in the set and dividing by the total number of elementary events in. This method of calculating the probability can be laborious when dealing with a large number of elementary events; additionally, it necessitates that the elementary events be equally likely.

Examine the likelihood that A = {the sum of the two dice's faces equals seven}. In the preceding section, we observed that $P(A) = 6/36 = 1/6 \approx 0.167$. $P(A^c) = 30/36 = 5/6 \approx 0.833$, since A^c contains 30 elementary events. We observe that, as is always the case, $P(A^c) = 1 - P(A)$.

4.2. Independent and Disjoint Events

We will now provide some formal definitions of disjoint and independent events. However, we must first define the symbols for the union and intersection of events.

- ***Definition 1***: Intersection. Let E and F be two events; then E ∩ F denotes the event G that is the intersection of E and F. G is the collection of elementary events that are contained in both E and F.

  We often say that G occurs only if both E and F occur. Let us define the union of two events.

- ***Definition 2***: Union. Let A and B be two events; then A∪ B denotes the event C that is the union of A and B. C is the collection of elementary events that are contained in both A and B or in either A or B.

In Example 4.2 (roll two dice independently), let E = {observe the same face on each die} and let F = {the first face is even}. Then E = [{1, 1}, {2, 2}, {3, 3}, {4, 4}, {5, 5}, and {6, 6}]. F = [{2, 1}, {2, 2}, {2, 3}, {2, 4}, {2, 5}, {2, 6}, {4, 1}, {4, 2}, {4, 3}, {4, 4}, {4, 5}, {4, 6}, {6, 1}, {6, 2}, {6, 3}, {6,

4}, {6, 5}, and {6, 6}]. Take G = E ∩ F. Because G consists of the common elementary events, G = [{2, 2}, {4, 4} and {6, 6}].

We see here that P (E) = 6/36 = 1/6, P(F) = 18/36 = 1/2, and P(G) = 3/36 = 1/12. When we intersect three or more events, for example, the events D, E, and F, we simply denote that intersection by K = D ∩ E ∩ F. This set is the same as taking the set H = D ∩ E and then taking K = H ∩ F, or taking G = E ∩ F and then finding K = D ∩ G.

An additional point: It makes no difference what order the sets are arranged in or the sequence in which the successive intersections are taken.

- ***Definition 3***: Mutual Independence. Let $A_1, A_2, \ldots, A_k$ be a set of k events (k is an integer greater than or equal to 2). Then these events are said to be mutually independent if P(A1 ∩ A2 ∩ . . . , A_k) = P(A_1)P(A_2) . . . P(A_k), and this equality of probability of intersection to product of individual probabilities must hold for any subset of these k events.

According to Definition 3, a set of events is mutually independent if and only if the product of each pair's probability and the probability of any set of three's intersection, up to the set of all k events, is equal. We'll quickly see how this definition ties in with our common understanding that independence denotes the ability of one event to not influence the outcome of subsequent ones.

In Example 4.2, events E and F are unrelated to each other. Keep in mind that E refers to observing the same face on both dice, and F refers to the first face being even. It is evident from common sense that the likelihood of the second face matching the first is not influenced by whether the first face is even or not. Using the formal definition as a guide, we confirm mutual independence by computing P (G) and comparing it to P(E) and P(F). As we previously saw, P (F) = 1/2, P(E) = 1/6, and P(G) = 1/12. P (E) P (F) = (1/6) (1/2) = 1/12 as a result. Therefore, by examining the definition, we have confirmed that E and F are independent.

- ***Definition 4***: Mutually Exclusive Events. Let A and B be two events. We say that A and B are mutually exclusive if $A \cap B = \varnothing$, or equivalently in terms of probabilities, if P (A ∩ B) = 0. In particular, we note that A and Ac are mutually exclusive events.

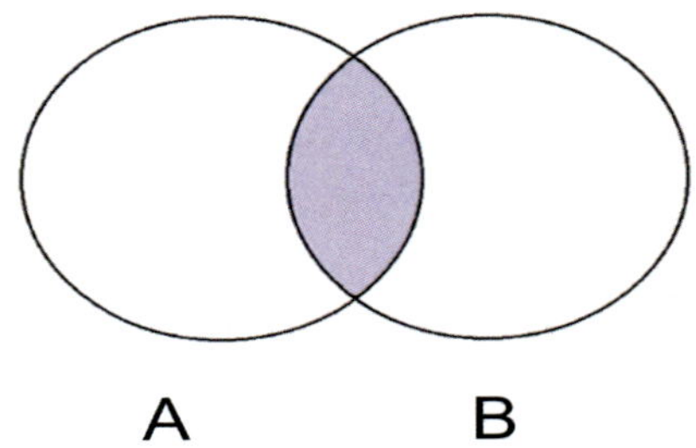

Figure 4.1. *Intersection.*

Source: https://www.pharmacy180.com/article/independent-and-disjoint-events-2908/.

Confusion frequently results from the distinction made between the ideas of independent events and mutually exclusive events. The only similarity between the two ideas is that they are both defined in terms of intersection probabilities.

Let us consider two nonempty events, A and B. Suppose A and B are independent. Now, P(A) > 0 and P(B) > 0, so P(A ∩ B) = P(A) P(B) > 0. Therefore, because P(A ∩ B) ≠ 0, A and B are not mutually exclusive.

Now consider two mutually exclusive events, C and D, which are also nonempty. So, P(C) > 0 and P(D) > 0, but P(C ∩ D) = 0 because C and D are mutually exclusive. Then, since P(C) P(D) > 0, P(C ∩ D) ∩ P(C)P(D); therefore, C and D are not independent

It is evident from this that two nonempty events cannot be independent if they are mutually exclusive. However, they cannot be mutually exclusive if they are independent. These two ideas are therefore diametrically opposed.

Venn diagrams are visual aids for representing sets in combinations, such as those that show intersections and unions. A Venn diagram showing where events A and B intersect is shown in **Figure 4.1**.

The individual events are represented by circles in the Venn diagram. Two circles with the labels A and B in **Figure 4.1** stand in for events A and B. The shaded area represents a third event, which is the point where events A and B intersect. In a similar vein, **Figure 4.2** offers a Venn diagram that shows how the same two events combine.

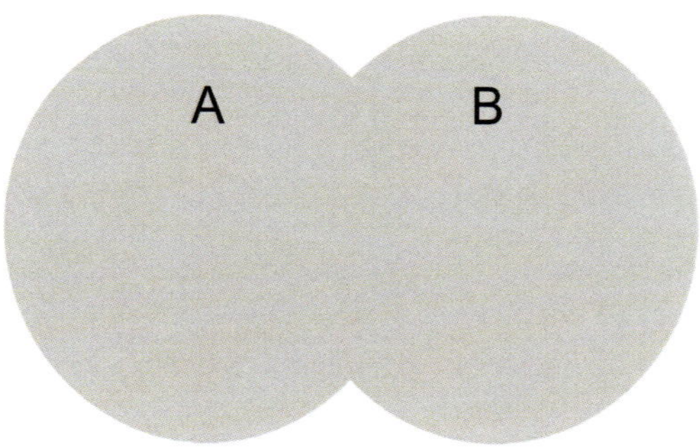

Figure 4.2. *Union.*

Source: https://www.pharmacy180.com/article/independent-and-disjoint-events-2908/.

To create this illustration, one must shade both the areas covered by each of the two separate sets and the areas where they overlap. (Olson et al., 2019) (Meyer et al., 2021).

4.3. Probability Rules

4.3.1. Product (Multiplication) Rule for Independent Events

If A and B are independent events, their joint probability of occurrence is given by the Formula 1:

$$P(A \cap B) = P(A) \times P(B) \quad (1)$$

Take into consideration the experiment where we roll two dice to see how this rule is applied. How likely is it that the first roll will be a 1, and the second roll will be a 2 or a 4?

Let B = {any outcome on one die and a 2 or a 4 on the second die}. First, since the result of the first roll is independent of the result of the second roll, define A = {get a 1-on-one die and any outcome on the second die}. A = [{1, 1}, {1, 2}, {1, 3}, {1, 4}, {1, 5}, {1, 6}] and B = [{1, 2}, {1, 4}, {2, 2}, {2, 4}, {3, 2}, {3, 4}, {4, 2}, {4, 4}, {5, 2}, {5, 4}, {6, 2}, {6, 4}] are the elementary events that make up A.

C = A ∩ B = [{1, 2}, {1, 4}] is the event. As per the independent event multiplication law, P(C) can be expressed as P(A) × P(B) = (1/6) × (1/3) = 1/18. You can verify this by looking at the basic occurrences connected to C. P(C) = 2/36 = 1/18 because there are two events, each with a probability of 1/36.

4.3.2. Addition Rule for Mutually Exclusive Events

If events A and B are mutually exclusive, then the probability of their union (meaning at least one of the events, A or B, occurs) can be calculated using Formula 2. Mutually exclusive events are also referred to as disjoint events. Symbolically, events A and B are disjoint if A ∩ B = Ø.

$$P(A \cup B) = P(A) + P(B) \quad (2)$$

Think about rolling dice once more. We roll two dice at a time. Let A represent the scenario where both dice yield an even number, and let B represent the scenario where both dice yield an odd number. Assume C = A U B. Then, event C is the outcome of rolling the dice, producing an even or odd number.

C appears in six elementary ways for the two dice together: {1, 1}, {2, 2}, {3, 3}, {4, 4}, {5, 5}, and {6, 6}. There are three basic ways that an occurs: {2, 2}, {4, 4}, and {6, 6}. Additionally, B can be found in three basic ways: {1, 1}, {3, 3}, and {5, 5}.

P(C) = 6/36 = 1/6, whereas P(A) = 3/36 = 1/12 and P(B) = 3/36 = 1/12. By the addition law for mutually exclusive events, P(C) = P(A) + P(B) = (1/12) + (1/12) = 2/12 = 1/6. Thus, we see that the addition rule applies.

An application of the rule of addition is the rule for complements, shown in Formula 3. Since A and Ac are mutually exclusive and complementary, we have $\Omega = A \cup A^c$ and $P(\Omega) = P(A \cup Ac) = P(A) + P(A^c) = 1$.

$$P(A^c) = 1 - P(A) \quad (3)$$

Generally speaking, non-disjoint events A and B can have the addition rule changed. Assume that the sets shown in **Figure 4.3**'s Venn diagram are A and B. Name the overlap region C = A ∩ B. Next, as indicated by the labels in the diagram, we can split the set A U B into three mutually exclusive sets: $A \cap B^c$, C, and $B \cap A^c$.

When we compute $P(A) + P(B)$, we obtain $P(A) = P(A \cap B) + P(A \cap B^c)$ and $P(B) = P(B \cap A) + P(B \cap A^c)$. Now $A \cap B = B \cap A$. So $P(A) + P(B) = P(A \cap B) + P(A \cap B^c) + P(B \cap A) + P(B \cap A^c) = P(A \cap B^c) + P(B \cap A^c) + 2P(C)$. But $P(A \cup B) = P(A \cap B^c) + P(B \cap A^c) + P(C)$ because it is the union of these three mutually exclusive events.

P(C) is counted twice in the summation formula, which is the issue. To fix this mistake, we subtract P(C) once. The generalized addition formula for the union of arbitrary events, represented as Formula 4, is obtained by subtracting this value.

$$P(A \cup B) = P(A) + P(B) - P(A \cap B) \quad (4)$$

Please take note that Formula 4 can also be applied to mutually exclusive events A and B, as for such events, P(A ∩ B) = 0. In the next step, we will discuss the generalization of the multiplication rule, but first we must establish the definition of conditional probabilities.

Let's say we have two events, A and B, and we wish to determine the likelihood that A will occur based on the likelihood that B will occur. This result is what we refer to as the conditional probability of A given B, and P(A|B) represents it. The formal mathematical definition of P(A|B) is given in Definition 5.

- ***Definition 5***: Conditional Probability of A Given B. Let A and B be arbitrary events. Then $P(A|B) = P(A \cap B)/P(B)$.

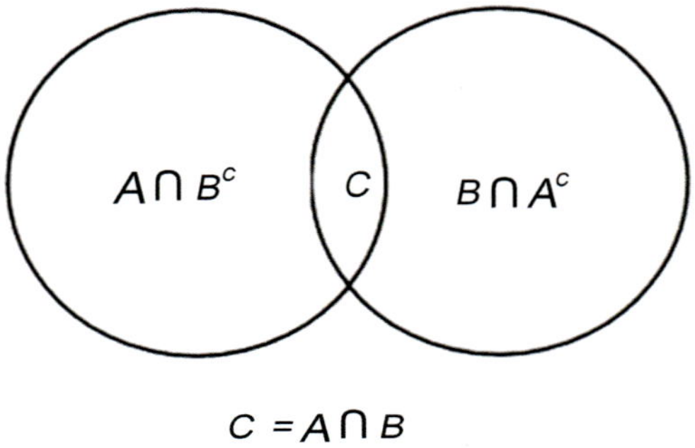

Figure 4.3. *Decomposition of AU B into disjoint sets.*

Source: https://www.pharmacy180.com/article/probability-rules-2909/.

Think about tossing one die. Let B = {an even number occurs} and let A = {a 2 occurs}. Afterwards, A = {2} and B = [{2}, {4}, {6}]. P(A B) = 1/6 since there is a 1 in 6 chance that 2 will occur and A ∩ B = A = {2}. Since there are three ways out of six for an even number to occur, P(B) = 1/2. Thus, P(A|B) = P(A ∩ B)/P(B) = (1/6)/(1/2) = 2/6 = 1/3 by definition.

Taking into account the limited possibilities provided that B occurs is another method to comprehend conditional probabilities. The only possible outcomes—{2}, {4}, and {6}—are those that have an equal chance of happening if we know that B occurs. Because each possible result has a 1/3 chance, the likelihood of a 2 is 1/3 as well. That's precisely what P(A|B) means.

The general law of conditional probabilities, or Formula 5, can be obtained directly from Definition 5.

$$P(A|B) = P(A \cap B)/P(B) \qquad (5)$$

After multiplying P(B) on both sides of the equation, we get $P(A|B)\ P(B) = P(A \cap B)$. The generalized multiplication law for the intersection of random events is represented by the following equation, designated as Formula 6:

$$P(A \cap B) = P(A|B)P(B) \qquad (6)$$

For random events A and B, the generalized multiplication formula is valid. As such, it applies to independent events as well.

Suppose now that A and B are independent; then, from Formula 1, $P(A \cap B) = P(A)\ P(B)$. On the other hand, from Formula 6, $P(A \cap B) = P(A|B)\ P(B)$. So $P(A|B)\ P(B) = P(A)\ P(B)$.

We obtain $P(A|B) = P(A)$ by dividing both sides of $P(A|B)\ P(B) = P(A)\ P(B)$ by $P(B)$ (because $P(B) > 0$). In other words, the probability of A given B is equal to the unconditional probability of A if A and B are independent.

This finding is consistent with our intuitive understanding of independence, which holds that conditioning on B influences the likelihood that A will occur. In a similar vein, it can be demonstrated that $P(B|A) = P(B)$ if A and B are independent.

4.4. Permutations and Combinations

We will use combinatorial mathematics to derive a few results. These findings will help expedite the computation of event probabilities associated with particular probability distributions.

By counting the potential ways for an event to happen and dividing the result by the total number of equally likely elementary outcomes, we can determine the probability of an event. We used straightforward examples with a maximum of 36 possibilities, so using this formula was not difficult.

But in many practical scenarios, there are so many possible ways for an event to happen that listing them all would be time-consuming or unfeasible.

Let's revisit the experiment of rolling dice. When we roll a die, there are six possible outcomes. If we roll the die three times independently, we want to determine the number of ways we can roll a number 4 or less on each roll without repeating any numbers.

Direct enumeration is an option, but there are 216 possible outcomes ($6 \times 6 \times 6$). Furthermore, it might not be clear how many outcomes are successful. As the space of potential outcomes—including successful outcomes—grows beyond the scope of this example, there is a shortcut solution that becomes even more crucial.

Our issue is not clearly defined as of yet. It is necessary to first clarify whether the distinct numbers' order is significant. We deal with permutations when order matters. We deal with combinations when order is irrelevant.

First, let's examine the scenario where order matters; as a result, we will count the number of possible combinations. The triple {4, 2, 3} is a successful result if order matters, but it is not the same as the triple {4, 2, 3} because order matters. The triples {4, 3, 2}, {4, 2, 3}, {3, 4, 2}, {3, 2, 4}, {2, 4, 3}, and {2, 3, 4} correspond to an outcome in which the three numbers 2, 3, and 4 occur once each, so when order matters, they are six distinct outcomes, but when order is irrelevant, they only count as one outcome.

Assume that a result of four or less is successful. In this instance, we have four options to select from: 1, 2, 3, and 4. This is because selecting 5 or 6 on any given trial results in an unsuccessful outcome. There are only three die rolls, and each trial must result in a different roll number, so we are interested in the total number of ways to choose three objects out of four when order matters. The number of possible permutations for choosing three objects out of four is the name given to this kind of selection.

Consider the issue of choosing the items to fill the available slots. After counting the number of ways in which the first slot can be filled, we will look at the number of ways in which the second slot can still be filled. After filling the first two slots, we finally take into account the number of ways left to fill the third slot. The number of ways that three objects can be chosen from a set of four objects can then be calculated by multiplying these three numbers together.

Why do we multiply these numbers together? This procedure is based on a simple rule of counting. To give an example, let's look at a slightly different case with two trials. On the first trial (designated as event A), we want to see an even number, and on the second trial, we want to see an even number. But the second trial's number needs to be different from the one selected on the first (let's call that event B).

We could get a 2, 4, or 6 on the first try. Therefore, there are three ways that A could happen. We can also receive a 2, 4, or 6 on the second trial, but the outcome of the first trial cannot be repeated. Therefore, the only possible outcomes for B are 4 and 6, assuming that 2 occurred for A. In a similar vein, if A experiences 4, then B can only experience 2 or 6.

Finally, if the third possible outcome for A occurred, namely 6, then only 2 and 4 are possible outcomes for B. Note that regardless of what number occurs for A, there are always two ways for B to occur. Since A does not depend on B, there are always three ways for A to occur.

The number of ways A and B can occur together is the product of the number of ways each can occur separately, according to the multiplication rule. In this instance, $3 \times 2 = 6$ methods. To verify that six is, in fact, the correct number, let us count these pairs.

We have {2, 4}, {2, 6}, {4, 2}, {4, 6}, {6, 2}, and {6, 4}. This set consists of the number of permutations of two objects taken out of three, as we have two slots to fill with three distinct even numbers: 2, 4, and 6.

Let's return to our initial, more complex problem: choosing three items from a set of four (since we are filling three slots): 1, 2, 3, and 4. We can demonstrate that the multiplication law extends to any number of slots by applying mathematical induction. Let's take this statement at face value. As we can see, our approach to solving the problem is to count the number of ways to choose three objects out of four; the multiplication rule informs us that this number is $4 \times 3 \times 2 = 24$.

These twenty-four cases are listed as follows: {4, 3, 2}, {4, 3, 1}, {4, 2, 3}, {4, 1, 3}, {4, 1, 2}, {3, 4, 2}, {3, 4, 1}, {3, 2, 4}, {2, 4, 3}, {2, 3, 4}, {2, 1, 4}, {1, 4, 3}, {1, 4, 2}, {1, 2, 4}, {1, 2, 4}, {1, 4, 3}, {1, 2, 4}, {1, 2, 4}, {3, 2, 1}, {3, 1, 2}, {2, 1, 2}, and {1, 2, 3}. Keep in mind that using a methodical approach to enumeration is crucial, as it can be easy to overlook certain cases or count them twice by mistake.

The system chooses the highest number that is available for the first slot, the next highest number that is available for the second slot, and the highest number that is still available for the third slot after the first slot is chosen. Until all cases with four in the first slot are used up, this process is repeated. Next, we take into account the cases where there are three in the first slot, the greatest number still available for the second slot, and the highest number still available for the third slot. We repeat the process with 2 in the first slot and, at last, with 1 in the first slot after the 3s have run out.

In general, let r be the number of objects to choose and n the number of objects available. We then denote by $P(n, r)$ the number of permutations of r objects chosen out of n. As an example of permutations, we denote the quantity $3 \times 2 = 3 \times 2 \times 1$ as 3! where the symbol "!" represents the function called the factorial. In our notation and formulae, 0! exists and is equal to 1. Formula 7 shows the permutations of r objects taken from n objects:

$$P(n, r) = n!/(n - r)! \qquad (7)$$

From Formula 7, we see that when $n = 3$ and $r = 2$, $P(3, 2) = 3!/(3 - 2)! = 3!/1! = 3! = 6$. This result agrees with our enumeration of distinct even numbers on two rolls of the die. Also, $P(4, 3) = 4!/(4 - 3)! = 4!/1! = 4! = 24$. This number agrees with the result we obtained for three independent rolls less than 5.

We will now look at combinations. We only take into account distinct subsets for combinations; their order is unconsidered. The triplets {2, 3, 4}, {2, 4, 3}, {3, 2, 4}, {3, 4, 2}, {4, 3, 2}, and {4, 2, 3} differ only in order and not in the objects included in the example of distinct outcomes of three rolls of the die where success means three distinct numbers less than 5 without regard to order.

Notice that for each different set of three distinct numbers, the common number of permutations is always 6. For example, the set 1, 2, and 3 contains the six triplets {1, 2, 3}, {1, 3, 2}, {2, 1, 3}, {2, 3, 1}, {3, 1, 2}, and {3, 2, 1}. Notice that the number six occurs because it is equal to $P(3, 3) = 3!/0! = 3! = 6$.

Because for every distinct combination of r objects selected out of n, there are P(r, r) orders for these objects, we have P(n, r) = C(n, r)P(r, r) where C(n, r) denotes the number of combinations for choosing r objects out of n. Therefore, we arrive at the following equation for combinations, with the far-right-hand side of the chain of equalities obtained by substitution, since P(r, r) = r! C(n, r) = P(n, r)/ P(r, r) = n!/ [(n − r)! P(r, r)] = n!/[(n − r)! r!]. Formula 8 shows the formula for combinations of r objects taken out of n:

$$C(n, r) = n!/[(n - r)!\ r!] \qquad (8)$$

In our example of three rolls of the die leading to three distinct numbers less than 5, we obtain the number of combinations for choosing 3 objects out of 4 as $C(4, 3) = 4!/[1!\ 3!] = 4$. These four distinct combinations are enumerated as follows: (1) 1, 2, and 3; (2) 1, 2, and 4; (3) 1, 3 and 4; and (4) 2, 3 and 4. (Korenstein et al., 2022) (Baghdadi et al., 2022).

4.5. Probability Distribution

The probability of events is described by probability distributions. Properties of probability distributions are called parameters. Random variables are another name for the statistics that we have employed to estimate parameters. We will use the distributions of these statistics to draw conclusions about the characteristics of the population.

By building confidence intervals or testing parameter hypotheses, we will be able to make deductions.

The statistic, or random variable, is indicated by a capital letter, most frequently "X.." We use a lowercase x for the value that the random variable X takes on in a specific experiment, so that we can distinguish it from the latter. Assume that A = [X = x]. Assume that the events mentioned earlier in this chapter are analogous to the event represented by A = [X = x]. Events of the form A = [X = x] have positive probabilities associated with some finite set of values for x and zero probability for all other values of x if X is a discrete variable that can only take on a finite set of values.

A variable that has distinct values for every measurement is called a discrete variable. Every number has a positive probability that we can determine. An infinite discrete set is made up of all the possible combinations of values that can result from the probabilities attached to each discrete variable's value. Additionally, the discrete set might be finite. A Poisson random variable, which gives all non-negative integers, including zero, a positive probability, is the most widely used illustration of an infinite discrete set. An example of a distribution used to depict rare events is the Poisson distribution (e.g., the frequency of light bulb failures). The rate parameter establishes the degree to which events occur. By infrequent, we mean that there can't be two events happening simultaneously in a brief period of time. For the binomial distribution, the random variable is the number of successes in n trials; it can take on the n + 1 discrete values 0, 1, 2, 3, . . . , n.

Another kind of random variable that we will encounter often is the absolutely continuous random variable. This variable has a continuous range of possible values. The range may consist of the whole set of real numbers or an interval like [0, 1]. A uniformly distributed random variable serves as an example of a distribution that employs a range of values within an interval, like [0, 1]. A dataset with uniform distribution is one in which each value has an equal probability of occurring. One example of an absolutely continuous distribution that takes values over the whole set of real numbers is the normal, or Gaussian, distribution.

Probability densities are associated with absolutely continuous random variables. These densities, as you will see, are the discrete random variable equivalents of the probability mass functions that we shall define.

Events such as A = P(X = x) for absolutely continuous random variables will be shown to be meaningless since P(X = x) = 0 for all values x. In order to derive significant probabilities for completely continuous random variables, we must discuss the likelihood that X falls within a range of values, such as $P(0 < X < 1)$. We can calculate positive probabilities for these random variables on such intervals.

Certain properties of probability distributions are applicable to both discrete and absolutely continuous distributions. A single example of this is symmetry. If a probability distribution has a center point, where a vertical line can be drawn, the distribution to the right of the line will have the same shape as the distribution to the left, indicating that the distribution is symmetric.

Several symmetric continuous and discrete distributions will be encountered. The normal distribution, Student's t distribution, Cauchy distribution, uniform distribution, and specific beta distribution are a few instances of symmetric, absolutely continuous distributions.

If and only if the success probability, p, equals 1/2, the binomial distribution is symmetric. To recap, there are two possible results when a fair coin is flipped: heads or tails. When we toss a coin and hope to get a head, that outcome is known as a "success." There is a 50% chance of a head.

Skewed distributions are probability distributions that lack symmetry. Positively and negatively skewed distributions are the two types of skewed distributions. Negatively skewed distributions have probability mass or density concentrated to the left with a long, declining tail to the left, whereas positively skewed distributions have a higher concentration of probability mass or density to the left and a long, declining tail to the right.

The probability densities in **Figure 4.4** are continuous and correspond to four different distributions: (1) symmetric normal, (2) symmetric bimodal, (3) negatively skewed, and (4) positively skewed. Positively skewed distributions include the chi-square distribution and the negative exponential distribution. Depending on the values of specific parameters, beta distributions and binomial distributions (both of which will be discussed in more detail later) can be symmetric, positively skewed, or negatively skewed. The binomial distribution, for example, is positively skewed if p. $< 1/2$, is symmetric if $p = 1/2$, and is negatively skewed if $p > 1/2$.

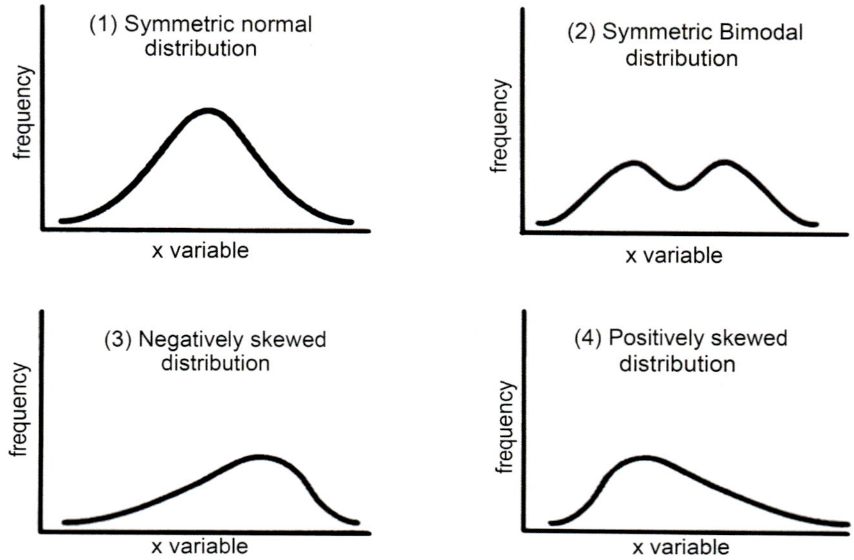

Figure 4.4. *Continuous probability densities.*

Source: https://www.pharmacy180.com/article/probability-distributions-2911/.

Assume for the purposes of the experiment that we will toss a fair coin three times in separate trials. There are eight elementary outcomes that we can list. The triplets are {H, H, H}, {H, H, T}, {H, T, H}, {H, T, T}, {T, H, H}, {T, H, T}, {T, T, H}, and {T, T, T}, where H stands for heads and T for tails. Eight elementary events can be categorized as follows: E_1 = {H, H, H}, E_2 = {H, H, T}, E_3 = {H, T, H}, E_4 = {H, T, T}, E_5 = {T, H, H}, E_6 = {T, H, T}, E_7 = {T, T, H}, and E_8 = {T, T, T}.

Z is the random variable that we want to represent the number of heads in the experiment. As you can see from the results above, Z can have the values 0, 1, 2, and 3. You also know that because the trials are independent and the coin is fair, all eight of the above elementary outcomes have an equal chance of occurring. Thus, the probability of each triplet is 1/8. You now understand that basic events are disjoint, or mutually exclusive. As a result, the probability of all elementary events combined is equal to the sum of each event's probability.

You are now ready to compute the probability distribution for Z. Since Z can be only 0, 1, 2, or 3, we know its distribution once we compute $P(Z = 0)$, $P(Z = 1)$, $P(Z = 2)$, and $P(Z = 3)$. Each of these events $\{Z = 0\}$, $\{Z = 1\}$, $\{Z = 2\}$, and $\{Z = 3\}$ can be described as the union of a certain set of these elementary events.

For example, Z = 0 only if all three tosses are tails. E_8 denotes the elementary event {T, T, T}. We see that $P(Z = 0) = P(E_8) = 1/8$. Similarly, Z = 3 only if all three tosses are heads. E_1 denotes the event {H, H, H}; therefore, $P(Z = 3) = P(E_1) = 1/8$.

Consider the event Z = 1. For Z = 1, we have exactly one head and two tails. The elementary events that lead to this outcome are E_4 = {H, T, T}, E_6 = {T, H, T}, and E_7 = {T, *T*, *H*}. So P(Z = 1) = *P*(E_4 *U* E_6 *U* E_7). By the addition law for mutually exclusive events, we have P(Z = 1) = P(E_4 U E_6 U E_7) = P(E_4) + P(E_6) + P(E_7) = 1/8 + 1/8 + 1/8 = 3/8.

Next, consider the event *Z* = 2. For *Z* = 2, we have exactly one tail and two heads. Again, three elementary events give three elementary events give this outcome. They are E_2 = {*H*, *H*, *T*}, E_3 = {*H*, *T*, *H*}, and E_5 = {*T*, *H*, *H*}. So, *P*(*Z* = 2) = *P*(E_2 U E_3 U E_5). By the addition law for mutually exclusive events, we have *P*(*Z* = 2) = *P*(E_2 U E_3 U E_5) = *P*(E_2) + *P*(E_3) + *P*(E_5) = 1/8 + 1/8 + 1/8 = 3/8.

This is the distribution for Z in Table 4.1. The likelihood mass function for Z is shown in the table's second column. The cumulative probability function is shown in column three. The first cell of the second column contains the value that is carried over to the first cell of the third column. The value displayed in cell one and all of the cells above cell two of the second column adds up to the value displayed in the second cell of the third column. Similarly, each of the remaining values indicated in the third column can be located, e.g., column 3 (0.875) = (0.125 + 0.375 + 0.375) is the third cell. Analogs for the distribution functions that are continuous will be discovered.

Remember another method to complete the computation. We studied how to quickly calculate these probabilities using permutations and combinations in the previous section. Let's try to use combinations to ascertain Z's distribution.

To obtain *Z* = 0, we need three tails for three objects. There are *C*(3, 3) ways to do this. *C*(3, 3) = 3!/[(3 – 3)! 3!] = 3!/[0! 3!] = 1. So *P*(*Z* = 0) = *C*(3, 3)/8 = 1/8 = 0.125.

Table 4.1. *The Probability Distribution for the Number of Heads in Three Coin Tosses*

Value for *Z*	*P*(*Z* = Value)	*P*(*Z* ≤ Value)
0	1/8 = 0.125	1/8 = 0.125
1	3/8 = 0.375	4/8 = 0.500
2	3/8 = 0.375	7/8 = 0.875
3	1/8 = 0.125	8/8 = 1.000

Source: https://www.pharmacy180.com/article/probability-distributions-2911/.

To find *Z* = 1, we need two tails and one head. Order does not matter, so the number of ways of choosing exactly two tails out of three is *C*(3, 2) = 3!/[(3 – 2)! 2!] = 3!/[1! 2!] = 3 × 2/2 = 3. So, *P*(*Z* = 1) = *C*(3, 2)/8 = 3/8 = 0.375.

Now for *Z* = 2, we need one tail and two heads. Thus, we must select exactly one tail out of three choices; order does not matter. So *P*(*Z* = 2) = *C*(3, 1)/8 and *C*(3, 1) = 3!/[(3 – 1)! 1!] = 3!/[2! 1!] = 3 × 2/2 = 3. Therefore, *P*(*Z* = 2) = *C*(3, 1)/8 = 3/8 = 0.375.

For *P*(*Z* = 3), we must have no tails out of three selections. Again, order does not matter, so *P*(*Z* = 3) = *C*(3, 0)/8 and *C*(3, 0) = 3!/[(3 – 0)! 0!] = 3!/[3! 0!] = 3!/3! = 1. Therefore, *P*(*Z* = 3) = *C*(3, 0)/8 = 1/8 = 0.125.

It's easier to compute permutations this way than it is to list every elementary result once you know how to do it. As the range of possible outcomes significantly expands, the time and effort savings become even more evident. Think about how time-consuming it would be to calculate the distribution of the number of heads after ten coins flips!

The binomial distribution is represented by the notation Bi(n, p). The distribution is determined by the two parameters, n, and p. We'll see that p is the chance of success on any given trial, and n is the total number of trials. The number of successes is the only thing that makes up the binomial random variable.

Since we have a fair coin in our example, we can see that p = 1/2 = 0.50 if we declare a head on a trial to be a success and a tail to be a failure. Since we threw the coin three times independently, n = 3. As a result, we obtained the distribution Bi(3, 0.50) from our exercise.

Consider a discrete random variable such as the binomial, which has a positive probability associated with a finite set of discrete values x_1, x_2, x_3, . . . , x_n. To each value, we associate the probability mass p_i for i = 1, 2, 3, . . . , n. The mean μ for this random variable is defined as $\mu = \Sigma^n_{i=1} p_i x_i$. The variance σ^2 is defined as $\sigma^2 = \Sigma^n_{i=1} p_i(x_i - \mu)^2$. For the Bi(n, p) distribution it is easy to verify that μ = np and σ^2 = npq, where $q = 1 - p$.

We have only talked about discrete distributions up to this point. We now wish to examine random variables with completely continuous. The uniform distribution on [0, 1] is the most basic illustration of an continuous distribution. The distribution we want for random number generation is represented by the uniform distribution. It is the distribution that assigns a "equal" chance of selection to every real number in the interval [0, 1], meaning that the probability of selection for each subinterval of length L is the same for all other subintervals of length L.

Let U be a uniform random variable on [0, 1]; then $P\{0 \le U \le x) = x$ for any x satisfying $0 \le x \le 1$. With this definition and using calculus, we see that the function $F(x) = P\{0 \le U \le x) = x$ is differentiable on [0, 1]. We denote its derivative by $f(x)$. In this case, $f(x) = 1$ for $0 \le x \le 1$, and $f(x) = 0$ otherwise.

Knowing that $f(x) = 1$ for $0 \le x \le 1$, and $f(x) = 0$ otherwise, we find that for any a and b satisfying $0 \le a \le b \le 1$, $P(a \le U \le b) = b - a$. So, the probability that U falls in any particular interval is just the length of the interval and does not depend on a. For example, $P(0 \le U \le 0.2) = P(0.1 \le U \le 0.3) = P(0.3 \le U \le 0.5) = P(0.4\ U \le 0.6) = P(0.7 \le U \le 0.9) = P(0.8 \le U \le 1.0) = 0.2$.

Numerous other distributions that are completely continuous arise organically. Two significant absolutely continuous distributions that will be covered later in the text are the normal distribution and the negative exponential distribution.

Defining continuous distributions is simple. To define a continuous function with a finite integral, g, either on an interval or the entire line is all that is required.

Assume the integral has a value of c. The density function f(x) is then obtained by defining f(x) = g(x)/c. The value 1 is then obtained by integrating f over the area where g is not zero. We will refer to the integral of as F. The cumulative distribution function is obtained by integrating it from the smallest value with a nonzero density to a given point x. It has the characteristic that, as we get closer to the largest value of x for which f > 0, it increases to 1 from zero at the first real value for which f > 0.

Let us examine a particular instance of the beta family, which is a family of continuous distributions on [0, 1]. The two parameters α and β are crucial for the beta family. We will examine a particular scenario in which α = 2 and β = 2. The beta density is generally given by $f(x) = B(\alpha, \beta)x^{a-1}(1 - x)^{b-1}$. The constant term B(α,β) is selected to ensure that the integral of the function g from 0 to 1 equal 1. The beta function is the name given to this function. To define g(x) = x(1 – x) for 0 ≤ x ≤ 1 and g(x) = 0 for all other values of x, we just need to know the special case. Refer to the integral of g as G.

By integral calculus, $G(x) = x^2/2 - x^3/3$ for all $0 \le x \le 1$, $G(x) = 0$ for $x > 0$, and $G(x) = 1/6$ for all $x > 1$. Now $G(1) = 1/6$ is the integral of g over the interval [0, 1]. Therefore, $G(1)$ is the constant c that we want.

Let $f(x) = g(x)/c = x(1 - x)/(1/6) = 6x(1 - x)$ for $0 \leq x \leq 1$ and $f(x) = 0$ for all 0th-er x. The quantity $1/G(1)$ is the constant for the beta density f. In our general formula it was $B(\alpha, \beta)$. In this case, since $\alpha = 2$ and $\beta = 2$ we have $B(2, 2) = 1/G(1) = 6$. This function f is a probability density function (the analog for absolutely continuous random variables to the probability mass function for discrete random variables). The cumulative probability distribution function is $F(x) = x^2(3 - 2x) = 6G(x)$ for $0 \leq x \leq 1$, $F(x) = 0$ for $x < 0$, and $F(x) = 1$ for $x > 1$. We see that $F(x) = 6G(x)$ for all x.

The mean (ρ) and variance (σ^2) of a continuous random variable can be defined by analogy with the definitions for discrete random variables. All we do is substitute the probability mass function with the density function f and the integration symbol for the summation sign. Thus, we have $\sigma=\int xf(x)dx$ and $\sigma^2=\int(x - \mu)^2f(x)$ dx for an continuous random variable X.

If you know some elementary integral calculus, you can verify that $\mu = 1/2$ and $\sigma^2 = 1/12$ for the uniform distribution on [0, 1].

4.6. The Binomial Distribution

When the probability of success on any given trial is p, the binomial random variable is the count of the number of successes in n independent trials. In scenarios where there are just two possible outcomes—success and failure, respectively—the binomial distribution is applicable.

These trials are all referred to as Bernoulli trials. For trial I, we will conveniently assume that X_i is a Bernoulli random variable. If the trial is successful, this random variable is assigned the value 1, and if the trial is unsuccessful, it is assigned the value 0.

For Z (the number of successes in n trials) to be Bi(n, p), we must have n independent Bernoulli trials with each trial having the same probability of success p. Z then can be represented as the sum of the n independent Bernoulli random variables X_i for i = 1, 2, 3, . . . , n. This representation is convenient and conceptually important when we are considering the Central Limit Theorem and the normal distribution approximation to the binomial.

In many problems, the binomial distribution naturally occurs. It could suitably depict, for instance, the distribution of boys in families of sizes 3, 4, or 5, or the number of heads in an n-time coin flip. In a clinical trial, it might stand for the total number of successful ablation procedures. It could be a representation of the number of victories your preferred baseball team has this year or the total number of hits your preferred batter has collected in his first 100 at-bats.

We will now calculate Bi(n, p), the general binomial distribution. We merely extend the combinatorial arguments for Bi(3, 0.50) that we employed in the preceding section. We examine $P(Z = r)$, where $0\leq r\leq n$. $C(n, r) = n!/[(n - r)!\, r!]$ is the number of elementary events that result in r successes out of n trials (that is, obtaining exactly r successes and n − r failures).

Recall our earlier example of filling slots. Applying that example to the present situation, we note that one such outcome that leads to r successes and n − r failures would be to have the r successes in the first r slots and the n − r failures in the remaining n − r slots. For each slot, the probability of a success is p, and the probability of a failure is 1 − p. Given that the events are independent from trial to trial, the multiplication rule for independent events applies, i.e., products of terms which are either p or 1 − p. We see that for this particular arrangement, p is multiplied r times and 1 − p is multiplied n − r times.

$P^r(1-p)^{n-r}$ is the probability that each of the first r trials will be successful and each of the subsequent trials will be unsuccessful. Any other arrangement could be supported with the same logic. In the product, the quantity p will appear r times, and 1 – p will appear n – r times. If the terms are rearranged in the multiplication formula, the result remains unchanged. As a result, the probability of occurrence of every combination of the r successes and n – r failures are equal to the one we just calculated.

The number of such arrangements is just the number of ways to select exactly r out of the n slots for success. This number denotes combinations for selecting r objects out of n, namely, C(n, r). Therefore, $P(Z = r) = C(n, r)(1-p)^{n-r} = \{n!/[r!(n-r)!]\}p^r(1-p)^{n-r}$. Because the formula for P(Z = r) applies for any value of r between 0 and n (including both 0 and n), we have the general binomial distribution.

Suppose Z has the distribution Bi(n, p); then $P(Z = r) = n!/[(n-r)!r!]p^r(1-p)^{n-r}$. Now suppose W has the distribution Bi(n, 1 – p). Let us consider P(W = n – r). $P(W = n-r) = n!/[\{n-(n-r)\}!(n-r)!](1-p)^{n-r}p^r = n!/[r!\,(n-r)!](1-p)^{n-r}p^r$. Without changing the product, we can switch terms around in the numerator and switch terms around in the denominator: $P(W = n-r) = n!/[r!\,(n-r)!](1-p)^{n-r}\,p^r = n!/[(n-r)!\,r!]p^r(1-p)^{n-r}$. But we recognize that the term on the far-right-hand side of the chain of equalities equals P(Z = r). So P(W = n – r) = P(Z = r). Consequently, for $0 \le r \le n$, the probability that a Bi(n, p) random variable equals r is the same as the probability that a Bi(n, 1 – p) random variable is equal to n – r. (Morgan et al., 2020) (Djulbegovic et al., 2015).

4.7. The Monty Hall Problem

Probability theory can be extremely subtle and misleading, despite its apparent simplicity and intuitiveness. Numerous outcomes in the field of probability defy common sense; examples include the Monty Hall Problem, Benford's Law of Lead Digits, the St. Petersburg Paradox, the Birthday Problem, and Simpson's Paradox.

Feller is a good resource for additional reading on the aforementioned issues. It covers Benford's Law, the Waiting Time Paradox, and the Birthday Problem. We also suggest reading the charming story, which is written in the Arthur Conan Doyle vein, in which Sherlock Holmes corrects Watson on a number of common misconceptions about probability.

Many years ago, The Monty Hall Problem became well-known and well-respected. In response to a query from a reader, Marilyn Vos Savant offered a solution to the issue in her Parade magazine column. There was a lot of controversy, and many readers questioned her response in writing—some of them in a very offensive way. Mathematicians and statisticians made up a large portion of those who presented the most challenging questions. Nevertheless, computer simulation makes it simple to illustrate Vos Savant's solution, which was accurate.

The Monty Hall Problem is this: After every episode of the television show "Let's Make a Deal," Monty Hall would give one of the contestants a chance to win the big prize. There were three options for showcase doors. The prize was hidden behind one of the doors, while the other two held "clunkers"—worthless prizes sometimes called "goats.."

There was a chance that a real goat was actually behind one of the doors on the stage! Monty would ask a contestant to select a door, then reveal another door that was concealing a dud. After that, a bribe of $500, $1000, or more would be made to the competitor to get them to open the door. The grand prize was always worth much more than the bribe, so most of the contestants opted to keep the door, especially if Monty offered a large sum of money in exchange for the bribe. The candidates began to suspect they had the right door the more Monty offered. Contestants believed Monty was pressuring them to forfeit the grand prize because he knew which door held it.

The well-known issue Vos Savant tackled in her column concerned a small variation, which Monty might or might not have really used. Once more, the competitor chooses one of the two still-open doors after one of the three doors is removed. Rather than giving the contestant money, the host (like Monty Hall) lets them keep the door they've chosen or choose another one. Marilyn advised the contestant to change doors because doing so increases his chances of winning by 2/3, compared to the 1/3 chance that the door he initially selected will be the correct one.

Those who disagreed claimed that it wouldn't matter if the competitor switched because there would still be two doors remaining, each with an equal 50% chance of being the correct door after one of the empty doors is removed. This appeared to some to be a straightforward conditional probability exercise.

A valid point would be that there is a 1/3 chance to choose the right door at first. Monty will reveal a door that conceals a clunker once a door has been chosen. Only because he is aware of which door contains the prize can he accomplish this. Monty is free to choose any of the two remaining doors if the first door chosen is the winner. But Monty has to reveal to the competitor the one door that still hides a clunker if the competitor doesn't have the right door.

With a switching strategy, however, the right door will be found two-thirds of the time. Therefore, switching will result in success in two-thirds of the cases and failure in only one-third of the cases. As such, switching all the time will win roughly 67 percent of the time, while sticking with the chosen door will only win 33 percent of the time.

A few mathematicians made a mistake by failing to take into account the contestant's choice of door, which had an impact on Monty's plan. The issue would have been different had Monty chosen at random one of the two "clunker" doors first. The competitor would then be aware that there is a 50% chance that any of the two still open doors will be the correct one. The contestant's chance of winning would then remain unchanged, regardless of which door they selected: 50% if they stayed, and 50% if they switched. The nuance here is that the game and the likelihood of the result are entirely altered by the variation in the decision-making sequence.

Create the game on a computer if you still don't think that switching increases your chances of winning. Select the winning door using a uniform random number generator, and instruct the computer to display a clunker door by Monty's rule. That is the best method to see that you will win approximately 67 percent of the time when you switch and only about 33 percent of the time when you keep the same door after playing the game numerous times (for example, at least 100 times using the switching strategy and 100 times using the staying strategy).

If you are not very good at programming computers, you can visit the Stanford University Statistics Department's Susan Holmes website. You can play the computerized version of the game that she has; she will keep track of how many wins you have from switching around and how many wins you have when sticking with your first option.

Susan shows you a cartoon with three doors to play the game. You start by clicking on the desired door. Her computer software then opens a door and displays a cartoon image of a donkey. Once more, you can click on your door to keep it in place or click on the other door to switch. The application then displays what's behind your door, giving you the option to either find another donkey or win.

You're then asked if you'd like to play once more. You are free to use any strategy you like and play the game as often as you would like. Lastly, the application displays the total number of times you have switched as well as the number of times you won when you decide to stop. Along with the total number of times you selected the staying strategy, the program also counts the number of times you won when you employed it.

4.8. A Quality Assurance Problem

One of the current authors advised a medical device manufacturer whose product was being distributed into the field. The business regularly puts the product through a series of quality control inspections prior to shipping. One item was found to have been shipped with an incorrect label in the field. Following an examination of the details, the business discovered that over 100 items had the incorrect item's label at the time of shipment. The purpose of sampling these 100 items was to check for label mismatches or malfunctions.

After testing 13 randomly selected samples out of 100, the company reported no failures. The company thought that this particular mismatch was a unique instance, but they couldn't be positive. They might have to take out all of the remaining items from the lot and check them all for inconsistencies. This would be an expensive and time-consuming procedure. However, they wouldn't have to carry out the recall if they could prove with a high enough degree of confidence that the likelihood of one or more mismatched labels in the field is extremely low.

The lot went through the following sequence of tests:

1. Thirteen out of 100 items were randomly selected for label mismatch checking.
2. No mismatches were found and the 13 were returned to the lot; two items were pulled and destroyed for other reasons.
3. Of the remaining 98 items, 13 were chosen at random and used for a destructive test (one that causes the item to be no longer usable in the field).
4. The remaining 85 items were then released.

In the field, it was discovered that one of these 85 had a mismatched label. A statistician (Chernick) was asked to determine the probability that at least one more of the remaining 84 items in the field could have a mismatch, assuming:

a) Exactly two are known to have had mismatches.
b) The mismatch inspection works perfectly and would have caught any mismatches.
c) In the absence of any information to the contrary, the two items pulled at the second stage could equally likely have been any of the 100 items.

Assuming that exactly three of the 84 items in the field have mismatched, the statistician was also asked to calculate the likelihood that at least one more could have a mismatch. To solve this problem, you must first calculate and add the following two probabilities: (1) the likelihood that all three mislabelled items passed inspection, and (2) the likelihood that one of the two pulled items was destroyed while the other two passed. Of the two probabilities, the first was the more important one. The statistician was also required to calculate the probability that, of the 100 items in the lot, 85 would pass the series of tests and, in the event that only one item was mismatched, for the purpose of establishing a baseline comparison. Since it is the simplest to compute, this probability will be obtained first.

If mismatch checking is completely accurate, the one mismatched label that passed with the 85 that made it through the series of inspections wouldn't have survived if it hadn't been chosen from the first 13 for label mismatch check. It is equivalent to drawing 13 at random, one at a time, without replacement, when 13 items are chosen at random from a pool of 100. The product of 13 probabilities is the likelihood that the item is not among these 13.

The probability that the item will not be drawn in any of the 13 draws is represented by each of these 13 probabilities. This probability on the first draw is 99/100. With just 99 items left to choose from in the second draw, there is a 98/99 chance that none of the items will be chosen. Continuing in this way and multiplying these probabilities together, we see that the probability of the item not being drawn in any one of the 13 draws is

1. (99/100)(98/99)(97/98)(96/97)(95/96)(94/95)(93/94)
2. (92/93)(91/92)(90/91)(89/90)(88/89)(87/88)

By eliminating common numerators and denominators to 87/100, we can significantly simplify this calculation and obtain the likelihood that the item will survive the initial inspection.

The first inspection is not related to the second or third inspections. The outcome of the second inspection determines the probability we compute for the third inspection. To get our final result, we multiply the three probabilities together after calculating the probability of surviving those inspections.

The thirteen items that passed the first inspection are changed in the second stage. Thus, there are 100 things to choose from once more. Now, one of the two items that were initially drawn cannot be the item with the mismatched label for it to avoid destruction. The probability that the item with the mismatched label is not drawn is the probability that it is not the first one drawn multiplied by the probability that it is not the second one drawn, given that it was not the first one drawn since we assumed that each item has an equal chance of being drawn. Its likelihood is (98/100)(97/99).

Just 98 items are remaining at the third stage, and 13 are randomly selected for destructive testing. As a result, the procedure for calculating the probability is the same as the one employed in the initial stage; the only difference is that the product's first term is 97/98 rather than 99/100. We get 85/98 after multiplication and cancellation.

The product of these three probabilities, or [(87/100)][(98/100)(97/99)][(85/98)], is the ultimate outcome. After cancellation, this reduces to (87/100)(97/100)(85/99). The outcome is 72.46 percent, or 0.72456. Keep in mind that a percentage can also be used to express a proportion.).

Next, we determine the likelihood that, out of the 100 items in the lot, there are two items with mismatched labels. Our goal is to ascertain the likelihood that each of them will be overlooked throughout the three inspection phases. Calculations of probability that resemble the ones mentioned previously are applicable. We multiply the three probabilities acquired in the first three stages collectively as a result.

To repeat, the probabilities obtained in the first three stages (the probability that both mismatched items are missed during inspection) are as follows:

- The first stage—(87/100)(86/99)
- The second stage, given that they survive the first stage—(98/100)(97/99)
- The third stage, given that they are among the remaining 98—(85/98)(84/97)

The final result is (87/100)(86/99)(98/100)(97/99)(85/98)(84/97). This result simplifies to (87/100)(86/99)(85/100)(84/99) = 0.54506 or 54.51%.

Out of the 100 items in the lot, if there are three with mismatched labels, we have to multiply the chance that two of the three will pass inspection by the chance that all three will pass. We need to eliminate exactly one of the three at stage two to calculate the latter probability. In contrast to the last computation, this one includes the possibility of two passes and one failure.

We multiply these probabilities together at each stage to determine the likelihood that every item with mismatched labels passes inspection.

4.9. Improved Diagnostic Accuracy Through Probability-Based Diagnosis

We outline the steps in the diagnostic pathway and the probabilistic knowledge and abilities required at each one. It shows the centrality of probabilistic understanding to making diagnoses at each of the following steps:

- ***Step 1: Chief complaint and initial differential diagnosis***

  A patient's main complaint starts the diagnostic process. Based on information about disease incidence in the population of interest, or the population the patient is from, the clinician makes an initial differential diagnosis. The first "pretest probability" is represented by this estimate."

- ***Step 2: Adjustment based on history and physical exam***

  A patient-specific differential diagnosis is reached by the clinician after conducting a physical examination and taking a history. Each of these steps helps to adjust the probabilities of diseases in the differential diagnosis. Understanding how each history and physical exam result affects probability (such as test accuracy), as represented by likelihood ratios or sensitivity and specificity, is necessary for this step.

- ***Step 3: Selection of diagnostic tests***

  The doctor then chooses to investigate potential diagnoses by running a specific diagnostic test (or series of tests). Depending on the clinical situation, the selected tests may correspond with the most likely diagnosis or the most concerning diagnosis. Knowing the likelihood that a test will help or hurt the patient is necessary when deciding whether to order one.

  Tests, like all other health services, will either benefit or harm patients, even though many clinicians do not frame diagnostic testing in terms of benefits and harms to the patient. For instance, a test may reveal a diagnosis for which treatment leads to better results, or it may expose a patient to hazardous materials, discomfort, or needless care, the benefits of which outweigh the risks. The magnitude of these benefits and harms varies greatly.

- ***Step 4: Test Interpretation***

  To determine the post-test probability, the clinician must evaluate the test results in light of the pre-test probability. To complete this step, you must grasp the Bayes Theorem, which incorporates test accuracy measures into the pre-test probability and demands that you reject the idea that test results are final.

Though it might not be possible to perform explicit calculations using the Bayes Theorem in clinical practice, clinical reasoning is informed by a conceptual understanding of the Theorem. For instance, an abnormal exercise stress test is found in a 40-year-old woman who has nonspecific chest pain and no cardiac risk factors. She still has a low pretest probability, which makes coronary artery disease unlikely to be her condition. When determining the final post test probability, the outcomes of each test should be taken into account if more than one is conducted.

- ***Step 5: Final diagnosis or further testing***

To finish the diagnostic phase, the clinician must finally determine when diagnostic closure is reached. To start management, this step entails assessing whether a diagnosis has been established, that is, if the post-test probability is high enough or the uncertainty is low enough. The likelihood of a disease developing at that point (referred to as the "treatment threshold") will differ depending on the disease's features, how it is treated, and the risk tolerance of the patient and clinician. More testing might be necessary if the chance of illness is less than the threshold.

Therefore, accurate estimations of pretest probability and knowledge of the impact of both positive and negative tests on that probability are essential for accurate diagnosis. Nonetheless, both before and after testing, doctors typically overestimate the likelihood that a patient has the illness they are looking into. This propensity probably results in false-positive test results leading to incorrect diagnosis of conditions and subsequent missed diagnoses that are causing symptoms, which could be harmful to the patient. (Morgan et al., 2021) (Cooper et al., 2021).

4.9.1. Reasons to Refocus Training on Probability

Although it is commonly acknowledged that weighing probabilities is fundamental to the diagnostic process, and medical students may be instructed in test accuracy, there is a deficiency in clinically integrated training in probabilistic diagnostic reasoning. Most of the time, learning about probability has consisted of learning the definitions of sensitivity and specificity and computing them using 2X2 tables derived from studies of test accuracy.

This approach may lead to errors in estimating the probability of disease because clinical medicine makes difficult use of mathematical calculations. The preclinical years of medical school are when most test interpretation and probability education take place, indicating that this approach to testing is distinct from that which is employed in regular clinical practice.

Additionally, the majority of medical decisions made in clinical practice are made quickly and intuitively, so it is essential for clinicians to accurately estimate the "gestalt" of pre-test probabilities of common disorders and to intuitively modify pre-test probabilities in response to test results. With every new test, these estimates need to be revised. At the same time, clinicians must rely on quantitative estimates when making decisions regarding less common presenting complaints or syndromes for which they lack intuition.

Presently, there is insufficient data to guide methods for instructing diagnostic reasoning, and trainees typically discuss diagnosis in relation to making differential diagnoses. Probabilistic understanding is not emphasized in these talks. In fact, by rewarding students for proposing uncommon diseases with incredibly low likelihood, they may undermine learners' intuitive understanding of prevalence and probabilistic reasoning.

4.9.2. Methods to Teach and Inform Probability for Diagnostic Decision-Making

Clinicians must possess both an intuitive understanding of probability and ready access to the variety of crucial quantitative data that is currently difficult to obtain to properly integrate probabilistic thinking into the diagnostic process. We present the current need to close the gap and the probabilistic information required at each stage of the diagnostic process.

- ***Step 1: Developing initial differential diagnosis***: Make incidence data for common diseases easily accessible. Clinicians require easy access to local incidence data when estimating an initial differential diagnosis based on the chief complaint. While getting this information might be difficult, it is still possible.
- ***Step 2: Adjustment based on history and physical***: Provide data from the physical examination and history with sensitivity and specificity. Clinicians require evidence of the sensitivity and specificity of clinical features and physical examination findings, which are generally unavailable when modifying the initial differential based on aspects of the history and physical examination. Furthermore, they must comprehend how to modify probability in response to test outcomes, be it physical examination techniques or blood or imaging tests.
- ***Step 3: Selection of a diagnostic test:*** Give patients access to up-to-date, absolute information on the likelihood of potential benefits and harms from common tests at the point of care. Although there are currently few clinicians who view tests in terms of benefits and harms, the way that screening tests are approached is an example of an exception. For instance, we can weigh the potential benefits (like a decrease in prostate cancer deaths or advanced disease) and harms (like erectile dysfunction and urine incontinence) when making decisions about PSA tests using the decision aids that are currently available. With improved information availability, a similar rationale might be used for testing in a broader sense.
- ***Step 4: Test interpretation:*** Use games or other creative ways to teach students about natural frequency interpretation when it comes to test accuracy. The most crucial thing is that physicians require a deeper intuitive grasp of probability. It is best to teach probability to students by exposing them to natural frequency figures.

Approaches based on patient populations can be used in place of tables with probability calculations. Students might be asked, for instance, to divide a group of 100 identical patients by the percentage that either has the disease (representing the pre-test probability) or does not. Based on incidence, sensitivity, and specificity, respectively, one could estimate the proportion of positive tests that would occur in patients with and without disease. Graphic pictures with grids or icons that represent risks out of 100 or 1,000 people can be used to illustrate these estimates; it has been observed that these illustrations are more effective than other representations when used with individuals who are less trained.

These methods have not, as far as we know, been extensively researched or used in medical education. Additionally, a time-tested and successful teaching strategy that can aid clinicians in gaining an intuitive understanding of probability is repeated practice combined with clear, actionable feedback.

- ***At Step 5: Final diagnosis or further testing or consideration of other diagnoses:*** Recognize ambiguity and impart threshold-setting techniques. In clinical medicine, diagnostic error can be attributed, in part, to the inherent uncertainty surrounding many diagnoses and the wide range of patient symptoms and findings. When doctors face this uncertainty, they rarely get feedback regarding the presumptions that guide their diagnosis, which can lead to incorrect reasoning being reinforced.

Educators themselves may require training in handling uncertainty. Geographically and individually specific probability thresholds for testing and treatment may differ, but survey studies can be used to estimate appropriate ranges. Incorporating probabilistic treatment thresholds into diagnostic testing plans is imperative in clinical discussions. The significance of probability can be emphasized by this information, and learners' perceptions of suitable thresholds for testing or treatment in various contexts can be improved with feedback. (Zipkin et al., 2014) (Stephens et al., 2021).

A Closer Look

Probability from Statistics: Frequentism

Imagine, for the first time, that you see a coin and realize it has two sides. This is how the frequentist approach to probability works. You want to know how likely it is that the coin will land heads when tossed. To answer this question, you can count the number of times you toss the coin and get a head. When you calculate that roughly half of the results were heads after a sufficient number of repetitions, you can deduce that the probability of getting a head at the next toss is ½ or 50%. Most importantly, you wouldn't feel comfortable making a judgment after just three, five, or twenty tosses. You can rely on the result to be accurate to a greater extent if your calculation is based on more instances.

As we can see, the frequentist method determines the likelihood of an event occurring by looking into how frequently it has occurred in the past. This kind of approach is referred to as "empirical" by philosophers, indicating that it is solely dependent on observation. Remember that David Hume's empiricist beginnings dictated that he only trusted knowledge that could be observed through our senses. You would then not need to know anything about the characteristics or hidden dispositions of the coin in order to determine the likelihood that it will land heads or tails. All you have to do is count the distribution of results after tossing the coin as many times as possible.

To determine the relative frequency of a particular outcome in a series of events, scientists employ statistical models and tools because, in practice, the computation of past events is typically far more complex than in the coin example.

Keep in mind that this strategy was created by considering games of chance, such as coin tossing, and that in order for it to be considered successful, it must meet two crucial requirements. First, the frequentist method assumes that an infinite number of repetitions is possible (at least in theory). Second, the same conditions must be repeated numerous times. This means that if a single case cannot be repeated, it is impossible to compute a frequentist probability for it. We can only infer the actual result from a single case; we cannot infer the percentage of similar results from a set of related trials.

Calculating the objective probability of an event based on the percentage of successful trials in a series is known as frequentism. The next step is to observe how frequently the same kind of event occurred in earlier, comparable cases in order to calculate probability.

Summary

- Probability is a mathematical construction that determines the likelihood of occurrence of events that are subject to chance.
- Based on mathematical axioms and theorems, probability also involves a mathematical model to describe the mechanism that produces uncertain or random outcomes.
- The probability of an event A is determined by first defining the set of all possible elementary events, associating a probability with each elementary event, and then summing the probabilities of all the elementary events that imply the occurrence of A. The elementary events are distinct and are called mutually exclusive.
- The elementary events are the building blocks (or atoms) of a probability model. They are the events that cannot be decomposed further into smaller sets of events.
- Venn diagrams are graphics designed to portray combinations of sets such as those that represent unions and intersections.
- Probability distributions describe the probability of events. Parameters are characteristics of probability distributions.
- Probability distributions have certain characteristics that can apply to both continuous and discrete distributions. One such property is symmetry.
- A probability distribution is symmetric if it has a central point at which we can construct a vertical line so that the shape of the distribution to the right of the line is the mirror image of the shape to the left.
- Probability distributions that are not symmetric are called skewed distributions. There are two kinds of skewed distributions: positively skewed and negatively skewed.
- The binomial random variable is the count of the number of successes in n independent trials when the probability of success on any given trial is p.
- The clinician performs a history and physical examination, each element of which informs adjustment of the probabilities of diseases in the differential diagnosis, ending in a patient-specific differential diagnosis.

References

1. Altman, D. G., & Bland, J. M. (1991). Improving doctors' understanding of statistics. *Journal of the Royal Statistical Society: Series A (Statistics in Society), 154*(2), 223–267.
2. Baghdadi, J. D., Korenstein, D., Pineles, L., Scherer, L. D., Lydecker, A. D., Magder, L., Stevens, D. N., & Morgan, D. J. (2022). Exploration of primary care clinician attitudes and cognitive characteristics associated with prescribing antibiotics for asymptomatic bacteriuria. *JAMA Network Open, 5*(5), e2214268.
3. Cooper, N., Bartlett, M., Gay, S., Hammond, A., Lillicrap, M., Matthan, J., & Singh, M.; UK Clinical Reasoning in Medical Education (CReME) consensus statement group. (2021). Consensus statement on the content of clinical reasoning curricula in undergraduate medical education. *Medical Teacher, 43*(2), 152–159.
4. Dempster, A. P. (1968). A generalization of Bayesian inference. *Journal of the Royal Statistical Society: Series B (Methodological), 30*, 205–232.

5. Diamond, G. A., Forrester, J. S., & Hirsch, M. (1980). Application of conditional probability analysis to the clinical diagnosis of coronary artery disease. *Journal of Clinical Investigation, 65*, 1210–1221.

6. Djulbegovic, B., van den Ende, J., Hamm, R. M., Mayrhofer, T., Hozo, I., & Pauker, S. G.; International Threshold Working Group (ITWG). (2015). When is rational to order a diagnostic test, or prescribe treatment: The threshold model as an explanation of practice variation. *European Journal of Clinical Investigation, 45*(5), 485–493.

7. Halkin, A., Reichman, J., Schwaber, M., Paltiel, O., & Brezis, M. (1998). Likelihood ratios: Getting diagnostic testing into perspective. *Quarterly Journal of Medicine, 91*, 247–258.

8. Hayden, S. R., & Brown, M. D. (1999). Likelihood ratio: A powerful tool for incorporating the results of a diagnostic test into clinical decision making. *Annals of Emergency Medicine, 33*, 575–580.

9. Jaeschke, R., Guyatt, G. H., & Sackett, D. L. (1994). Users' guide to the medical literature III: How to use an article about a diagnostic test. *Journal of the American Medical Association, 271*, 703–707.

10. Korenstein, D., Scherer, L. D., Foy, A., Pineles, L., Lydecker, A. D., Owczarzak, J., Magder, L., Brown, J. P., Pfeiffer, C. D., Terndrup, C., Leykum, L., Stevens, D., Feldstein, D. A., Weisenberg, S. A., Baghdadi, J. D., & Morgan, D. J. (2022). Clinician attitudes and beliefs associated with more aggressive diagnostic testing. *The American Journal of Medicine, 135*(7), e182–e193.

11. McColl, A., Smith, H., White, P., & Field, J. (1998). General practitioners' perceptions of the route to evidence-based medicine: A questionnaire survey. *British Medical Journal, 316*, 361–365.

12. Meyer, A. N. D., Giardina, T. D., Khawaja, L., & Singh, H. (2021). Patient and clinician experiences of uncertainty in the diagnostic process: Current understanding and future directions. *Patient Education and Counseling, 104*(11), 2606–2615.

13. Morgan, D. J., Pineles, L., Owczarzak, J., Magder, L., Scherer, L., Brown, J. P., Pfeiffer, C., Terndrup, C., Leykum, L., Feldstein, D., Foy, A., Stevens, D., Koch, C., Masnick, M., Weisenberg, S., & Korenstein, D. (2021). Accuracy of practitioner estimates of probability of diagnosis before and after testing. *JAMA Internal Medicine, 181*(6), 747–755.

14. Morgan, D. J., Scherer, L. D., & Korenstein, D. (2020). Improving physician communication about treatment decisions: Reconsideration of "risks vs benefits." *JAMA, 324*(10), 937–938.

15. Morris, R. W. (2002). Does EBM offer the best opportunity yet for teaching medical statistics? *Statistics in Medicine, 21*(7), 969–977.

16. Noguchi, Y., Matsui, K., Imura, H., Kiyota, M., & Fukui, T. (2002). Quantitative evaluation of the diagnostic thinking process in medical students. *Journal of General Internal Medicine, 17*(11), 839–844.

17. Oliveri, R. S., Gluud, C., & Wille-Jorgensen, P. A. (2004). Hospital doctors' self-rated skills in and use of evidence-based medicine—a questionnaire survey. *Journal of Evaluation in Clinical Practice, 10*(2), 219–226.

18. Olson, A., Rencic, J., Cosby, K., Rusz, D., Papa, F., Croskerry, P., Zierler, B., Harkless, G., Giuliano, M. A., Schoenbaum, S., Colford, C., Cahill, M., Gerstner, L., Grice, G. R., & Graber, M. L. (2019). Competencies for improving diagnosis: An interprofessional framework for education and training in health care. *Diagnosis (Berlin, Germany), 6*(4), 335–341.

19. Palmer, C. R. (2002). Discussion: Teaching hypothesis tests: Time for significant change? *Statistics in Medicine, 21*(7), 995–999.
20. Stephens, G. C., Rees, C. E., & Lazarus, M. D. (2021). Exploring the impact of education on preclinical medical students' tolerance of uncertainty: A qualitative longitudinal study. *Advances in Health Sciences Education: Theory and Practice, 26*(1), 53–77.
21. Windish, D. M., Huot, S. J., & Green, M. L. (2007). Medicine residents' understanding of the biostatistics and results in the medical literature. *Journal of the American Medical Association, 298*(9), 1010–1022.
22. Winglee, M., Valliant, R., Brick, J. M., & Machlin, S. (2000). Probability matching of medical events. *Journal of Economic and Social Measurement, 26*, 129–140.
23. Xu, H., Ang, B. W. G., Soh, J. Y., & Ponnamperuma, G. G. (2021). Methods to improve diagnostic reasoning in undergraduate medical education in the clinical setting: A systematic review. *Journal of General Internal Medicine, 36*(9), 2745–2754.
24. Zipkin, D. A., Umscheid, C. A., Keating, N. L., Allen, E., Aung, K., Beyth, R., Kaatz, S., Mann, D. M., Sussman, J. B., Korenstein, D., Schardt, C., Nagi, A., Sloane, R., & Feldstein, D. A. (2014). Evidence-based risk communication: A systematic review. *Annals of Internal Medicine, 161*(4), 270–280.

Chapter 5

CONFIDENCE INTERVAL ESTIMATES

Contents

Introduction 127
5.1. Understanding Estimation 129
5.2. Choosing Effect Measures and Computing Estimates of Effect 137
Summary 160
References 161

Introduction

In public health practice, confidence intervals are used to show the level of uncertainty in estimates resulting from random error. Given that relationships in the sample are unlikely to precisely reflect relationships in the true population, even in cases where sampling is random, this makes intuitive sense when estimates are based on data from a sample of a larger population. Error is bound to happen—random error, at the very least.

Confidence intervals, however, are occasionally omitted from official reports when data are provided for the entire population. This is acceptable when the total number of cases is so high that random error is minimal (e.g., as in extensive nationwide summaries). Smaller numbers, on the other hand, are occasionally left out on the grounds that the observed rates are measurements rather than population estimates, and as a result, random error is not necessary to take into account because the statistics accurately depict the population's behavior.

Orientation and Directional Terms

Term	Definition	Illustration
Random error	Random error is a chance difference between the observed and true values of something (e.g., a researcher misreading a weighing scale records an incorrect measurement).	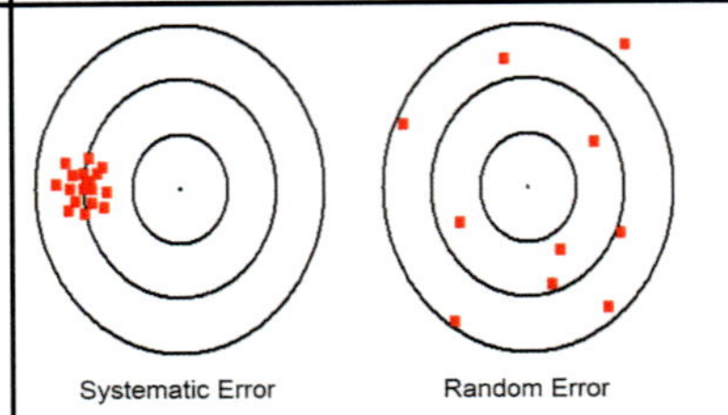
Confidence intervals	A confidence interval (CI) is an interval which is expected to typically contain the parameter being estimated.	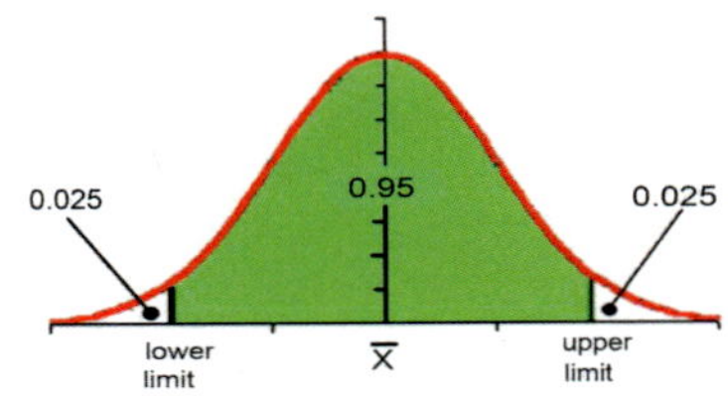
Population	Population is defined as all nationals present in, or temporarily absent from a country, and aliens permanently settled in a country.	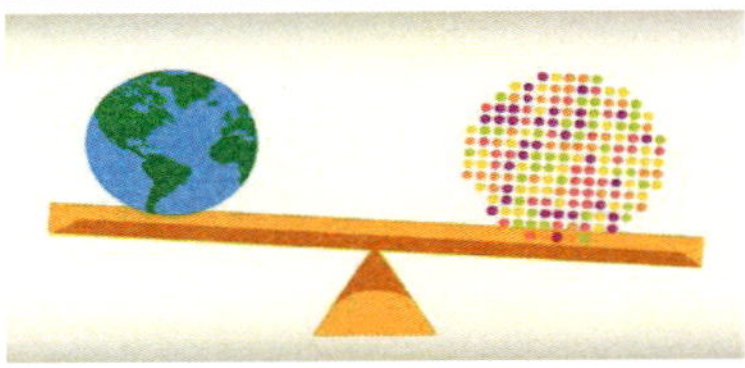
Surveillance	Surveillance is the monitoring of behavior, many activities, or information for the purpose of information gathering, influencing, managing or directing.	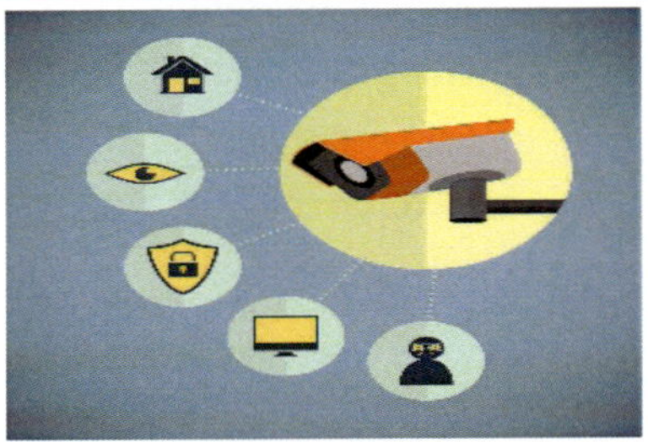

5.1. Understanding Estimation

Indicators of global health are essential for tracking the accomplishment of globally recognized objectives, such as the Sustainable Development Goals, and for helping donors decide where to focus their financial efforts. However, the data are of low quality and scarce in some countries. For instance, the cause of slightly less than half of all deaths worldwide is known. Data on national death registrations are limited to four African nations. There are even fewer useful population-level data on the incidence or prevalence of injury and disease.

International agencies and scholars prepare estimates of important health indicators that are comparable across nations and/or time periods using statistical models in order to address data gaps. The agencies use reported or published data from various national sources, including population surveys, health management information systems, and civil registration, to calculate these estimates.

Global estimates can be helpful to nations in the following ways:

- analyzing their values in comparison to peer nations;
- tracking their progress toward regional and global goals and targets;
- reporting to donors and development partners, such as for performance-based grants; and
- evaluating the accuracy and completeness of empirically reported data.

5.1.1. Common Sources of Bias

These are the sources of bias in country data that a group of agencies found.

5.1.1.1. Inconsistent Case Definitions or Diagnostic Criteria

Individuals who meet a specific case definition can be identified by looking up their health information. The comparability of case definitions may be limited by differences in data sources. Variations in the qualifications of assessors may result in discrepancies in the condition's estimated prevalence. Even in cases where case definitions have not changed, laboratory procedures can alter over time, making comparisons less accurate. Case identification may be significantly impacted by modifications to the sensitivity or specificity of detection techniques as well as by the choice of whether to modify for either one.

5.1.1.2. Self-report Biases

Systematic biases in certain survey instruments can result from challenges in getting precise responses from survey participants. Social desirability bias and recall bias are two instances of self-report biases. Since some cases do not interact with the health system or are not diagnosed, self-reports of prior diagnoses frequently underestimate the true incidence or prevalence of a condition. These biases might change over time and systematically across populations.

5.1.1.3. Incomplete Population-based Surveillance

Systems for registration and surveillance that aim to record every event in a population are frequently deficient. Quantifying the degree of completeness of events like the incidence of infectious diseases may be challenging. For other kinds of events, estimation of completeness might be possible through the use of demographic or capture-recapture techniques.

5.1.1.4. Non-representative Population Bias

Certain data types are purposefully gathered for a portion of the overall population, such as e. g. when information is gathered from volunteers or clinic attendees, or when information is specific to urban or rural populations only. There may be systematic differences in health status and health determinants between the general population and these chosen populations.

5.1.2. Types of Modelling

A theoretical framework that depicts and measures the causal pathways and mechanisms connecting determinants and health outcomes is established by mathematical models. These models use parameter estimates obtained from multiple data sources to predict health outcomes, which can be challenging to measure. A basic mathematical model was employed in the first GBD Study. A mathematical modeling framework was also employed by the WHO in the early 2000s when developing the Comparative Risk Assessment methodology.

The most common method used by analysts to create global estimates is statistical modeling. Using empirical data on the outcome and correlated variables, or covariates, statistical models estimate or predict outcome indicators. Regression techniques are frequently used in statistical models to find a functional form that both fits the data and provides a sufficient summary of the variation in the data. Prediction modeling only attempts to predict outcomes, whereas explanatory modeling attempts to precisely characterize relationships between variables in the data.

To increase predictive validity, statistical models can calculate and make use of the correlation between data observations and covariates. This method is used by statisticians to produce values for indicators in situations where there is little to no primary data available on the outcome of interest, such as trends and levels of maternal mortality and other causes of death. Causality concerns are unimportant with these kinds of models. It is important to caution users not to read the associations as causal, and analysts not to limit their selection of covariates to those they consider to be causal. Accurate prediction is the goal.

5.1.3. Uses

5.1.3.1. Improve Accuracy and Comparability

Enhancing the accuracy and comparability of raw data is a primary goal of statistical modeling. Surveillance or registration data incompleteness is a significant source of bias that estimates need to address. This is a challenge because evaluations of completeness require the use of external data in addition to primary data. A priori bias resulting from definitional and measurement problems can be addressed by analysts by modifying the data before statistical modeling and utilizing outside data. For instance, utilizing a known or presumptive relationship between threshold and cumulative prevalence, it is possible to adjust the prevalence of hearing loss measured using various loudness decibel thresholds to a common threshold. Alternatively, data adjustment through various measurement strategies could be done statistically within the model. According to a common definition, this is called cross-walking. For instance, analysts can use statistical models to estimate the relationships between thresholds and prevalence for multiple hearing loss surveys with different thresholds and to estimate a standard set of thresholds for each population.

5.1.3.2. Synthesise Data from Multiple Sources

When all the data meet inclusion criteria, statistical modeling can produce indicator values that are consistent and comparable across populations and/or time. For instance, several nations have several sources of information on mortality among children under five, including household surveys and the census. By utilizing all currently available, high-quality data, synthesis eliminates the need for an analyst to choose the best single data source arbitrarily—a difficult task given the existence of measurement error. Rather than selecting the treatment effect from a single trial, this method is akin to estimating a treatment effect through a meta-analysis of multiple randomized trials.

5.1.3.3. Fill Data Gaps in Time Series

Completing data gaps in time series and projecting toward a shared goal year or range of years. In the case of most raw data types, different populations have different dates for the most recent data available. A projection component is typically included in the model by analysts because they aim to estimate trends to a common recent year for all populations. The information used in these imputation techniques is frequently taken from neighboring data, which could come from other time points in a country's primary data series or from nations in the same region. Incorporating predictor variables, or covariates, into the model that correlate with the quantity of interest can also help analysts with imputations and projections.

5.1.3.4. Estimate Quantities that Cannot be Directly Measured

Measuring intermediate outcomes and using a model to extrapolate to the final result may be more practical when measuring the health outcome proves to be challenging or expensive. These models typically entail simulating the causal chain mathematically. For instance, the World Health Organization bases its estimates of measles mortality on multiplying measles case estimates by independently estimated case fatality rates.

5.1.3.5. Evaluate Large Scale Interventions

When it is not feasible or ethical to conduct a randomized controlled trial. Researchers track changes in the target outcome while the program is running and create a counterfactual model to calculate the results if the program doesn't exist. This method can also be applied to evaluate the suggested interventions' possible effects and economic viability.

5.1.3.6. Forecast Indicators

Use a forward-looking (and occasionally backward-looking) projection component for a standard time frame (base year to latest target year). In certain situations, longer-term forecasting or projection is the primary goal of the modeling. These models can be divided into two primary categories:

- Projections that are deterministic and driven by covariates, typically based on scenarios. These enable the modeling of alternative future interventions or policies using modifiable parameter assumptions, such as covariates.
- Statistical projections that extrapolate past trends using time-series projection techniques. Hybrid models incorporate multilevel modeling, covariate drivers, and stochastic time series projections.

5.1.4. Statistical Modelling

5.1.4.1. Estimation using Covariates

When using covariates, especially when outcome data is sparse, there is a risk that estimated trends will reflect changes in covariates rather than changes in the estimated outcome indicator. Maternal mortality prediction models, for instance, frequently incorporate covariates like GDP per capita, which is subject to change based on commodity prices. For brief periods, rising GDP per se might have almost no effect on maternal health. However, a model that takes GDP into account as a covariate will forecast lower rates of maternal death.

Regressions that include data type covariates are frequently used when dealing with datasets or nations where data are available by multiple definitions. By adding indicator variables for each alternative data type in a regression analysis and then setting the data type to the preferred type for generating regression estimates, it is possible to cross-walk to the preferred definition. Alternatively, performing the cross-walking as a pre-processing step based on a different regression analysis might be more practical. An illustration of this is a recent study on the prevalence of diabetes mellitus, which included data sources that measure fasting plasma glucose and others that identify diabetes using HbA1c measurements.

The WHO model for estimating national homicide rates across countries is an example of how covariates are used for cross-walking between two data types as well as for level and trend prediction. Following cross-validation, the final model included covariates for infant mortality rate, gender inequality index, percentage of the population living in urban areas, percentage of males aged 15 to 30 years, and pattern of alcohol consumption. An extra covariate for data type accounted for the distinctions between data obtained from death registration and data from police and criminal justice systems.

5.1.4.2. Frequentist versus Bayesian Estimation Methods

Probabilities are interpreted as objective summaries of repeated trials of the same process in frequentist statistical methods. Ordinary least squares regression and other frequentist statistical modeling techniques rely on maximizing a likelihood function that expresses the conditional probability of the actual observations as a function of the parameters that need to be estimated.

According to the Bayesian paradigm, probabilities are arbitrary judgments based on prior information (prior probability distributions) that are revised in response to new information. In general, Bayesian methods enable more appropriate uncertainty characterization, permit the fitting of more complex and flexible models that aim to make numerous internal adjustments, and avoid the approximations necessary for many classical frequentist methods. More computation is needed for these techniques than for frequentist techniques. As computing power increases, Bayesian methods are becoming more and more tractable for almost all parametric methods. As a result, they are being used more and more for modeling global health issues. For instance,

UN agencies are now using Bayesian methods to track maternal and child mortality.

5.1.5. Uses of Statistical Modelling

5.1.5.1. Complex Curve Fitting

To generate smooth estimates across several observations, complex curve fitting is used. Multiple and occasionally overlapping data inputs are used in complex curve smoothing, also known as time series projections, to allow for flexibility in curve fitting.

To estimate trends in child mortality for a nation over a standard time period, for instance, the UN Interagency Group on Mortality Estimation (UN-IGME) previously used the loess regression method. To interpolate and extrapolate a smooth curve for a single population, this method only used data specific to a given country. Rather than using loess regression, UN-IGME now models time trends using Bayesian bias-adjusted B-splines, which allows for more objective curve fitting. We explain this case to show how statistical modeling is becoming more and more complex.

The B3 model, which is based on multiple observations from multiple surveys at uneven intervals, is used by the UN-IGME to estimate a best-fit trend line for the under-five mortality rate (U5MR) using the B-splines model. A data model built into the B-splines model simultaneously accounts for statistically estimated biases specific to each kind of measurement technique (e.g., direct versus indirect birth history).

Assume that indirect birth history observations were, on average (across all country data) 10% lower than the final estimates of child mortality based on all data types. When estimating the final child mortality rate curve, the model will make an upward adjustment in response to the indirect birth history observations. This implies that the final estimated U5MR curve for a nation is dependent upon data that is not country-specific but rather country-wide. The final estimates may completely deviate from the original, raw data observation if a nation solely has observations from skewed data sources. Users of the statistics frequently find it difficult to understand this.

5.1.5.2. Multilevel Modelling

Using multilevel modeling, estimates based on comparatively sparse data can be made more stable and of higher quality. Regression models that are multilevel or hierarchical enable the simultaneous modeling of parameters that vary at multiple levels (e.g., country, region, and global). By using a hierarchical modeling approach, estimation for countries with incomplete or missing data can be informed by data from neighboring countries as well as from other regions. To estimate the variation between groups as a fixed effect, a group dummy variable could be included in non-hierarchical regression models. Additionally, random effects can be included in hierarchical models, allowing the model to more fully share information from higher levels of the hierarchy in situations where the quality of the data from lower levels is lacking.

5.1.5.3. Complex Predictive Models

To extrapolate and interpolate outside of the available data, utilize sophisticated predictive models. Time-varying covariates, multilevel structures, and temporal smoothing techniques are among the methods that are used by most statistical models in combination.

For instance, the UN system employs a multilevel Bayesian regression model with time series modeling, covariates, and random effects to estimate maternal mortality trends by nation. Using a multinomial regression model with covariates and fixed effects, the Maternal Child

Health Epidemiology Estimation collaboration with WHO models a full set of cause of death fractions simultaneously.

The IHME's use of Gaussian process regression to borrow strength and smooth across space and time is one example of another complex statistical model. With health indicators imputed to intricate spatial-temporal grids, such as five km x 5 km grids for the world over 15 years, relatively sparse data can now become large estimates thanks to the use of these statistical imputation and prediction techniques combined with predictive covariates.

5.1.6. Model Frameworks and Validation

Validation of explanatory models is not the same as validation of predictive models.

By determining whether the model fits the data and whether its structure accurately depicts the data, analysts validate explanatory models. An explanatory model's validation, for instance, would look at whether adding more covariates, changing the covariates, or including more nonlinear terms would materially boost the model's explanatory power. Goodness-of-fit tests and model diagnostics like residual analysis are used to evaluate the fit of the model.

On the other hand, in cases of predictive modeling where observations are lacking for specific populations or periods, the validation process centers around the model's capacity to forecast the absent data. This is commonly referred to as out-of-sample predictive validation or cross-validation, and it entails withholding part of the data from the model fitting process and then comparing the accuracy of the model predictions against the withheld data. The type of data being used and the question being asked determine the predictive validity of the analysis. Thus, there isn't a common metric to assess model performance.

One possible use for a model would be to estimate the results for every country for a target year that is not included in the dataset. This will necessitate that the model has exceptional out-of-time prediction capabilities. The model predicts well out-of-sample across countries if the goal is to make predictions for those without primary data.

The withheld data included a combination of five different types of missing data that were used to evaluate the predictive validity of the cause-of-death models used in the GBD 2010 study: countries without data, countries with missing data years within the available data, countries with missing data years at earlier periods, countries with missing data for later periods, and countries with missing data for specific age groups.

Developments in other fields have shown that an ensemble modeling strategy can provide more predictive validity than a single model. The field of global health has recently employed ensemble models, which are composed of various models that have been weighted together. Usually, two sets of withheld data are needed for validation of such ensemble modeling. The individual models' predictive validity is evaluated using the first set, and the ensemble average's predictive validity is evaluated and maximized using the second set.

5.1.7. Presenting Results

The techniques employed to generate the estimates determine their accuracy. More importantly, the basis upon which they are based determines the quantity and caliber of data. Inadequate data quality or accessibility can cause final estimates from alternative methods to differ significantly. This may cause a great deal of confusion among donors and international organizations.

5.1.7.1. GATHER

The best practices for reporting health estimates were agreed upon by a group of agencies in 2016. An 18-item checklist that needs to be included in every report that is released with new global health estimates was part of the Guidelines for Accurate and Transparent Health Estimates Reporting (GATHER) statement that was released. Important items on this list consist of:

- A thorough explanation of all the steps involved in the analysis,
- the different types of uncertainty quantified,
- the procedures used to obtain the analytic or statistical source code used,
- the reasons for any changes made when updating an earlier set of estimates, are all provided
- a discussion of the modeling assumptions and data limitations that impact the interpretation of the estimates is included.

An attainable standard for reporting health estimates is offered by GATHER. However, there are numerous implementation challenges. A study's complete documentation usually necessitates extensive technical appendices. It also needs unrestricted access to computer code and input data. This suggests that publishing estimates will involve more reporting requirements. Understanding estimates requires more than just a fair discussion of the limitations and a clear explanation of the methods used. however, are difficult to supply or validate.

5.1.7.2. Uncertainty Estimation

The GATHER working group believed that reporting results required quantifying uncertainty around modeled health estimates, usually by calculating and reporting uncertainty intervals. GATHER encouraged this approach. Users can better grasp the accuracy of the estimates with the use of uncertainty ranges, which are essential for comparison-making. However, significant statistical knowledge and processing power are typically needed to include the primary sources of uncertainty.

Random errors, sampling errors, non-sampling errors (caused by measurement errors, missing data, coverage errors, and other systematic biases), errors in the model covariates, parameter uncertainty, model specification uncertainty, fundamental uncertainty, and uncertainty from different data transformation steps and externally derived parameters are some examples of potential sources of uncertainty. In actuality, the majority of quantitative uncertainty estimates only take into account a portion of the sources of uncertainty that could exist.

Certain types of uncertainty cannot be estimated using a standard methodology. Analysts employ various techniques or create original techniques. They might accept this as a limitation of their analysis and choose to ignore the source of the uncertainty. The information and data required to quantify uncertainty are frequently lacking. Certain sources of uncertainty, for instance, might not exist or might be hard to quantify. This indicates that the uncertainty of some modeling techniques is greater than that of others. This might just be the case because some people are identifying more sources of ambiguity. Generally speaking, Bayesian approaches make it easier to account for various sources of uncertainty and accurately reflect these sources in the resulting estimates. For modeled indicators, uncertainty in covariate values is usually not available or included in quantitative uncertainty ranges. As an illustration, consider covariates like average per capita income or denominator values like population estimates.

5.1.7.3. Sensitivity Analysis

Assumptions are a part of every estimation process. These cover topics like the functional form of a model and inclusion criteria for data. Sensitivity analysis is a tool that some analysts use to evaluate how much the final values of the estimates depend on these assumptions. The results of the sensitivity analysis might indicate that estimates from different analytical techniques are comparable. This reinforces the findings and gives the estimations more validity. However, the sensitivity analysis can indicate that the estimates are heavily influenced by the modeling strategy or by the inclusion or exclusion criteria for the data. This might contribute to informing future research and encourage readers to carefully review the analytical presumptions.

5.1.7.4. Transparency, Replicability and Complexity

At the center of disagreements regarding global health estimates is transparency. An outsider will have a harder time comprehending and replicating the results the more varied the raw data that is available, the ways in which the raw data has been modified, and the statistical model. Analysts must also take the advantages of creating intricate models into account. A more basic model that is easier for others to duplicate and apply is probably more effective if their estimated results are comparable.

Moreover, although providing more technical documentation under the GATHER guidelines is beneficial, it might not be sufficient to educate users about proper interpretation on its own. Many lack the technical know-how to comprehend the limitations of the methods. A fair discussion of the limitations and a description of the methods in simple terms are required by GATHER. On the other hand, users and researchers cannot agree on what defines plain language. Some believe that open communication about limitations undermines the reliability of the estimates.

5.1.7.5. Communicating Estimates

Frequently, agencies fail to explicitly identify estimates that are mostly imputed. Moreover, they do not offer comprehensive user-friendly documentation of statistical procedures. Researchers should ideally provide estimates along with confidence intervals or uncertainty ranges. For users and decision-makers, however, the usefulness of these uncertainties is frequently unclear.

For instance, the WHO employs a four-color coding scheme for its estimates of mortality by cause. The underlying data's strength is indicated by this system. Additionally, it indicates whether country-specific data or strength from other countries or covariates has been primarily used in the models and data.

5.1.8. Challenges

For many health indicators, there are currently multiple global health estimates available. There are representatives from academic institutions and the UN system. International users like donor organizations and national governments may find this concerning. Dissonant health statistics can be cut both ways, much like international rankings. Sometimes they are discouraging. They may make it more difficult for donors to fund initiatives whose achievements are not yet shown in international statistics. In other instances, they have sparked national discussion and increased federal funding for data gathering and analysis.

The data needs of health statistic users vary. Their opinions on the reliability and applicability of various statistical types differ greatly. Users of national and subnational data frequently favor empirically measured data that can assist in national and subnational decision-making. Comparability with other national estimates or international standards is not as important to these users. Global users value estimates that are comparable across nations and over time, including international agencies, donors, and development partners. This results in differences between the kinds of statistics that are regarded as most reliable at various levels of government. This in turn influences the possibility that policy will be informed by statistics.

The fact that each revision usually entails a full re-estimation of the entire time series rather than the addition of new values for recent years presents a challenge for users of these estimates. These adjustments to the time series can occasionally be explained by new empirical data. Take child mortality rates, for instance, which take into account survey replies with at least 15 years' worth of historical memory. In other instances, significant variations in the estimated series result from modifications to the estimation techniques. This is true even if the data doesn't change. This may be unclear. For instance, if baseline estimates fluctuate, it could have an impact on how quickly and even in which way time trends and shifts away from or possibly even over ultimate targets. Even though the differences are typically within uncertainty bounds, it can be challenging to explain these shifts to decision-makers.

Political purposes can be served by globally produced statistics that significantly deviate from data reported by individual countries. Positive estimates can be used by governments to bolster support for ongoing initiatives. On the other hand, negative assessments support political opposition and civil society critiques of the administration. Due diligence in establishing a more comprehensive understanding of the rationale behind global modeling modifications to raw input data is especially crucial in light of this. Estimates of global health do not take the place of nations' ongoing, consistent, and accurate collection of empirical data. Estimating data gaps, however, can deceive users into believing that empirical data are accessible and lessen the need for information systems to be improved. Utilizing advanced modeling techniques to produce estimates remotely could potentially compromise a nation's comprehension and control over its indicators. There is a risk that projected statistics will be used to assess progress in an era of global target-setting. The creation of estimates and the growth of a nation's ability to generate, analyze, and interpret data should go hand in hand.

5.2. Choosing Effect Measures and Computing Estimates of Effect

For every type of data, there are multiple approaches to compare outcome data (also known as "effect measures") between two intervention groups. For example, a risk ratio, odds ratio, risk difference, or number needed to treat can be used to compare dichotomous outcomes between intervention groups. One can use a mean difference or a standardized mean difference to compare continuous outcomes between groups receiving an intervention. Ratio measures are the two types of effect measures. g. risk ratio, odds ratio, or measures of differences (e.g., mean difference, risk difference). Usually, a logarithmic scale is used to analyze ratio measures. It could be necessary to transform the results taken from study reports into a format that is consistent or useful for analysis.

5.2.1. Types of Data and Effect Measures

5.2.1.1. Types of Data

Selecting the appropriate data type for the outcome measurements is a crucial first step in analyzing the findings of effectiveness research.

Take into consideration outcome data of five common types:

1. dichotomous (or binary) data, where each individual's outcome is one of only two possible categorical responses;
2. continuous data, where each individual's outcome is a measurement of a numerical quantity;
3. ordinal data (including measurement scales), where each individual's outcome is one of several ordered categories, or generated by scoring and summing categorical responses;
4. counts and rates are calculated by counting the number of events experienced by each individual; and
5. time-to-event (typically survival) data that analyze the time until an event occurs, but where not all individuals in the study experienced the event (censored data).

5.2.1.2. Effect Measures

Statistical constructs that compare outcome data between two intervention groups are referred to as effect measures. Examples are mean differences (comparing the mean values between two groups) and odds ratios (comparing the odds of an event between two groups). The two main categories of effect measures are ratio measures and difference measures (also referred to as relative and absolute measures, respectively). As an illustration, the mean differences is a measure of difference and the odds ratio is a ratio measure.

Effect estimates quantify the impact of an intervention by measuring the difference in outcome data between two groups. For ratio measures, a value of 1 signifies no difference, while a value of 0 for difference measures indicates the same. Values above or below these benchmarks may signal the benefit or harm of the intervention, depending on how they are compared (e.g., A versus B or B versus A) and the specific outcome being evaluated.

The actual impact of interventions is never known for sure; the studies that are currently available can only provide an estimate. A measure of that uncertainty, such as a confidence interval or standard error (SE), should always be included with any estimate.

1. Ratio Measures of Intervention Effect: The Use of Log Scales

The odds ratio, risk ratio, rate ratio, and hazard ratio are examples of ratio measures of intervention effect whose values are typically log-transformed before analysis. Occasionally, these values are expressed in terms of their log-transformed values (e.g., log odds ratio). Typically the *natural* log transformation (log base *e*, written 'ln') is used.

The lowest value that ratio summary statistics can take is 0, the highest value that they can take is infinity, and the value 1 denotes no intervention effect. These are the common features shared by all ratio summary statistics. There is an asymmetry in this number scale. For instance, even though an odds ratio (OR) of 2 (a doubling) and 0 (a halving) are opposites and should average to zero, the average of 0 and 2 is 1.25 rather than 1. The scale is made symmetric by the log transformation: the log of 0 is equal to minus infinity, the log of 1 is equal to zero, and the log of infinity is equal to infinity. The example shows that the log of the OR of 2 is 0.69 and the log of the OR of 0.5 above is –0.69. The log-transformed value of an OR of 1 is 0 for the average of –0.69 and 0.69, which appropriately implies no average intervention effect. A log scale is typically used in graphic displays for meta-analyses carried out on ratio scales. For the same reasons, this has the effect of making the confidence intervals appear symmetric.

2. Effects of Interest

In any given analysis of a randomized trial, the effect of interest is typically the result of either the "intention-to-treat" effect or the "per-protocol" effect, which is the result of adhering to the intervention. Depending on the effect of interest, different calculations will be made for the data gathered for a systematic review and for producing effect estimates.

5.2.2. Study Designs and Identifying the Unit of Analysis

5.2.2.1. Unit-of-Analysis Issues

The level of randomization must be considered in the analysis, which is a fundamental tenet of randomized trials. The majority of the time, the number of randomized "units" and the number of observations in the analysis should coincide. A single measurement is taken and analyzed for each outcome in a clinical trial with a basic parallel group design where participants are randomly assigned to one of two intervention groups. There are, however, a lot of variations on this design. You ought to think about whether each study:

- Individual groups were randomly assigned to the same intervention (i.e., trials with cluster randomization);
- People received multiple interventions (e.g., in a crossover trial, which involves treating several sites on a single person at once); and
- For the same result, there were several observations (e.g., measurements taken repeatedly, events that repeat, and measurements taken on various body parts).

5.2.2.2. Cluster-randomized Trials

A cluster-randomized trial involves randomly assigning participant groups to various interventions. The groups could be families, medical practices, schools, villages, or the patients of a single physician.

5.2.2.3. Crossover Trials

In a crossover trial, participants take on the role of their control and receive all interventions in the order that they are assigned at random.

5.2.2.4. Repeated Observations on Participants

Long-term studies may present results for multiple follow-up periods (e.g., six months, a year, and two years). A standard meta-analysis cannot include data from more than one-time point for each study without incurring unit-of-analysis error. The following are some choices for choosing and calculating effect estimates:

- Acquire individual participant data and run an analysis using the entire follow-up for each participant (e.g., time-to-event analysis). As an alternative, calculate an effect measure (such as the total number of events, the overall mean, or a trend over time) for each individual participant that takes into account all time points.
- Determine a number of distinct outcomes based on various follow-up times and schedule

distinct analyses. Time frames could be established, for instance, to account for follow-up that is short-, medium-, and long-term.

- For studies in which the data is presented, pick a single time point and analyze only the data at this point. This ought to be a clinically significant moment.
- Choose the study's longest follow-up from each one. Heterogeneity could result from a lack of consistency between studies as a result of this.

5.2.2.5. Events that May Re-occur

A unit-of-analysis error must be carefully avoided if the outcome of interest is an event that has multiple possible outcomes. It is not appropriate to handle count data like dichotomous data.

5.2.2.6. Multiple Treatment Attempts

Similarly, a unit-of-analysis error may result from a participant receiving multiple treatments. Confidence intervals should only be calculated using the number of randomized participants, not the number of treatment attempts. For instance, women may experience multiple cycles in subfertility studies; therefore, researchers may mistakenly use cycles rather than women as the denominator. Except the fact that each participant is the "cluster," this is comparable to the setup in cluster-randomized trials.

5.2.2.7. Body Parts receive the Same Intervention

Some randomized studies involve multiple sites or body parts receiving the same intervention; an independent outcome judgment is made for each site, and the number of sites is used as the denominator in the analysis. For instance, eyes can be erroneously used as the denominator without taking into account the non-independence between them. With the exception that the participants are the "clusters," this is comparable to the circumstances of cluster-randomized studies.

5.2.2.8. Body Parts Receive Different Interventions

An alternative scenario involves randomly assigning different interventions to different body parts. This type of "split-mouth" design occurs in oral health, where various interventions are applied to different parts of the mouth. These trials are similar to crossover trials in that participants receive multiple interventions at different sites, as opposed to receiving multiple interventions at different times in crossover studies.

5.2.2.9. Multiple Intervention Groups

Care must be taken when conducting studies that compare more than two intervention groups. By performing multiple pairwise comparisons between every possible pair of intervention groups, such studies are frequently included in meta-analyses. If the same participants are included twice in the same meta-analysis, there is a serious unit-of-analysis issue (for instance, if the same placebo patients are included in both comparisons for "Dose 1 vs. Placebo" and "Dose 2 vs. Placebo").

5.2.3. Extracting Estimates of Effect Directly

However, there are times when it is necessary or appropriate to take an effect estimate straight out of a study report (this is sometimes referred to as "contrast-based" data extraction instead of "arm-based" data extraction). This is true in a few instances, such as the following:

- ***For specific types of randomized trials:*** Individual matching or clustering should be taken into consideration in analyses of crossover trials and cluster-randomized trials.

- ***For specific analyses of randomized trials:*** Other scenarios in which extracting effect estimates directly makes sense include those in which analyses were conducted to account for variables utilized in stratified randomization or minimization, or in which covariance analysis was employed to account for baseline measures of an outcome. Additional instances of complex analyses are those conducted to manage missing data, lower the possibility of bias, or use instrumental variables analysis to estimate a "per-protocol" effect.
- ***For specific types of outcomes:*** It is typically more convenient to extract hazard ratios rather than use summary statistics from each intervention group to summarize time-to-event data. Similarly, extracting effect estimates might be useful for ordinal and rate data.
- ***For non-randomized studies:*** Adjusted effect estimates may be available when extracting data from non-randomized studies (e.g., modified rate ratios from Poisson regression analysis or adjusted odds ratios from logistic regression analyses). They are usually better than analyses based on summary statistics since they lessen the likelihood of confounding. It is necessary to keep track of the variables that have been adjusted.
- ***When summary data for each group are not available:*** Occasionally, it may be possible to look for but not extract summary data for every intervention group. If an effect estimate is taken straight out of the study report, it might still be feasible to include the study in a meta-analysis (using the generic inverse variance method) in these kinds of circumstances.

A P value or a confidence interval may be shown with an effect estimate. Since software procedures for performing meta-analyses using generic inverse-variance weighted averages typically take input data in the form of an effect estimate and its SE from each study, it is usually necessary to obtain a SE from these numbers. It is necessary to determine whether the effect measure is an absolute measure (e.g., mean difference, risk difference, or standardized mean difference) or a ratio measure (e.g., rate ratio, odds ratio, risk ratio, and hazard ratio).

One drawback of this methodology is that, even in cases where the other studies in the meta-analysis provide summary data by intervention group, estimates and SEs of the same effect measure have to be computed for each of them. For instance, ORs would need to be determined for the first set of studies to facilitate meta-analysis with the second set of studies when numbers in each outcome category by intervention group are known for some studies but only ORs are available for other studies. These ORs can be determined using statistical software like RevMan (in this case, by first analyzing the data as dichotomous data), and the resulting confidence intervals can then be converted to SEs.

5.2.3.1. Obtaining Standard Errors from Confidence Intervals and P Values: Absolute (Difference) Measures

The availability of a 95% confidence interval (CI) for an absolute effect measure (e.g., standardized mean difference, rate difference, and risk difference), the SE can be computed as follows:

$$(\text{Upper limit} - \text{Lower limit}) / 3.92$$

It is recommended to substitute 2.29 for 90% confidence intervals and 5.15 for 99% confidence intervals in place of 3.92.

For continuous outcome data, particular considerations must be made before extracting mean differences. This is due to the fact that t distributions should have been used to compute confidence intervals, particularly in cases where sample sizes are small.

SEs can be derived when precise P values are provided with estimates of the intervention effect. Although P values are produced by all statistical significance tests, different tests employ different mathematical techniques. This approach, which statisticians often refer to as a Wald test, assumes that P values have been obtained by a particularly straightforward method of dividing the effect estimate by its SE and comparing the result (denoted Z) with a standard normal distribution.

To begin, find the Z value that matches the given P value in a standard normal distribution table. Next, calculate the standard error (SE):

SE = Intervention effect estimate / Z.

Consider the following scenario: an estimate of a risk difference of 0.03 (P = 0.008) is presented in a conference abstract. Z = 2.652 is the Z value that translates to a P value of 0.008 in this case. This can be obtained using a computer program (e.g., by typing =abs(norms in (0.008/2)) into any cell in a Microsoft Excel spreadsheet) or a table of the standard normal distribution. The risk difference (0.03) is divided by the Z value (2.652) to obtain the SE of the risk difference, which equals 0.011. The estimated SEs and true SEs may not coincide precisely in cases where different mathematical techniques were used in significance tests.

5.2.3.2. Obtaining Standard Errors from Confidence Intervals and P Values: Ratio Measures

SE for ratio measures can be obtained in a manner akin to that of absolute measures, albeit with an extra preliminary step. Ratio measure analyses are done on the natural log scale. For a ratio measure, such as a risk ratio, odds ratio, or hazard ratio (which we refer to as RR in this case), first compute

- Lower limit = ln (lower confidence limit given for RR)
- Upper limit = ln (upper confidence limit given for RR)
- Intervention effect estimate = lnRR.

5.2.4. Dichotomous Outcome Data

5.2.4.1. Effect Measures for Dichotomous Outcomes

When each participant's outcome can be classified as either dead or alive, or as either no clinical improvement or a clinical improvement, dichotomous (binary) outcome data are produced. If the desired outcome takes on a binary form, this section examines potential summary statistics to employ. Effect measures that are most frequently employed in randomized trials with dichotomous data are as follows.

1. the risk ratio (RR; also called the relative risk);
2. the odds ratio (OR);
3. the risk difference (RD; also called the absolute risk reduction); and
4. the number needed to treat for an additional beneficial or harmful outcome (NNT).

Apart from that, it would be better to use a more neutral term than risk (like probability) since events of interest might be desirable rather than undesirable; however, for the sake of convention, we will use the terms risk ratio and risk difference throughout. For consistency with other terminology, we also refer to "risk ratio" rather than "relative risk.." Both can be used interchangeably and conveniently shortened to "RR.." Also take note of the fact that we have used the terms "risk" and "rates" with caution. These terms are frequently used interchangeably. Nonetheless, we have made an effort to limit the usage of the term "rate" to data types that describe counts and rates—that is, events that occur frequently over a specified amount of time.

1. Calculation of Risk Ratio (RR), Odds Ratio (OR), and Risk Difference (RD) from a 2×2 table

A 2x2 table can be used to show the outcomes of a two-group randomized trial with a dichotomous outcome (see **Table 5.1**).

Table 5.1. *Results of a Two-Group Randomized Trial with a Dichotomous Outcome*

	Event ('**S**uccess')	No event ('**F**ail')	Total
Experimental intervention	S_E	F_E	N_E
Comparator intervention	S_C	F_C	N_C

Source: Higgins JPT, Li T, Deeks JJ (editors). Chapter 6: Choosing effect measures and computing estimates of effect. In: Higgins JPT, Thomas J, Chandler J, Cumpston M, Li T, Page MJ, Welch VA (editors). Cochrane Handbook for Systematic Reviews of Interventions version 6.4 (updated August 2023). Cochrane, 2023. Available from www.training.cochrane.org/handbook.

where $S_{E,}$ $S_{C,}$ F_E and F_C are the numbers of participants with each outcome ('S' or 'F') in each group ('E' or 'C'). The following summary statistics can be calculated:

$$RR=\frac{\text{Risk of event in experimental group}}{\text{Risk of event in comparator group}}=\frac{S_E/N_E}{S_C/N_C}$$

$$OR=\frac{\text{Odds of event in experimental group}}{\text{Odds of event in comparator group}}=\frac{S_E/F_E}{S_C/F_C}=\frac{S_E F_C}{F_E S_C}$$

$$RD=\text{Risk of event in experimental group-Risk of event in comparator group}$$

$$=\frac{S_E}{N_E}-\frac{S_C}{N_C} \qquad (5.1)$$

2. Risk and Odds

   Together with the terms "chance," "probability," and "likelihood," the terms "risk" and "odds" are frequently used interchangeably in everyday speech to refer to the same quantity. However, in statistics, odds and risk are computed differently and have distinct meanings. Ignoring their differences could lead to incorrect interpretations of the results.

The idea of *risk* is one that the general public and health professionals are more familiar with. Risk is the likelihood that a health consequence will materialize. Risk is typically expressed in research as a decimal number between 0 and 1, though it can also occasionally be expressed as a percentage. It is frequently stated in "Summary" as the number of people per 1000. The relationship between a risk and the likelihood of events occurring is easy to understand: in a sample of 100 people, the average number of events observed will be the risk multiplied by 100. For instance, if the risk is 0.1, roughly 10 persons out of 100 will experience the event; if the risk is 0.5, roughly 50 people out of 100 will experience the event. These figures are 100 and 500 in a sample of 1000 individuals, respectively.

Gamblers may be more familiar with the concept of *odds*. The term "odds" can refer to any integer between zero and infinity that represents the ratio of the likelihood that a specific event will occur to the likelihood that it won't. In the world of gambling, odds refer to the ratio of the potential winnings to the wager; in the context of health care, odds represent the ratio of those who experience an event to those who do not. A ratio of two integers is a common way to express it. It is common practice to write the odds of 0.01 as 1:100, 0.33 as 1:3, and 3 as 3:1. The following formulas can be used to convert odds to risks and risks to odds.

$$\text{Risk}=\frac{\text{Odds}}{1+\text{Odds}};\text{Odds}=\frac{\text{Risk}}{1\text{-Risk}}.$$

Odds interpretation is more intricate than risk interpretation. Changing the odds into a risk is the first step towards ensuring that the interpretation is accurate. For instance, at odds of 1:10, or 0.1, the risk of the event is 0.1/(1+0.1)=0.091, meaning that one person will experience the event for every ten who do not. Nine people out of a sample of 100 will experience the event, while the remaining 91 will not. In a sample of 100, 100×1/(1+1)=50 will have the event and 50 will not, since one person will have the event for every person who does not when the odds are equal to 1.

The difference between odds and risk is small when the event is rare (as illustrated in the example above where a risk of 0.091 was seen to be similar to an odds of 0.1). When events are common, as is often the case in clinical trials, the differences between odds and risks are large. For example, a risk of 0.5 is equivalent to an odds of 1; and a risk of 0.95 is equivalent to odds of 19.

In randomized trials with dichotomous outcomes, effect measures involve comparing risks or odds between two intervention groups. This comparison can be done by analyzing the ratio (risk ratio or odds ratio) or the difference in risk (risk difference) between the groups.

3. Measures of Relative Effect: The Risk Ratio and Odds Ratio

Relative effect measures convey the expected result in one group in comparison to the other. While the odds ratio (OR) represents the ratio of the odds of an event, the risk ratio (RR, or relative risk) represents the risk of an event in the two groups. A value of 1 for any of the two measures denotes that the estimated effects for each intervention are the same.

If there are no events in the comparator group, neither the risk ratio nor the odds ratio can be calculated for a study. Dividing by zero is not possible, as shown in the equation 5.1. Similarly, the odds ratio cannot be calculated if all individuals in the intervention group experience an event. In such cases, and when standard errors cannot be determined, it is common practice to add ½ to each cell of the 2x2 table. If no events occur in both groups, or if all events occur in both groups, the study does not provide any useful information on the relative probability of the event and should be excluded from the meta-analysis. This is especially relevant in scenarios where the event of interest is rare, such as unintended adverse outcomes.

The risk that multiplies when an experimental intervention is used is expressed using risk ratios. An intervention, for instance, has a risk ratio of three, meaning that events involving the intervention are three times more likely than events not involving the intervention. An alternative way to put it is that intervention raises the probability of events by 200%, or 100×(RR–1)%. Likewise, a risk ratio of 0:25 indicates that the likelihood of an event involving intervention is equivalent to one-fourth that of an event without intervention. An alternative way to put this would be that intervention reduces the risk of events by 100×(1–RR)%, or 75%. This is referred to as the reduction in relative risk. Without knowledge of the typical risk of events without intervention, it is impossible to interpret the clinical significance of a given risk ratio. For example, a risk ratio of 0.75 may indicate a small, less significant reduction in events from 4% to 3% or a clinically significant reduction in events from 80% to 60%. The definition of what is clinically significant will vary depending on the population or individual's values and preferences as well as the outcome.

The observed risk ratio's numerical value must always lie between 0 and 1/CGR, where CGR is the comparator group's observed risk expressed as a number between 0 and 1. CGR is an acronym for "comparator group risk," also known as the control group risk or the control event rate. This implies that it is impossible to have high risk ratio values for typical occurrences. For instance, the observed risk ratio cannot be greater than 1.5 when the observed risk of events in the comparator group is 0.66, or 66%. This boundary only applies to increases in risk, which can lead to issues when an analysis's findings are extrapolated to a population where risks in comparator groups are higher than those found in the study.

Like odds, odds ratios are more challenging to understand. The odds of the outcome multiplied by the use of the intervention are represented by odds ratios. It is easiest to convert an odds ratio into a risk ratio first, then interpret the risk ratio in the context of a typical comparator group risk, as described here, to understand what an odds ratio means in terms of changes in the number of events. There are situations when it makes sense to compute the RR for multiple assumed comparator group risks.

4. Warning: OR and RR are not the same

When events are common, not only do risk and odds change, but so do the risk ratio and the odds ratio. Since both approaches are legitimate for characterizing an intervention effect, this non-equivalence does not imply that one is incorrect. However, if the odds ratio is mistaken for a risk ratio, issues could occur. The misinterpretation will tend to overestimate the intervention effect, especially when events are common (with, say, risks of events more than 20%). This is because, for interventions that increase the chances of events, the odds ratio will be larger than the risk ratio. Again, misinterpretation overestimates the impact of the intervention because the odds ratio for interventions that lower the likelihood of events will be smaller than the risk ratio.

5. Measure of Absolute Effect: The Risk Difference

The difference between the two groups' observed risks—that is, the percentages of people who have the desired outcome—is known as the risk difference. Even in studies where neither group experiences any events, the risk difference can be computed. It is simple to understand how to interpret the risk difference: for an individual, it represents the estimated difference in the probability of experiencing the event. It describes the difference in the observed risk of events between experimental and comparator interventions. However, the underlying risk of events in the population may determine the clinical significance of a risk difference. A risk difference of 0.02, or

2%, for instance, could indicate a relatively larger and potentially significant change from 1-3%, or a small, clinically insignificant change from a risk of 58% - 60%. When interpreting a risk difference, it is still crucial to consider the underlying risk of the events and their consequences, even though the risk difference offers more directly relevant information than relative measures. Absolute metrics, like the risk difference, are especially helpful when weighing the possible advantages and disadvantages of an intervention.

Similar to the risk ratio, the risk difference is inherently limited, which could make it challenging to generalize the findings to different patient populations and environments. For instance, a group with an initial risk of, say, 7% will have an impossible estimated negative probability of −3% if a study or meta-analysis estimates a risk difference of −0.1 (or −10%). At the other end of the risk spectrum, similar situations arise. Only when the findings are applied to populations with different risks from those seen in the studies can such issues occur.

The risk difference yields the number that has to be treated. NNTs cannot be combined in a meta-analysis, even though they are frequently used to summarize clinical trial results. However, when analyzing the findings of a meta-analysis, odds ratios, risk ratios, and risk differences may be helpfully converted to NNTs.

6. What is the event?

Healthcare interventions are designed to either lower the likelihood of an unfavorable outcome or raise the likelihood of a favorable outcome when dealing with dichotomous outcomes. In the analysis of dichotomous data, the term "event" is frequently used to characterize any outcome or state of interest. For example, the event of interest is typically recovery or cure when participants begin the study with specific symptoms. The event is the onset of disease or the occurrence of an adverse outcome if participants are well at the start of the study or if they are at risk of some adverse outcome. It is feasible to reverse the order of events and non-events and instead analyze the percentage of patients who do not recover or who do not encounter the event. This switch has little bearing on meta-analyses that use odds ratios or risk differences because it only modifies the sign of a risk difference, indicating the same effect size in the opposite direction, whereas for odds ratios, the new odds ratio is equal to the reciprocal (1/x) of the original odds ratio.

For risk ratios, on the other hand, changing the outcome can have a significant impact on the effect estimate, its statistical significance, and the consistency of intervention effects amongst studies. This is because there are significant differences in the precision of a risk ratio estimate between scenarios with low risk and those with high risk. The impact of this reversal is difficult to forecast in a meta-analysis. It is crucial to determine which risk ratio is most likely to be the most pertinent summary statistic before conducting data analysis. Selecting to concentrate on the event that signifies a shift in condition is frequently practical. For instance, it might be more natural to concentrate on "cure" as the event in treatment studies where everyone begins in an unfavorable state and the goal is to "cure" this. On the other hand, it might make more sense to focus on the term "adverse event" as the event in prevention studies where everyone begins in a "healthy" state and the goal is to prevent an adverse event. As a general rule of thumb, the event of interest should be the less common state. This may result in less heterogeneity between studies and fewer issues with extrapolation. Empirical evidence suggests that risk ratios of the adverse event are more consistent than risk ratios of the non-event when interventions are aimed at lowering the incidence of the adverse event.

5.2.4.2. Data Extraction for Dichotomous Outcomes

The only information needed for a dichotomous outcome is the number of participants in each intervention group who experienced and did not experience the outcome of interest (the numbers needed to fill in a standard 2×2 table). This information is then used to calculate summary statistics and include the result in a meta-analysis. These can be entered as the total sample sizes for the two groups as well as the outcome numbers in RevMan. It is not always clear whether the reported total numbers represent the entire sample size or just those for whom the outcome was measured or observed, even though in theory this is equivalent to gathering the total numbers and the numbers experiencing the outcome. It is better to get the total number of observations rather than making assumptions about participants for whom the outcome was not measured. Sometimes percentages must be used to determine the number of participants who experienced the event (though it's not always obvious which denominator to use because rounded percentages can work with multiple numerators). When participant and event counts are unavailable, an effect estimate, such as an odds ratio or risk ratio, may be provided instead. When such data are accompanied by measures of uncertainty like a SE, 95% confidence interval, or exact P value, they can be included in meta-analyses (using the generic inverse variance method).

5.2.5. Continuous Outcome Data

5.2.5.1. Effect Measures for Continuous Outcomes

In statistics, a variable that can have any value within a given range is referred to as "continuous." This implies that a number can be measured and reported to any number of decimal places when working with numerical data. Volume, weight, and area are a few instances of truly continuous data. The same statistical techniques can be applied in practice to other kinds of data, most notably measurement scales and counts of a large number of events.

One characteristic of continuous data that unites them is the measurement of a participant's outcome at baseline, or prior to the administration of interventions. This opens up the possibility of using change from baseline (also known as a change score) to compute effects. When effect measures are derived from changes from the baseline, each participant receives a unique measurement that is obtained by deducting either the post-intervention measurement or the baseline measurement from the post-intervention measurement. After that, analyses continue just like they would for any other kind of continuous outcome variable.

For meta-analysis of continuous data, two summary statistics are frequently utilized: the mean difference and the standardized mean difference. These can be computed regardless of whether each person's data are change-from-baseline or post-intervention measurements. Other methods, such as calculating ratios of means, can also be used to quantify effects.

It may occasionally take into account dichotomizing continuous outcome measures in order to express the trial's outcome as an odds ratio, risk ratio, or risk difference. This may be done because most studies present results after dichotomizing a continuous measure, or it may be done to improve the interpretation of the results. Under certain presumptions, results presented as means and SDs may be translated into risks. For each intervention group, an outcome variable with a normal distribution is typically assumed.

1. The Mean Difference (or Difference in Means)

A common statistic used to quantify the absolute difference in mean values between two groups in a randomized trial is called the mean difference (MD), or more accurately, "difference in means." It calculates the average change in outcome that the experimental intervention brings when compared to the comparator intervention. When all studies use the same scale for their outcome measurements, this statistic can be used as a summary in a meta-analysis.

2. The Standardized Mean Difference

When studies report the same result but use different metrics to measure it (e.g., all studies measure depression but use different psychometric scales), the standardized mean difference (SMD) is used as a summary statistic in the meta-analysis. In this case, standardizing the study results to a common scale is a prerequisite for combining them. The study's between-participant variability in outcome measurements is expressed by the SMD, which indicates the magnitude of the intervention effect in each study. (Once more, the intervention effect is a mean difference rather than a mean of differences.)

$$\text{SMD} = \frac{\text{Difference in mean outcome between groups}}{\text{Standard deviation of outcome among participants}}.$$

Therefore, independent of the actual scales used to make the measurements, studies for which the difference in means is the same proportion of the standard deviation (SD) will have the same SMD.

The approach, however, assumes that variations in SDs across studies are due to variations in measurement scales rather than actual variations in population variability. The SMDs will differ if the true effect (as determined by the mean difference) in two trials is the same but the SDs differ. In certain situations, where actual variations in participant variability across studies are anticipated, this could pose a challenge. For instance, pragmatic trials may contain a larger range of participants and, as a result, have higher SDs when early explanatory trials are merged with later pragmatic trials in the same review. Since the overall intervention effect is reported in SD rather than in any of the measurement scales used in the review, it can also be challenging to interpret; however, there are several options to help.

In the social sciences, the phrase "effect size" is commonly employed, especially to meta-analyses. Usually, but not always, effect sizes relate to SMD versions. It should be mentioned that variations in the scale's direction are not corrected for by the SMD method. To ensure that all the scales point in the same direction before standardization, multiply the mean values from one set of studies by –1 (or subtract the mean from the maximum possible value for the scale) if some scales increase with disease severity (for example, a higher score indicates more severe depression) and others decrease (a higher score indicates less severe depression).

Depending on the specific SD option selected for the denominator, several SMD variations are possible. The effect size referred to as Hedges' (adjusted) g in social science is the specific definition of SMD. Assuming that the SDs in the two groups are comparable, this uses a pooled SD in the denominator, which is an estimate of the SD based on outcome data from both intervention groups. On the other hand, Glass' delta (Δ) solely employs the standard deviation from the comparator group, reasoning that if the experimental intervention influences inter-individual variation, it shouldn't have an impact on the effect estimate.

It may occasionally be preferable to standardize using an external estimate of SD to get around issues with estimating SDs within small studies and with actual differences in between-person variability across studies. External estimates could come from a cross-sectional analysis of several people evaluated with the same continuous outcome measure, for instance (the sample of people could come from a large cohort study). The external estimate would normally be taken to be known without error, and if it is based on a large number of people, it is probably reasonable. The statistical techniques for MDs would be applied under this supposition, with the externally derived SD being divided by both the MD and its SE.

3. The Ratio of Means

A less frequently used statistic that compares the means of two groups in a randomized trial is called the ratio of means (RoM). It calculates the coefficient of multiplicity of the average outcome value for participants on the experimental intervention relative to the comparator intervention. An intervention with a RoM of 2, for instance, indicates that participants obtaining the experimental intervention had mean scores that were, on average, twice as high as those of the group that did not receive the intervention. When outcome measurements in a meta-analysis can only be positive, this statistic can be used as a summary. As a result, it works well for individual assessments (post-intervention), but not for measures that alter from baseline (which may have negative effects).

One benefit of the RoM is its utility in meta-analysis for merging findings from studies employing different measurement scales. Nonetheless, these scales must share comparable lower thresholds. For instance, it is feasible to combine results from a study utilizing a scale of 0 to 10 with those ranging from 1 to 50 using the RoM. However, merging RoM outcomes from a study with a scale of 0 to 10 with one ranging from 20 to 30 is not advisable, as RoM values outside the range of 0.67 to 1.5 cannot be derived in the latter study, while they can be in the former study. Consequently, the RoM is unsuitable as an effect measure for the latter study.

When the outcome is a physical measurement that can only take positive values—that is, when different studies use different measurement approaches that are difficult to convert from one to another—the RoM might be an especially good choice for an effect measure. It was applied, for instance, in a meta-analysis where studies evaluated urine output using measures that did not account for body weight.

4. Other Effect Measures for Continuous Outcome Data

For continuous outcome data, additional effect measures consist of the following:

- ***Standardized difference in terms of the minimally important differences (MID) on each scale.*** In this way, the MD is expressed as a percentage of the change on a scale that is thought to be clinically significant.
- ***Prevented fraction.*** This represents the mean difference (MD) in change scores compared to the comparator group mean change. As a result, it indicates the extent to which the experimental intervention may have stopped the comparator group from changing. It has been applied frequently in dentistry.
- ***Difference in percentage change from baseline.*** In this version of the MD, the mean change divided by the mean baseline level is used to summarize each intervention group and express the results as a percentage. For instance, the metric has been frequently applied to outcomes like blood pressure, glaucoma, and cholesterol levels. Making sure the

SE accurately takes into account the correlation between the pre- and post-intervention values requires attention.

- ***Direct mapping from one scale to another.*** Should conversion factors that translate one scale to another be available (e.g., pounds to kilograms), then utilize these measurements. There are also techniques available for estimating these conversion factors.

5.2.5.2. Data Extraction for Continuous Outcomes

To conduct a meta-analysis of continuous data with ratios of means, SMDs, or MDs, a review should look for:

- the number of participants for whom the outcome was measured in each intervention group;
- the mean value of the outcome measurements in each intervention group; and
- the standard deviation of the outcome measurements in each intervention group.

Owing to incomplete and inconsistent reporting, it might be hard or impossible to extract these figures from the provided data summaries. The statistics used by different studies to summarize the variance and average vary (sometimes using ranges, interquartile ranges, confidence intervals, and SEs instead of SDs). Additionally, they differ in the scale used to analyze the data (e.g., measurements taken after the intervention compared to baseline changes; logarithmic scale versus raw scale).

The mistake of mistaking a SE for an SD is especially deceptive. Unfortunately, it's not always obvious which is being reported, so it might be necessary to compare the results with those of other studies and use some critical thinking. The terms SDs and SEs are sometimes used interchangeably in study reports, leading to misunderstandings.

There are situations when an effect estimate, such as an MD or SMD, has been reported but the participant count, means, and SDs are not available. When such data are accompanied by measures of uncertainty like a SE, 95% confidence interval, or exact P value, they can be included in meta-analyses that employ the generic inverse variance method.

1. Extracting Post-intervention Versus Change from Baseline Data

The fact that baseline and post-intervention measurements may have been reported for different numbers of participants owing to missed visits and study withdrawals presents a final issue with deriving information on change from baseline measures. Finding the subset of participants who report baseline and post-intervention measurements so that change scores can be calculated for them may prove to be challenging.

2. Obtaining Standard Deviations from Standard Errors and Confidence Intervals for Group Means

From the SE of a mean, one can calculate the standard deviation by multiplying it by the square root of the sample size.

$$SD = SE \times \sqrt{N}$$

The SE of the mean difference between two intervention groups cannot be used to compute the SE when performing this transformation; instead, it must come from within a single intervention group.

The SD can also be computed from the confidence interval for a mean. Once more, the confidence interval for a mean value determined within an intervention group is covered by the following; estimates of differences between interventions are not covered by it. The majority of confidence intervals that are published are

95% confidence intervals. If each group has a sample size greater than 100, the 95% confidence interval has a width of 3.92 SE (3.92=2×1.96). Each group's standard deviation (SD) is found by multiplying the square root of the sample size in that group by 3.92, which is the width of the confidence interval in that group.

$$D=\sqrt{N}\times(\text{Upper limit - Lower limit})/3.92$$

For 90% confidence intervals, 3.92 should be replaced by 3.29, and for 99% confidence intervals it should be replaced by 5.15.

A value from a t distribution should have been used to compute confidence intervals if the sample size was small—less than 60 people in each group, for example. The slightly larger t distribution-specific numbers that take the place of 3.92, 3.29, and 5.15 can be found in tables of the t distribution with degrees of freedom equal to the group sample size minus 1. For instance, entering =tinv (1-0.95,25-1) in a cell of a Microsoft Excel spreadsheet will yield the t statistic for a 95% confidence interval from a sample size of 25 (the result is 2.0639). In the above formula, 2×2.0639=4.128 would take the place of the divisor, 3.92.

A normal distribution or a t distribution might have been applied for moderate sample sizes (roughly 60–100 in each group).

As an example, consider data presented as follows:

Group	Sample size	Mean	95% CI
Experimental intervention	25	32.1	(30.0, 34.2)
Comparator intervention	22	28.3	(26.5, 30.1)

Based on t distributions with 24 and 21 degrees of freedom, respectively, the confidence intervals ought to have been calculated. 4.128 is the divisor for the experimental intervention group. This group's SD is √25×(34.2–30.0)/4.128=5.09. Similar computations are carried out for the comparator group.

Verifying that the confidence interval is symmetrical about the mean—that is, that the distance between the mean and the upper limit and the lower limit is equal—is crucial. If not, it's possible that transformed values were used to calculate the confidence interval.

3. Obtaining Standard Deviations from Standard Errors, Confidence Intervals, t Statistics and P Values for Differences in Means

One can calculate standard deviations using a variety of methods such as a SE, confidence interval, t statistic, or P value that pertains to the difference between means in two groups (the MD). The MD is necessary for calculating the t statistic or P value. It is assumed that the SDs of outcome measurements are equal in both groups. This assumption allows for the use of the same SD for both intervention groups. The process involves obtaining a t statistic from a P value, then a SE from a t statistic or confidence interval, and finally a SD from the SE. Care must be taken to select the appropriate steps based on the available results. Similarly, SDs can be derived from certain F statistics by taking the square root, which may produce the same t statistic. It is important to ensure the correct F statistic is used, and seeking advice from a statistician is recommended.

- From P value to t statistic

The corresponding t statistic can be found in a table of the t distribution when actual P values from t-tests are quoted. N_E+N_C-2, where N_E and N_C represent the sample sizes in the experimental and comparator groups, yields the degrees of freedom. We'll use an example to clarify. Examine a trial in which a comparator intervention (N_C=22) with an MD=3.8 is compared to an experimental intervention

(N_E=25). A two-sample t-test yielded P=0.008 as the comparison's P value. T=2.78 is the t statistic that is associated with a P value of 0.008 and 25+22−2=45 degrees of freedom. This can be found on a computer (for instance, by typing =tinv(0.008, 45) into any cell in a Microsoft Excel spreadsheet) or in a table of the t distribution with 45 degrees of freedom.

There are challenges when reporting significance levels (like P. <0.05 or even P=N_S ('not significant,' which usually implies P> 0.05) as opposed to precise P values. A prudent course of action would be to use the P value at the maximum value (e.g., for P<0.05 take P=0.05, for P<0.01 take P=0.01 and for P<0.001 take P=0.001). However, this is not a solution for results that are reported as P=NS, or P> 0.05.

- From t statistic to standard error

The SE of the MD can thus be found by dividing it by the t statistic, which is the ratio of the MD to the SE of the MD.

$$SE=\left|\frac{MD}{t}\right|,$$

where $|X|$ denotes 'the absolute value of X.' In the example, where MD=3.8 and t=2.78, the SE of the MD is obtained by dividing 3.8 by 2.78, which gives 1.37.

- From confidence interval to standard error

The same SE can be computed as follows if the MD's 95% confidence interval is available.

SE = (Upper limit – Lower limit) / 3.92,

as long as there is a big trial. Divide the 90% confidence intervals by 3.29, not 3.92, and the 99% confidence intervals by 5.15. In cases where the sample size is small, with less than 60 participants in each group, a t distribution should have been used to calculate the confidence intervals. Larger numbers unique to the t distribution and sample size are used in place of 3.92, 3.29, and 5.15. These larger numbers can be found in tables of the t distribution with degrees of freedom equal to N_E+N_C-2, where NE and NC represent the sample sizes in the two groups. To obtain the t statistic for a 95% confidence interval, for instance, one can enter =tinv(1-0.95,25+22-2) in a cell of a Microsoft Excel spreadsheet and compare a sample size of 25 with a sample size of 22.

- From standard error to standard deviation

The formula below can be used to extract the within-group SD from the SE of the MD.

$$SD=\frac{SE}{\sqrt{\frac{1}{N_E}+\frac{1}{N_C}}}.$$

In the example,

$$SD=\frac{1.37}{\sqrt{\frac{1}{25}+\frac{1}{22}}}=4.69.$$

It should be noted that this SD should be entered into RevMan twice, once for each intervention group. This SD is the average of the SDs of the experimental and comparator arms.

4. Transformations and Skewed Data

Studies may display summary statistics that were computed following the raw data's transformation. Logarithmic value means and standard deviations, for instance, could be accessible (or, equivalently, a geometric mean and its confidence interval). These findings ought to be gathered since they could be utilized in meta-analyses or, under certain conditions, converted back to the original scale.

For instance, a trial that used the meningitis C vaccine and a control vaccine revealed meningococcal antibody responses 12 months later as geometric mean titres of 24 and 4.2, respectively, with 95% confidence intervals of 17 to 34 and 3.9 to 4.6, respectively. The aforementioned summaries were produced by calculating the natural logs of the antibody responses (mean and confidence intervals for vaccine 3.18 (95% CI 2.83 to 3.53) and control 1.44 (1.36 to 1.53)) and obtaining their exponentials, or anti-logs). Alternatively, the scale of these natural log antibody responses could be used for a meta-analysis instead of the geometric means.

5. Interquartile Ranges

Interquartile ranges show the location of the central 50% of participants' results. The interquartile range's width is roughly 1.35 standard deviations when sample sizes are high and the outcome distribution resembles a normal distribution. In other cases, estimating a standard deviation (SD) from an interquartile range is not feasible, particularly when the outcome's distribution is skewed. Keep in mind that using interquartile ranges rather than standard deviations can frequently reveal a skewed outcome distribution.

6. Ranges

In contrast to other measures of variation, ranges are extremely unstable and rise with sample size. Rather than describing the average variation, they characterize the extremes of observed outcomes. Utilizing the reality that 95% of values in normally distributed data fall within 2×SD of the mean has been a popular strategy. As a result, it is possible to estimate the SD to be roughly 25% of the typical data value range.

7. No Information on Variability

Meta-analyses of continuous outcome data frequently contain missing standard deviations. If the trialists are unable to provide the information needed to calculate the standard deviations from the trial report using any of the aforementioned methods, the study may have to be imputed, or "filled in," with the missing data in order to be included in the meta-analysis.

Using the SD from one or more other studies is the most straightforward method of imputation. Furukawa et al. discovered that in two case studies, imputed SDs from studies in the same meta-analysis or studies in a different meta-analysis produced roughly accurate results. Choose whether to use the average, the highest, a "reasonably high" value, or another tactic if there are multiple candidate SDs available. Selecting a higher SD down weights a study and produces a wider confidence interval in meta-analyses of MDs. Selecting a larger SD, however, will skew the results of SMD meta-analyses in favor of no effect. There are more advanced options available for using several candidate SDs. For instance, because there is a strong linear relationship between the two, Marinho and colleagues implemented a linear regression of log(SD) on log(mean).

It is advisable to stay away from imputation techniques whenever possible because they all entail making assumptions about statistics that are not known. These values shouldn't be imputed if the majority of the studies in a meta-analysis have missing SDs. For the synthesis, a narrative approach might then be required. Imputation, however, might make sense for a tiny percentage of studies that only include a small percentage of the data, provided it makes it possible to combine those studies with others for which complete data are available. Sensitivity analyses ought to be employed to evaluate the effects of altering the presumptions.

5.2.6. Ordinal Outcome Data and Measurement Scales

5.2.6.1. Effect Measures for Ordinal Outcomes and Measurement Scales

When each participant is assigned to a category and those categories exhibit a natural ordering, ordinal outcome data are produced. An instance of an ordinal type outcome is a "trichotomous" one, such as the division of disease severity into "mild," "moderate," and "severe.." Ordinal outcomes become more like continuous outcomes as the number of categories rises, and they were most likely examined as such in a randomized trial.

One specific kind of ordinal outcome that is widely used to measure hard-to-quantify conditions like behavior, depression, and cognitive abilities is measurement scales. A set of questions or tasks are usually used in measurement scales; each is scored, and the sum of the scores produces the final "score." Should the items be deemed unequal in significance, a weighted total could be employed.

There are techniques for analyzing data on ordinal outcomes that express effects as proportional odds ratios. Assume that there are three categories, with 1 being the best and 3 being the worst, arranged according to desirability. Two possible dichotomies for the data exist: either category 1 represents a success and categories 2 and 3 represent failures, or categories 1 and 2 represent successes and category 3 represents failures. According to a proportional odds model, the odds ratios for the two data dichotomies are equal. Consequently, regardless of how the ordered categories are split into success and failure, the odds ratio derived from the proportional odds model can be understood as the odds of success on the experimental intervention relative to the comparator. Approaches for estimating study estimates of the log odds ratio and its SE are available, specifically polychotomous logistic regression models.

When there are many categories, ordinal data-specific methods become cumbersome and superfluous. In actuality, shorter ordinal scales are typically converted into dichotomous data by merging adjacent categories until there are only two, whereas longer ordinal scales often take on characteristics of continuous outcomes and are analyzed as such. The latter is particularly suitable if there is a recognized, tenable cut-point at hand. However, selecting the wrong cut-point in a randomized trial can lead to bias, especially if the cut-point is selected to maximize the difference between two intervention arms.

One of the two sets of grouped categories is defined as the event and the intervention effects are described using risk ratios, odds ratios, or risk differences when ordinal scales are summarized using techniques for dichotomous data. The mean score in each group is determined when ordinal scales are summarized using techniques for continuous data, and the intervention effect is expressed as an MD, SMD, or potentially a RoM. If studies have used medians to summarize their findings, then problems will arise.

5.2.6.2. Data Extraction for Ordinal Outcomes

The method of extracting data for ordinal outcomes will vary based on how the ordinal scale will be used in the analysis – either dichotomized, treated as continuous, or analyzed directly. It may be difficult to determine in advance whether data extraction will involve counting participants above and below a certain threshold or calculating mean values and standard deviations.

When dichotomizing ordinal data and there are multiple options for choosing a cut-point, or the cut-point is chosen arbitrarily, it makes sense to plan and conduct a sensitivity analysis to examine the effects of the cut-point choice. To prevent the need to repeatedly extract data from a paper, it is necessary to record the numbers in each category of short ordinal scales to gather the data that would be used for each alternative dichotomization. Recording all categorizations is a reasonable approach when studies employ slightly different short ordinal scales, and it's unclear if a common cut-point can be utilized for dichotomization across all studies.

When using the proportional odds ratio method, it is also required to record the numbers for each intervention group in each category of the ordinal scale.

5.2.7. Count and Rate Data

5.2.7.1. Effect Measures for Counts and Rates

Certain events can occur multiple times for an individual, such as a heart attack, a negative reaction, or a hospital stay. It is important to consider the frequency of these events rather than just focusing on if a person experienced them or not. This is known as count data, which can be divided into rare and common event counts for practical purposes.

In statistics, counts of uncommon occurrences are frequently referred to as "Poisson data.." Rates are a common focus of analyses of uncommon events. Rates establish a relationship between the counts and the possible time frame for them to occur. For instance, the outcome of one clinical trial arm might be that, over the course of 314 person-years of follow-up—that is, the total number of years that all participants were followed together—18 myocardial infarctions (MIs) were experienced by all participants in that arm. 5.7 per 100 person-years, or 0.057 per person-year, is the rate. The rate ratio, also known as RR, is a summary statistic that is frequently used in meta-analyses. It divides the rate of events in each group by the other to compare the rates in the two groups.

Suppose E_E events occurred during T_E person-years of follow-up in the experimental intervention group, and E_C events during T_C person-years in the comparator intervention group. The rate ratio is:

$$\text{Rate Ratio} = \frac{E_E / T_E}{E_C / T_C} = \frac{E_E T_C}{E_C T_E}.$$

This rate ratio should then be log transformed for analysis purposes as a ratio measure. The log rate ratio's approximate SE can be found by:

$$\text{SE of ln rate ratio} = \sqrt{\frac{1}{E_E} + \frac{1}{E_C}}.$$

If there are no events, each count may have a correction of 0.5. Be aware that the selection of time unit (i.e., patient-months, woman-years, etc.) is not significant because it is not included in the SE and is subtracted from the rate ratio. When presenting the study results, the units should still be visible. A rate difference, or difference in rates, can also be used as a summary statistic, though this is much less common:

$$\text{Rate Difference} = \frac{E_E}{T_E} - \frac{E_C}{T_C}.$$

An approximate SE for the rate difference is:

$$\text{SE of Rate Difference} = \sqrt{\frac{E_E}{T_E^2} + \frac{E_C}{T_C^2}}.$$

The treatment of counts of more frequent occurrences, like the number of decayed, missing, or filled teeth, is frequently the same as that of continuous outcome data. The MD will be utilized as the intervention effect, comparing the variation in the mean number of events (possibly standardized to a unit period) that participants in the intervention group and participants in the comparator group experienced.

5.2.7.2. Data Extraction for Counts and Rates

There are various methods to analyze naturally countable data.

There are situations when comprehensive information on incidents and person-years at risk is unavailable, but the conclusions drawn from it are. One could present an estimate of a rate difference or ratio, for instance. Only when such data are accompanied by measures of uncertainty, like a 95% confidence interval—from which a SE can be derived—and the generic inverse variance method—which is employed for meta-analysis, can they be included in meta-analyses?

1. Extracting Counts as Dichotomous Data

Treating count data as dichotomous data is a common mistake. Assume that in the previously given example, 157 patients were observed for an average of two years, giving rise to 18 MIs in 314 person-years. The results might be quoted as 18/157 or even 18/314. This is not appropriate if the total of 18 MIs could have been attributed to more than one MI from the same patient (for example, if the 18 came from 12 patients with single MIs and 3 patients each with two MIs).

There may be more events than patients, in which case the results would be meaningless. For instance, 35 epileptic study participants may have 63 seizures in total during a year.

5.2.8. Time-to-event Data

5.2.8.1. Effect Measures for Time-to-Event Outcomes

When attention is drawn to the amount of time that passes before an event occurs, time-to-event data are generated. Because death is frequently the event of interest, especially in cases of cancer and heart disease, they are generally referred to as survival data in the medical statistics literature. Time-to-event data are made up of two sets of observations for every person: the first is the amount of time that passed without any events being noticed, and the second is a signal that indicates whether or not an event occurred at the end of the time period. Those who participate for a duration that does not culminate in an event are considered to have been "censored." They are incorporated into the analysis and their event-free time provides information. Time-to-event data can be based on non-fatal events as well, like the return of a disease event (e.g., the duration of a period without epileptic fits) or hospital discharge.

Dichotomous data analysis can occasionally be applied to time-to-event data. This necessitates knowing each patient's status in a study at a predetermined point in time. For example, a 2x2 table can be created and the intervention effects expressed as risk ratios, odds ratios, or risk differences if all patients have been followed for at least 12 months and the percentage of patients who experienced the event before 12 months is known for both groups.

Analyzing time-to-event data with techniques meant for continuous outcomes (e.g., since the pertinent times are only known for the subset of participants who have experienced the event (using mean times-to-event). Participants who have been censored must be disqualified, which will almost definitely introduce bias.

Using survival analysis techniques to summarize time-to-event data and express the intervention effect as a hazard ratio is the most appropriate approach. Though the concepts of risk and hazard are similar, the hazard is slightly different in that it quantifies instantaneous risk and is subject to constant change (for instance, a person's chance of dying changes when they cross a busy road). A hazard ratio indicates the number of times that a participant is more (or less) likely to experience an event at a specific moment if they receive the experimental intervention as opposed to the comparator intervention. The hazard ratio is frequently assumed to be constant throughout the follow-up period when comparing interventions in a study or meta-analysis, despite the possibility that the hazards themselves could change over time. The proportional hazards assumption is what is meant by this.

5.2.8.2. Data Extraction for Time-to-Event Outcomes

Getting individual patient data from the original investigators, reanalyzing the data to get estimates of the hazard ratio and its statistical uncertainty, and then conducting a meta-analysis are common steps in the meta-analysis of time-to-event data. It can be difficult to perform a meta-analysis using summary data from trial reports or published papers because the most relevant summary statistics are frequently omitted.

Two methods can be used to extract estimates of hazard ratios and their uncertainty from study reports where summary statistics are provided so that the generic inverse variance methods can be used to include the results in a meta-analysis. When trialists have analyzed the data using a Cox proportional hazards model (or some other regression models for survival data), they can employ the first strategy. The log hazard ratio and its SE are directly estimated by Cox models, and these estimates are adequate for a general inverse variance meta-analysis. An estimate of the SE can be obtained if a report quotes the hazard ratio along with a confidence interval or P value.

The second method uses statistics calculated during a log-rank analysis to approximate the hazard ratio. If this method is used, working with an experienced statistician is suggested. The log hazard ratio (experimental relative to comparator) is estimated by $(O-E)/V$, which has $SE=1/\sqrt{V}$, where O is the observed number of events on the experimental intervention, E is the log-rank expected number of events on the experimental intervention, O−E is the log-rank statistic and V is the variance of the log-rank statistic.

Sometimes, survival curves and quoted statistics can be used to extract these numbers. As an alternative, aggregated data for every intervention group in every trial may occasionally be used. Imagine, for instance, that the data includes the number of participants who experience the event in their first, second, third, etc. year, as well as the number of participants who do not experience any events and are still being monitored at the end of each year. To obtain the O-E and V values from these data, a log-rank analysis can be carried out; however, the handling of censored times requires careful consideration. The log hazard ratio is only roughly estimated due to coarse grouping.

5.2.8.3. Conditional Outcomes Only Available for Subsets of Participants

A portion of participants may be the only ones who benefit from certain study outcomes. For instance, doctors are frequently interested in the percentage of clinical pregnancies that miscarry after treatment in subfertility trials. The comparison is not of all randomized participants because by definition this outcome excludes those who do not reach an interim state (clinical pregnancy). Redefining such outcomes generally makes sense to include all randomized participants in the analysis. The result in this case might be whether the woman becomes pregnant and carries the pregnancy to term, or whether it ends in a "successful pregnancy." It is rarely possible to conduct appropriate analysis using summary data if the outcome of interest is miscarriage; however, this can be done with individual participant data. An additional illustration is offered by a morbidity outcome assessed over a medium- or long-term period (e.g., development of chronic lung disease), when there is a clear risk of death that would make it impossible to determine the morbidity. Combining the outcomes, such as "death or chronic lung disease," is a practical way to handle such circumstances.

Problems occur when a continuous outcome (such as a functional ability or quality of life score after a stroke) is assessed exclusively on individuals who make it through the duration of the follow-up. There are two unsatisfactory options: (i) analyzing the available data (which must be interpreted as a non-randomized comparison applicable only to survivors) and (ii) imputing zero functional ability scores for those who die (which may not appropriately represent the death state and will severely skew the outcome). Any discrepancy in the percentage of deaths between the two intervention groups must be taken into consideration when interpreting the results of these analyses. (Agresti et al., 2002) (Altman et al., 2000).

A Closer Look

Overcoming the Limitations of Interpreting P-Values: Magnitude of Effect

In order to get around this restriction, you should take into account two things: (1) whether the pre-established statistical plan indicates that the p-value of a comparison is significant, and (2) how much the treatment effects are (usually expressed as an effect estimate with 95% confidence intervals). For continuous outcomes, like visual acuity on the logMAR scale, the magnitude of effect is typically expressed as the mean difference between groups; for dichotomous/binary outcomes, like the occurrence of adverse events, the risk or odds ratio is used to indicate the magnitude of the effect. These metrics show the effect that was observed and measured by the study comparison. As was mentioned in the previous section, knowing the real size of the difference in the study comparison helps interpret the findings in a way that a p-value alone cannot. When interpreting study results, one should move away from a simple binary interpretation of "significant" or "not significant" and instead concentrate on making a more critical assessment of the observed effect's clinical relevance.

A number of crucial metrics are available to help assess whether a difference between groups is significant enough to have clinical significance, such as the Minimally Important Difference (MID). A clinician is far more equipped to comprehend the effects of a treatment and further explain the benefits and drawbacks of a treatment option to patients with reference to treatment effects that can be deemed clinically valuable when they are able to (1) identify the magnitude of effect within a study and (2) the MID (smallest change in the outcome that a patient would deem meaningful).

Summary

- Global health indicators are vital to track progress towards internationally agreed goals – e.g. the Sustainable Development Goals – and for donors to prioritize their investments. But in some countries, the data are sparse and of poor quality.
- Health data often identify persons who test positive for a particular case definition. Case definitions may vary by data source, limiting their comparability.
- Mathematical models set up a theoretical framework that represents and quantifies the causal pathways and mechanisms linking determinants and health outcomes. These types of models make predictions of health outcomes (which may be difficult to measure) based on parameter estimates derived from various data sources.
- One major purpose of statistical modeling is to process raw data to improve its accuracy and comparability. Incompleteness of Surveillance or registration data is an important source of bias that estimates must address and is a challenge because assessments of completeness cannot use primary data alone, and must employ external data.
- When using covariates, there is a danger that estimated trends reflect changes in covariates rather than changes in the estimated outcome indicator, particularly when there is little outcome data.
- Complex curve smoothing, or time series projections allow flexibility in curve fitting, and use multiple and sometimes overlapping data inputs.
- Analysts validate explanatory models by examining whether their structure adequately represents the data and if the model fits the data. For example, validation of an explanatory model would examine whether the addition of extra covariates to the model, transformations of covariates, or additional nonlinear terms significantly increase its explanatory power. Model fit is assessed using goodness-of-fit tests and model diagnostics such as residual analysis.
- The accuracy of the estimates depends on the methods used to create them. More importantly, the amount and quality of data depend upon which they are based.
- Multiple global health estimates are now available for many health indicators. One from the UN system and others from academic institutions. This can be of concern to international users such as donor agencies and national governments.
- There are several different ways of comparing outcome data between two intervention groups ('effect measures') for each data type. For example, dichotomous outcomes can be compared between intervention groups using a risk ratio, an odds ratio, a risk difference, or a number needed to treat. Continuous outcomes can be compared between intervention groups using a mean difference or a standardized mean difference. Effect measures are either ratio measures (e.g., risk ratio, odds ratio) or difference measures (e.g., mean difference, risk difference).
- An important principle in randomized trials is that the analysis must take into account the level at which randomization occurred. In most circumstances, the number of observations in the analysis should match the number of 'units' that were randomized.
- Dichotomous (binary) outcome data arise when the outcome for every participant is one of two possibilities, for example, dead or alive, or clinical improvement or no clinical improvement.

- The term 'continuous' in statistics conventionally refers to a variable that can take any value in a specified range. When dealing with numerical data, this means that a number may be measured and reported to an arbitrary number of decimal places. Examples of truly continuous data are weight, area, and volume.
- Ordinal outcome data arise when each participant is classified in a category and when the categories have a natural order. For example, a 'trichotomous' outcome such as the classification of disease severity into 'mild,' 'moderate,' or 'severe,' is of ordinal type.
- Some types of events can happen to a person more than once, for example, a myocardial infarction, an adverse reaction or a hospitalization. It may be preferable, or necessary, to address the number of times these events occur rather than simply whether each person experienced an event or not (that is, rather than treating them as dichotomous data). We refer to this type of data as count data.

References

1. Agresti, A. (2002). Categorical Data Analysis (2nd ed.). New York: John Wiley & Sons.
2. Altman, D. G. (2005). Why we need confidence intervals. World Journal of Surgery, 29, 554–556. https://doi.org/10.1007/s00268-005-7911-0
3. Altman, D. G., Machin, D., Bryant, T. N., & Gardner, M. J. (Eds.). (2000). Statistics with Confidence (2nd ed.). Bristol: BMJ Books.
4. Bolstad, W. M. (2007). Introduction to Bayesian Statistics (2nd ed.). Hoboken, NJ: Wiley.
5. D'Agostino, R. B., Sullivan, L. M., & Beiser, A. (2004). Introductory Applied Biostatistics. Belmont, CA: Duxbury-Brooks/Cole.
6. Du, S., Dong, J., Zhang, H., et al. (2015). Taichi exercise for self-rated sleep quality in older people: A systematic review and meta-analysis. International Journal of Nursing Studies, 52(1), 368–379.
7. Efron, B. (2013). Bayes' theorem in the 21st century. Science, 340, 1177–1178. https://doi.org/10.1126/science.1236536
8. Fineout-Overholt, E. (2014). EBP, QI, and research: Strange bedfellows or kindred spirits? In C. Hedges & B. Williams (Eds.), Anatomy of Research for Nurses (pp. 23–44). Indianapolis, IN: Sigma Theta Tau International.
9. Fineout-Overholt, E., Melnyk, B. M., Stillwell, S. B., & Williamson, K. M. (2010). Evidence-based practice, step by step: Critical appraisal of the evidence: Part II: Digging deeper—examining the "keeper" studies. American Journal of Nursing, 110(9), 41–48.
10. Gill, C. J., Sabin, L., & Schmid, C. H. (2005). Why clinicians are natural Bayesians. BMJ, 330, 1080–1083. https://doi.org/10.1136/bmj.330.7499.1080
11. Gray, K., Hampton, B., Silveti-Falls, T., McConnell, A., & Bausell, C. (2015). Comparison of Bayesian credible intervals to frequentist confidence intervals. Journal of Modern Applied Statistical Methods, 12, 43–52. https://doi.org/10.22237/jmasm/1430453220
12. Greenland, S., Senn, S. J., Rothman, K. J., Carlin, J. B., Poole, C., Goodman, S. N., et al. (2016). Statistical tests, P values, confidence intervals, and power: A guide to misinterpretations. European Journal of Epidemiology, 31, 337–350. https://doi.org/10.1007/s10654-016-0149-3

13. Hoekstra, R., Morely, R. D., Rouder, J. N., & Wagenmakers, E. J. (2014). Robust misinterpretation of confidence intervals. Psychonomic Bulletin & Review, 21, 1157–1164. https://doi.org/10.3758/s13423-013-0572-3

14. Lee, J. J., & Chu, C. T. (2012). Bayesian clinical trials in action. Statistics in Medicine, 31, 2955–2972. https://doi.org/10.1002/sim.5404

15. Little, R. J. A. (2006). Calibrated Bayes. The American Statistician, 60, 213–223. https://doi.org/10.1198/000313006X117837

16. Melnyk, B. M., & Fineout-Overholt, E. (2010). ARCC (Advancing Research and Clinical Practice through Close Collaboration): A model for system-wide implementation and sustainability of evidence-based practice. In J. Rycroft-Malone & T. Bucknall (Eds.), Models and Frameworks for Implementing Evidence-Based Practice: Linking Evidence to Action. Indianapolis, IN: Wiley-Blackwell & Sigma Theta Tau International.

17. Morey, R. D., Hoekstra, R., Rouder, J. N., Lee, M. D., & Wagenmakers, E. J. (2016). The fallacy of placing confidence in confidence intervals. Psychonomic Bulletin & Review, 23, 103–123. https://doi.org/10.3758/s13423-015-0947-8

18. O'Mathúna, D. P., & Fineout-Overholt, E. (2015). Critically appraising quantitative evidence for clinical decision making. In B. M. Melnyk & E. Fineout-Overholt (Eds.), Evidence-Based Practice in Nursing and Healthcare: A Guide to Best Practice (3rd ed., pp. 81–134). Philadelphia: Lippincott Williams & Wilkins.

19. Plichta, S. B., & Kelvin, E. (2013). Munro's Statistical Methods for Health Care Research (6th ed.). Philadelphia, PA: Lippincott, Williams & Wilkins.

20. Ponikowski, P., Voors, A. A., Anker, S. D., Bueno, H., Cleland, J. G., Coats, A. J., et al. (2016). 2016 Guidelines for the diagnosis and treatment of acute and chronic heart failure. European Heart Journal, 37, 2129–2200. https://doi.org/10.1093/eurheartj/ehw128

21. Rosner, B. (2006). Fundamentals of Biostatistics. Belmont, CA: Duxbury-Brooks/Cole.

22. Rothman, K. J., Greenland, S., & Lash, T. L. (2008). Precision and statistics in epidemiologic studies. In K. J. Rothman, S. Greenland, & T. L. Lash (Eds.), Modern Epidemiology (3rd ed., pp. 148–167). Philadelphia: Lippincott Williams & Wilkins.

23. Schenker, N., & Gentleman, J. F. (2001). On judging the significance of differences by examining the overlap between confidence intervals. The American Statistician, 55(3), 182–186.

24. Sedgwick, P. (2015). Uncertainty in sample estimates: Sampling error. BMJ, 350, h1914. https://doi.org/10.1136/bmj.h1914

25. Tiwari, R. C., Clegg, L. X., & Zou, Z. (2006). Efficient interval estimation for age-adjusted cancer rates. Statistical Methods in Medical Research, 15(6), 547–569.

26. van Belle, G., Fisher, L. D., Heagerty, P. J., & Lumley, T. (2004). Statistical inference: Populations and samples. In G. van Belle, L. D. Fisher, P. J. Heagerty, & T. Lumley (Eds.), Biostatistics: A Methodology for Health Sciences (2nd ed., pp. 61–116). Hoboken, NJ: Wiley.

27. Wasserstein, R. L., & Lazar, N. A. (2016). The ASA statement on p-values: Context, process, and purpose. The American Statistician, 70, 129–133. https://doi.org/10.1080/00031305.2016.1154108

Chapter

HYPOTHESIS TESTING PROCEDURES

6

Contents

Introduction 163
6.1. Hypothesis Testing 166
6.2. Hypothesis Testing: P Values, Confidence Intervals, and Significance 174
6.3. Chi-Square (X2) Test 178
6.4. Reliability of the Estimates 183
Summary 191
References 191

Introduction

Procedures for testing hypotheses are essential for assessing interventions, therapies, and other elements that could affect people's health. These processes are essential to epidemiology, public health, clinical research, and many other areas in the healthcare industry. Fundamentally, hypothesis testing in health is the process of developing theories regarding how certain behaviours, exposures, treatments, or other factors may affect health outcomes, and then evaluating the evidence to support these theories using statistical techniques. The null hypothesis (H0) and the alternative hypothesis (H1) are the two competing hypotheses that are usually put forth at the start of the process. The alternative hypothesis in health research proposes that there is a particular effect or difference of interest, whereas the null hypothesis frequently states that there is no effect or difference in health outcomes between groups or conditions. For instance, in a clinical trial evaluating a new drug's efficacy, the alternative hypothesis would contend that the drug improves health outcomes while the null hypothesis would claim that there is no difference in health outcomes between patients receiving the drug and those receiving a placebo. Following the establishment of hypotheses, data is gathered by researchers using cohort studies, randomized controlled trials, observational studies, and other research designs. Measures of health outcomes and details on possible predictors, confounders, and other pertinent variables are usually included in these data. Next, depending on the specific hypotheses being tested, the type of data being collected, and the study design, researchers choose an appropriate statistical test. Numerous non-parametric tests as well as t-tests, chi-square tests, regression analysis, and survival analysis are frequently employed as statistical tests in health research. The test selection is influenced by various elements, including the type of outcome variable (e.g., categorical, or continuous), the research design (e.g., observational study, randomized controlled trial), as well as presumptions regarding the data's underlying distribution.

Researchers determine a test statistic that measures the degree of agreement or disagreement between the observed data and what would be predicted under the null hypothesis after choosing the appropriate test. Assuming that the null hypothesis is true, this test statistic has a particular probability distribution. For instance, the test statistic in a t-test comparing the mean health outcomes of two groups follows a t-distribution, with the sample size and other factors determining the degrees of freedom. Assuming that the null hypothesis is true, researchers calculate the probability of observing a test statistic that is as extreme as or more extreme than the one derived from the sample data. This probability, sometimes referred to as the p-value, shows how likely it is that the observed results were the result of pure chance. Strong evidence against the null hypothesis is indicated by a small p-value, which implies that it is unlikely that the observed results would occur if the null hypothesis were true. A large p-value, on the other hand, indicates that there is insufficient evidence to refute the null hypothesis and that the observed data are fairly consistent with what would be predicted under it.

Using the p-value and a predetermined level of significance (e.g., 0.05), researchers choose whether to reject the null hypothesis or not. The alternative hypothesis is accepted and the null hypothesis is rejected if the p-value is less than the significance level, indicating that there is enough data to support the claim of interest. In contrast, the null hypothesis is not rejected and it is determined that there is insufficient evidence to support the claim if the p-value exceeds the significance level. It is significant to remember that hypothesis testing in health research has several restrictions and factors to take into account. These include problems with sample size, measurement error, confounding variables, study design, and statistical significance interpretation. Furthermore, hypothesis testing evaluates the strength of evidence based on sample data rather than offering definitive proof or disproof of a hypothesis. As a result, while interpreting the results of hypothesis testing, researchers should take the larger context of the research question into account as well as other pertinent data.

Orientation and Directional Terms:

Term	Definition	Illustration
Null hypothesis	Null hypothesis is a type of statistical hypothesis that proposes that no statistical significance exists in a set of given observations.	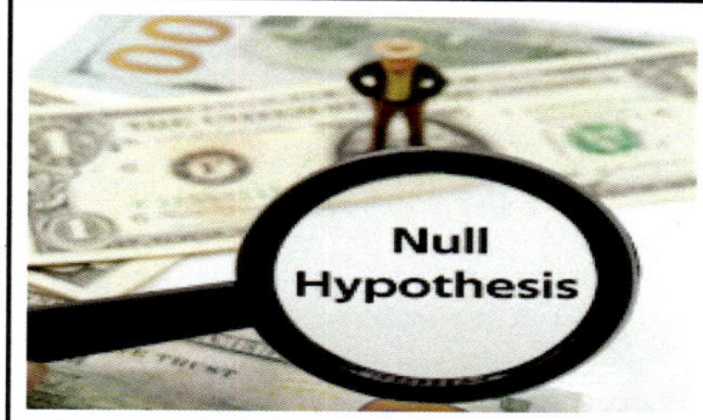
Mortality rate	A measure of the number of deaths in a particular population, scaled to the size of that population, per unit of time.	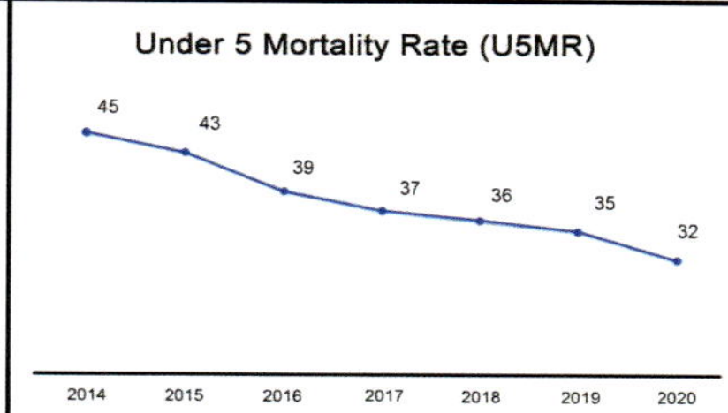
Sampling error	A statistical error that occurs when an analyst does not select a sample that represents the entire population of data.	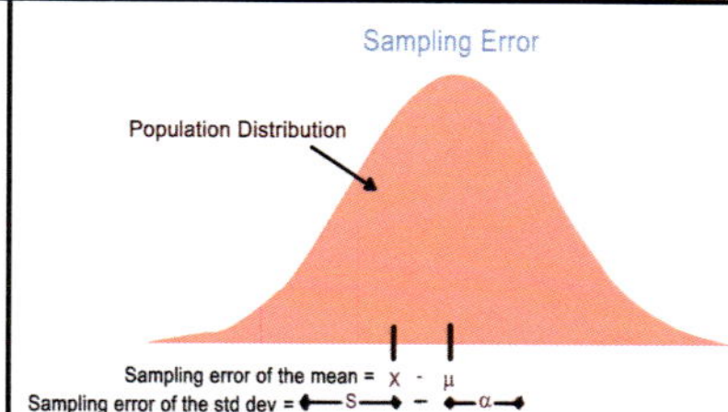
Blood Pressure	Blood pressure is the pressure of blood pushing against the walls of your arteries. Arteries carry blood from your heart to other parts of your body.	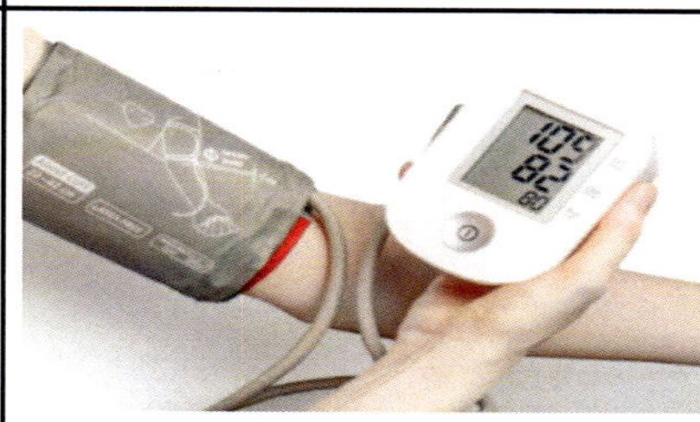
Data Analysis	The process of systematically applying statistical and/or logical techniques to describe and illustrate, condense and recap, and evaluate data.	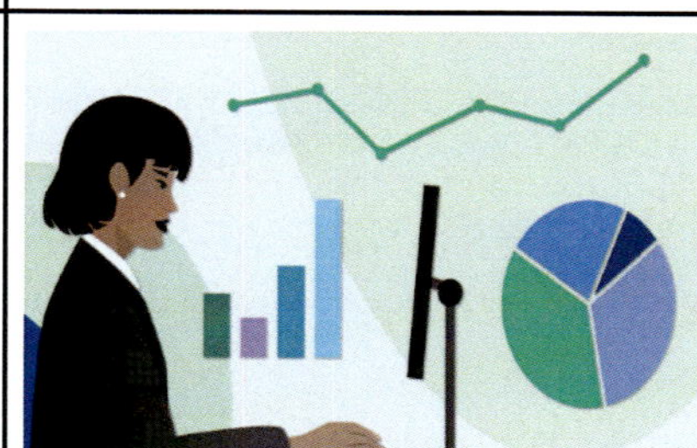

6.1. Hypothesis Testing

The process of ascertaining the likelihood that an observed event is the result of pure chance is known as hypothesis testing. Something else, such as the treatment's impact on the observed event (the outcome) that was measured, must have been the cause of the event if chance was not the cause. The majority of statistical analyses for individual research projects revolve around this process of testing a hypothesis. In an experimental research study, the subjects are divided into two groups, and one group receives treatment or medication that is not given to the other group. There is a comparison between the treatment and control groups' outcomes. If the results differ, the researcher aims to determine, with a reasonable degree of certainty, whether the difference is significant enough to be attributed to a systematic variation in the groups (i.e., treatment effect) as opposed to an effect of the treatment itself. e. error in random sampling). It is customary to test the null hypothesis even though the investigator is typically attempting to identify a difference between the two groups. According to the null hypothesis, there is no distinction between the groups under comparison. The null hypothesis asserts that, in the presence of a control and a treatment group, the treatment had no discernible impact on the dependent variable (i.e., the outcome). (e.g., death rate). Therefore, for both the control and treatment groups, the average mortality rate is the same.

In hypothesis testing, the main research question is reduced to one of two potential hypothesis types: the research hypothesis (sometimes referred to as the alternative hypothesis; denoted H1) or the null hypothesis (sometimes referred to as H0). Since it is typically simpler to reject a false statement (null hypothesis), we typically assume the opposite of the research question that interests us. Next, to support our research hypothesis, we test if we can reject the null hypothesis. Testing hypotheses merely indicates that the research hypothesis is plausible rather than proving it to be true.

6.1.1. Steps for Hypothesis Testing

In general, regardless of the research question, there are four hypothesis-testing steps:

- Formulate the null and research hypotheses.
- Select a significance level.
- Calculate the test statistic.
- Analyze and state conclusion based on H_0 (null hypothesis).
- ***Step 1: Formulate the Null and Research Hypotheses***

The investigator aims to address the research question, even though we initially assume the null hypothesis to be true. We would define our null and research hypotheses as follows. For instance, in a clinical trial of a new drug, our research question might be, "Is the new drug more effective (i.e., decrease mortality) than a placebo (sugar pill)?."

- o H_0: The average mortality rate does not differ between the treatment and control groups
- o H_1: The average mortality rate does differ between the treatment and control groups

Relationships that are suspected across the whole population of interest are referred to as research hypotheses. In this case, the researcher's hypothesis would be that all transported patients who meet the inclusion criteria—that is, the population of interest—would respond better to the new medication. In practice, though, an investigator tests a hypothesis by doing a statistical analysis on a small sample and extrapolating the results to the population of interest.

- ***Step 2: Select a Significance Level***

The probability that the researcher is willing to acknowledge that he or she has mistakenly rejected the null hypothesis is determined by the significance or alpha level (a). Put another way, if a = .05, the researcher is prepared to concede that, in 5% of cases, the choice to reject the null hypothesis will be incorrect (i.e., claiming that the treatment significantly lowers mortality when it doesn't). The alpha levels .05 and .01 are the most frequently used. The cutoff probability (of seeing a sample mean, for example) that is so high that we believe it is extremely unlikely that we would see a sample mean associated with that probability by chance is also defined by the significance level, which is the criterion level used in this process. Step 4 goes into detail about this cutoff probability, also known as the critical value, which is used to decide whether the null hypothesis should be rejected. Essentially, the alpha level is determined a priori (i.e., before the statistical test is conducted) to determine the statistical significance of the results.

- ***Step 3: Calculate the Test Statistic***

Having established the significance level to test the hypothesis, the investigator can now collect data and conduct the statistical test that has been selected.

- ***Step 4: Analyze and State the Conclusion based on H_0***

The critical value, which is partly determined by the significance level chosen in step 2, is then compared with the test statistic computed in step 3. The set of test statistic values (the critical region) for which the null hypothesis should be rejected is defined by the critical value. Stated differently, values of the obtained test statistic that fall within the critical region and/or equal or exceed the critical value are deemed unlikely to occur due to chance or sampling error alone. After that, the researcher can reasonably conclude that there is a "statistically significant difference" or that the treatment was responsible for the test statistic's extreme value. Given a true null hypothesis, we use the probability value (p-value) of a hypothesis test to calculate the likelihood that, through chance alone, we will obtain an equal or more extreme value of the test statistic than that computed in step 3. We contrast the p-value found in step 3 using our test statistic with the significance level specified in step 2 (a = .05). We reject H0 if the obtained p-value is less than .05 ($p \alpha .05$). We are unable to reject H0 if the p-value is greater than .05 ($p < .05$). Consequently, there is less than 5% chance that a sample taken from a given population (ALL transported patients who meet your inclusion criteria) will result in a test statistic value greater than or equal to the critical value. Test statistic values that are as extreme or more extreme than the test statistic you obtained are only produced by 5% of samples taken from a population. Smaller p-values support the research hypothesis by showing that it is more likely than not that the null hypothesis is correct.

One way to perform hypothesis testing is by assessing the impact of a drug on hypertension control. In this scenario, the researcher would analyze blood pressure as the dependent variable. Blood pressure is influenced by various factors, causing it to fluctuate over time. It is normal for an individual's blood pressure to deviate by 10 mmHg or more from one point to another. Therefore, if there is a 10 mmHg decrease in blood pressure at the second time point, the researcher must determine whether this change is due to random variation or the drug's effects. The four steps of hypothesis testing can guide the investigator in addressing this question.

- ***Step 1: Formulate the Null and Research Hypotheses***

- H_0: The average change in blood pressure does not differ from time 1 to time 2
- H_1: The average change in blood pressure does differ from time 1 to time 2

- ***Step 2: Select a Significance Level***

Upon meticulous analysis of the ramifications of committing type I and type II errors, we have concluded that our research project is suitable for a significance level of a = .05. This indicates that we are prepared to accept the possibility that, in 5% of cases, we will reject the null hypothesis in error and come to the incorrect conclusion that the investigational medication significantly lowered blood pressure when in fact it did not.

- ***Step 3: Calculate the Test Statistic***

Given that we are comparing the average change in blood pressure from time 1 to time 2 for our entire sample, the appropriate test statistic for our research design is a repeated measure or dependent samples *t*-test.

Based on data analysis, our obtained test statistic value is t_{obt} = .90.

- ***Step 4: Analyze and State Conclusion Based on H_0***

Now that we have our test statistic value (t_{obt} = .90), we can compare it to the critical value of t (t_{crit} = 1.697), which is partly based on the significance level that was established in step 2. Due to t_{obt} α t_{crit} (90 ± 1.697), the null hypothesis does not fall within the critical region, we cannot reject it. The researcher would conclude that the average change in blood pressure between times 1 and 2 is not significantly different. Any variations in the average blood pressure change differ only by the amount that could be predicted by chance or sampling error.

6.1.2. Potential Errors

Two possible mistakes can occur during hypothesis testing. One may determine that a difference exists between the two groups when in fact none does, or one may determine that no difference exists between the two groups when in fact none does (fail to measure a difference). Type I, or alpha, errors are the first kind of errors, and type II, or beta, errors are the second. Because the researcher can make choices regarding the study design and data analysis that will reduce one or both of these errors, type I and type II errors are significant to the researcher.

Table 6.1. *Possible Results for any Hypothesis Test*

Truth			
		H_0 No Treatment Effect	H_1 Treatment Effect
	H_0 No Treatment Effect	Correct	Type II error
Decision			
	H_1 Treatment Effect	Type I error	Correct

Source: https://www.airmedicaljournal.com/article/S1067-991X(09)00068-6/fulltext#:~:text=Hypothesis%20testing%20is%20the%20method,the%20outcome)%20that%20was%20measured.

This is crucial because the investigator can't know if they have interpreted the data incorrectly in one of these two ways. Another challenge is that the likelihood of a type II error rises and vice versa when the likelihood of a type I error falls. There are two possibilities for reality or truth given our choice to reject or not reject the null hypothesis. The four outcomes that can come from any hypothesis test are listed in the following table (see **Table 6.1**).

6.1.2.1. Type I Errors

Overconfidence in the difference between two groups' findings is reflected in type I errors. The investigator's alpha is directly correlated with the frequency of type I errors (step 2). If the researcher decides to set their alpha at .05, for instance, then all p-values that fall below .05 will be deemed statistically significant. This indicates that, given the results, there is only a 1 in 20 chance that the results would have been obtained in the absence of population group differences. The researcher is allowed to select any alpha (p-value) that seems suitable for a given investigation. It is simpler to achieve statistical significance when the p-value is higher, but there is a higher likelihood of a type I error. As a result, when an investigator claims that a treatment has an effect when, in fact, none existed and the differences observed were merely the product of chance, they are using a high alpha.

6.1.2.2. Type II Errors

Type II errors happen when the researcher failed to identify a real difference between two or more groups. The investigator's alpha is inversely correlated with the frequency of type II errors, which is inversely correlated with the frequency of type I errors. The likelihood of a type II error increases with decreasing alpha. The term "beta" describes the likelihood of committing a type II error. The probability of detecting an actual difference is known as power, which is beta's inverse. Sample size is one of several factors that affect the power of significance tests. This value needs to be chosen carefully because the alpha level affects both type I and type II errors. An excessively high alpha can lead to statistical significance even in cases where there was no real difference in the data. However, true differences in the data might go unnoticed if the alpha is set too low. The investigator ought to ascertain the suitable alpha by considering the ramifications of committing a type I or type II error. When researching a novel treatment for a deadly illness, researchers may look for anything that could genuinely benefit patients. As a result, the researcher would prefer to set the alpha at .05 or even .10 and commit a type I error, claiming something worked when it didn't. Nonetheless, even in cases where a novel medication for a mild illness has unfavorable side effects, the researcher would prefer to declare it ineffective—a mistake known as a type II error. The investigator would lower the alpha in this scenario (. 01).

Hypothesis Testing Formula

$Z = (\bar{x} - \mu 0) / (\sigma / \sqrt{n})$

- Here, $\bar{x}$ is the sample mean,
- $\mu 0$ is the population mean,
- σ is the standard deviation,
- n is the sample size.

6.1.3. Hypothesis Testing Works

An analyst tests the null hypothesis using a statistical sample to provide evidence supporting its plausibility. To test a theory, measurements, and analyses are performed on a random sample of the population. To test the null and alternative hypotheses, analysts take a random sample of the population. Usually, the null hypothesis asserts that two population parameters are equal; for instance, it might state that the population mean return is equal to zero. In essence, the alternative hypothesis is the null hypothesis's opposite (e.g., the population indicates that the return is non-zero). They are therefore incompatible, meaning that only one of them can be true. Nonetheless, there is always going to be one of the two true answers.

6.1.4. Null Hypothesis and Alternate Hypothesis

The presumption that the event won't happen is known as the null hypothesis. Unless it is rejected, a null hypothesis does not affect the study's conclusion. It is represented by the symbol H0, which is pronounced H-naught. The logical opposite of the null hypothesis is the alternate hypothesis. After the null hypothesis is rejected, the alternative hypothesis is accepted. The symbol for it is H1. Let's use an example to better understand this. According to a sanitizer manufacturer, their product typically eliminates 95% of germs. Establish a null and alternate hypothesis to test the assertion made by this company. H0 (Null Hypothesis): 95 percent on average. Hypothesis 1 (alternative): The mean is below 95 percent. Finding the fair and balanced position of a coin is another simple way to visualize this idea. The probability of a show of heads is equal to the likelihood of a show of tails, according to the null hypothesis. The alternative theory, on the other hand, claims that there would be a significantly different chance of a heads-and-tails show.

6.1.5. Hypothesis Testing Calculation with Examples

Let's consider a hypothesis test for the average height of women in the United States. Suppose our null hypothesis is that the average height is 5'4." We gather a sample of 100 women and determine that their average height is 5'5." The standard deviation of the population is 2.

To calculate the z-score, we would use the following formula:

- $z = (\bar{x} - \mu0) / (\sigma / \sqrt{n})$
- $z = (5'5'' - 5'4'') / (2'' / \sqrt{100})$
- $z = 0.5 / (0.045)$
- $z = 11.11$

We will reject the null hypothesis as the z-score of 11.11 is very large and conclude that there is evidence to suggest that the average height of women in the US is greater than 5'4."

6.1.6. Steps of Hypothesis Testing

- ***Step 1: Specify Your Null and Alternate Hypotheses***

To test your original research hypothesis (the prediction you want to investigate), you must rephrase it as a null (Ho) and alternative (Ha) hypothesis to conduct a quantitative analysis. Usually, your alternate hypothesis is your first hypothesis, which postulates a relationship between variables. No relationship between the variables of interest is predicted by the null hypothesis.

- ***Step 2: Gather Data***

For a statistical test to be legitimate, sampling and data collection must be done in a way that is meant to test your hypothesis. You cannot draw statistical conclusions about the population you are interested in if your data is not representative.

- ***Step 3: Conduct a Statistical Test***

Other statistical tests are available, but they are all based on comparing the within-group variance, which measures how the data are distributed within a category, with the between-group variance, which measures how distinct the categories are from each other. Your statistical test will show a low p-value to indicate this if the between-group variation is significant enough to cause little to no overlap between groups. This implies that it is unlikely that these groups' differences happened by chance. In contrast, a high p-value will be displayed by your statistical test if there is a high within-group variance and a low between-group variance. Any variation between groups is probably the result of chance. The range of variables and the degree of measurement in the data you collect will affect which statistical test you choose.

- ***Step 4: Determine Rejection Of Your Null Hypothesis***

The outcome of your statistical test must be used to decide whether or not to reject your null hypothesis. Generally, you will use the p-value that the statistical test provides as the foundation for your decision. Generally, when there is less than a 5 percent chance that these data would be observed if the null hypothesis were true, your preset level of significance for rejecting the null hypothesis will be 0.05. In other situations, scientists employ a lower significance level, like 0.01 (1 percent). This lessens the chance of rejecting the null hypothesis incorrectly.

- ***Step 5: Present Your Results***

Talk about whether or not your initial hypothesis was supported by your results during the conversation. In hypothesis testing, the formal term for rejecting or failing to reject the null hypothesis is used. Your statistics assignments probably require this.

6.1.7. Types of Hypothesis Testing

6.1.7.1. Z Test

To determine whether a discovery or relationship is statistically significant, hypothesis testing uses a z-test. It usually checks to see if two means are the same (the null hypothesis). Only when the population standard deviation is known and the sample size is 30 data points or more, can a z-test be applied.

6.1.7.2. T Test

A statistical test called a t-test is employed to compare the means of two groups. To determine whether two groups differ or if a procedure or treatment affects the population of interest, it is frequently used in hypothesis testing.

6.1.7.3. Chi-Square

To determine whether your data matches the predictions, you use the Chi-square test as a hypothesis test. With a random sample, the Chi-square test examines the differences between categorical variables to see if the observed and expected results are well-fitted. The basic idea of the test is to compare the observed values in your data with the values that would be expected if the null hypothesis were true.

6.1.8. Hypothesis Testing and Confidence Intervals

Inferential methods that rely on approximating the sample distribution include confidence intervals and hypothesis testing. Using confidence intervals, a population parameter is estimated from sample data. In hypothesis testing, a given hypothesis is investigated using data from a sample. To perform hypothesis testing, we need a postulated parameter. Comparable simulation methods are used to create randomization and bootstrap distributions. Whereas the null hypothesis value is the focal point of a randomization distribution, the observed sample statistic serves as the focal point of a bootstrap distribution. Confidence ranges include several reasonable population parameter estimates. Only two-tailed confidence intervals were created in this lesson. These two-tail hypothesis tests are directly related to these two-tail confidence intervals. Two-tailed confidence intervals and two-tailed hypothesis tests usually yield the same results. Put differently, if the predicted value is included in the 95 percent confidence interval, a hypothesis test conducted at the 0.05 level will almost always fail to reject the null hypothesis. Should the 95 percent confidence interval exclude the proposed parameter, a hypothesis test at the 0.05 level will almost definitely reject the null hypothesis.

6.1.9. Simple and Composite Hypothesis Testing

Depending on the population distribution, you can classify the statistical hypothesis into two types.

- **Simple Hypothesis:** A simple hypothesis specifies an exact value for the parameter.

- **Composite Hypothesis:** A composite hypothesis specifies a range of values.

Example: A company is claiming that their average sales for this quarter are 1000 units. This is an example of a simple hypothesis.

Suppose the company claims that the sales are in the range of 900 to 1000 units. Then this is a case of a composite hypothesis.

6.1.9.1. One-Tailed and Two-Tailed Hypothesis Testing

A directional test, also known as a one-tailed test, looks at a critical region of the data that, if the test sample falls inside it, would inevitably lead to the acceptance of the alternative hypothesis and the rejection of the null hypothesis. A one-tailed test has a one-sided critical distribution area, which indicates that the test sample is either larger or smaller than a given value. In a two-tailed test, the test sample is examined to see if it is greater or less than a range of values, suggesting that the critical distribution area is bimodal. The null hypothesis will be rejected and the alternative hypothesis accepted if the sample falls within this range.

6.1.9.2. Right-Tailed Hypothesis Testing

If the larger than (>) sign appears in your hypothesis statement, you are using a right-tailed test, also known as an upper test. Or, to put it another way, the disparity is to the right. For instance, you can contrast the battery life before and after a change in production. Your hypothesis statements can be the following if you want to know if the battery life is longer than the original (let's say 90 hours):

- The null hypothesis is (H0 <= 90) or less change.
- A possibility is that battery life has risen (H1) > 90.

The crucial point in this situation is that the alternate hypothesis (H1), not the null hypothesis, decides whether you get a right-tailed test.

6.1.9.3. Left-Tailed Hypothesis Testing

Alternative hypotheses that assert the true value of a parameter is lower than the null hypothesis are tested with a left-tailed test; they are indicated by the asterisk "<."

Example:

- Suppose H0: mean = 50 and H1: mean not equal to 50

According to the H1, the mean can be greater than or less than 50. This is an example of a Two-tailed test.

In a similar manner, if H0: mean >=50, then H1: mean <50 Here the mean is less than 50. It is called a One-tailed test.

6.1.10. Type 1 and Type 2 Error

A hypothesis test can result in two types of errors.

- Type 1 Error: A Type-I error occurs when sample results reject the null hypothesis despite being true.
- Type 2 Error: A Type-II error occurs when the null hypothesis is not rejected when it is false, unlike a Type-I error.

Example: Suppose a teacher evaluates the examination paper to decide whether a student passes or fails.

- H0: Student has passed
- H1: Student has failed

Type I error will be the teacher failing the student [rejects H0] although the student scored the passing marks [H0 was true].

Type II error will be the case where the teacher passes the student [do not reject H0] although the student did not score the passing marks [H1 is true].

6.1.11. Level of Significance

One way to assess if a test statistic is statistically significant is to look at its alpha value. Alpha in a statistical test denotes a reasonable chance of a Type I error. Since alpha is a probability, its value can range from 0 to 1. As a percentage of the chance of a Type I error, 0.01, 0.05, and 0.1 are the most often used alpha values in practice (i.e., 1 percent, 5 percent, and 10 percent). e. dismissing the null hypothesis even when it is true).

6.1.12. P-Value

The probability that an observed difference could have happened by chance is expressed by a p-value. The statistical significance of the observed difference rises as the p-value falls. The null hypothesis is rejected if the p-value is too low. Here, you've chosen an example to demonstrate your attempt to determine whether the new marketing initiative has improved sales of the product. The probability that the null hypothesis, which claims that the new advertising campaign does not affect sales, is correct is known as the p-value. There is a 30% chance that there won't be any change in the product's sales if the p-value is .30. There is a 3% chance that the new advertising campaign will not result in an increase or decrease in sales value if the p-value is 0.03. As you can see, the likelihood that the alternative hypothesis is correct rises with a lower p-value, indicating that the new advertising campaign either increases or decreases sales.

6.1.13. Why is Hypothesis Testing Important in Research Methodology?

Hypothesis testing is crucial in research methodology for several reasons:

1. Provides evidence-based conclusions: It allows researchers to make objective conclusions based on empirical data, providing evidence to support or refute their research hypotheses.
2. Supports decision-making: It helps make informed decisions, such as accepting or rejecting a new treatment, implementing policy changes, or adopting new practices.
3. Adds rigor and validity: It adds scientific rigor to research using statistical methods to analyze data, ensuring that conclusions are based on sound statistical evidence.
4. Contributes to the advancement of knowledge: By testing hypotheses, researchers contribute to the growth of knowledge in their respective fields by confirming existing theories or discovering new patterns and relationships.

6.1.14. Limitations of Hypothesis Testing

Hypothesis testing has some limitations that researchers should be aware of:

1. It cannot prove or establish the truth: Hypothesis testing provides evidence to support or reject a hypothesis, but it cannot confirm the absolute truth of the research question.
2. Results are sample-specific: Hypothesis testing is based on analyzing a sample from a population, and the conclusions drawn are specific to that particular sample.
3. Possible errors: During hypothesis testing, there is a chance of committing type I error (rejecting a true null hypothesis) or type II error (failing to reject a false null hypothesis).
4. Assumptions and requirements:

Different tests have specific assumptions and requirements that must be met to accurately interpret results.

6.2. Hypothesis Testing: P Values, Confidence Intervals, and Significance

Evidence-based medicine is frequently used by medical professionals as a guide when making decisions in the field. A test is frequently conducted on a research hypothesis, and the results are reported with p values, confidence intervals, or both. The investigators also estimate or determine the statistical or research significance. Regrettably, varying degrees of comfort among healthcare providers may exist when interpreting these results, potentially impeding the appropriate implementation of the information. It may be difficult for healthcare professionals to make clinical decisions that go beyond simply considering the level of significance determined by research investigators if they lack a fundamental understanding of hypothesis testing, p values, confidence intervals, and the distinction between statistical and clinical significance. To enable medical professionals to use their expertise to assess whether study outcomes are clinically appropriate for application in healthcare practice and whether results are sufficiently reported, an overview of these concepts is provided.

6.2.1. Process of Hypothesis Testing

To direct analyses, researchers undertaking studies require research questions and hypotheses. Researchers first formulate broad research questions (RQs) and then determine a gap in the literature or clinical practice. Any research question or claim is based on a deeper comprehension of the connections between two or more variables. We'll use the following research question example for this article:

6.2.1.1. Research Question: Is Drug 23 An Effective Treatment for Disease A?

Research hypotheses must be developed because research questions do not directly imply particular assumptions or forecasts. A hypothesis is a preconceived statement about the research question in which the researcher or researchers make a precise, well-informed estimate about the study's outcome. This is also referred to as the alternative hypothesis, and it ultimately enables the researcher to adopt a position based on knowledge gained from medical literature or personal experience. Below is an illustration of a hypothesis. Research Hypothesis: When compared to Drug 22, Drug 23 will significantly lessen the symptoms related to Disease A. According to the stated research hypothesis, the null hypothesis asserts that there is no statistically significant difference between the groups. When deciding how to report p values, researchers should be mindful of journal guidelines, and their manuscripts should maintain internal consistency. In terms of p values, the probability of discovering a statistically significant effect rises with the number of participants in a study (the sample size). The p-value for the differences between Drug 23 and Drug 22 in terms of the reduction of Disease A symptoms can be very small, even with very large sample sizes. Up until a study produces substantial evidence to support rejecting the null hypothesis is assumed to be true. The investigators will either fail to reject the null hypothesis (they could not provide proof that there were significant differences or associations) or reject it if they find significant differences or associations based on the results. To test a hypothesis, scientists gather information on a representative sample and decide whether to reject the null hypothesis or not. It is not possible to collect data for the entire population in most research studies. Although there is a chance of error, statistical inference can be made by using a sampling procedure. Errors of Type I and Type II can occur when deciding whether to reject or fail to reject the null hypothesis. Even though it is hard to guarantee that these mistakes haven't happened, researchers should reduce the likelihood that they have.

6.2.2. Significance

The substantive importance of medical research is referred to as significance. The probability that results are random is known as statistical significance. When evaluating biomedical research, healthcare professionals frequently make the mistake of confusing statistical significance with clinical significance. Healthcare professionals shouldn't just accept study findings and conclusions without taking the clinical significance into account when classifying findings as significant or not significant. To reduce dependency on the researchers for significance determination, healthcare practitioners should take into account the clinical relevance of findings and have a working knowledge of both p values and confidence intervals. Using p values is one common criterion for assessing statistical significance.

6.2.3. P Values

To ascertain whether the sample estimate differs significantly from a hypothesized value, researchers employ P values. The p-value represents the likelihood that the study's observed effect would have happened by chance if there had been no real effect at all. Generally speaking, information with a p-value of less than 0.05 or less than 001 is deemed statistically significant. Although there has been discussion about lowering the 0.05 threshold, it is still widely used. The size of the effect can be ascertained through hypothesis testing.

An example of findings reported with p values is below:

- **Statement:** Drug 23 reduced patients' symptoms compared to Drug 22. Patients who received Drug 23 (n=100) were 2.1 times less likely than patients who received Drug 22 (n = 100) to experience symptoms of Disease A, $p<0.05$.

Or

- **Statement:** Individuals who were prescribed Drug 23 experienced fewer symptoms (M = 1.3, SD = 0.7) compared to individuals who were prescribed Drug 22 (M = 5.3, SD = 1.9). This finding was statistically significant, p= 0.02.

The null hypothesis (that there was no relationship) should be rejected for both statements if the threshold had been set at 0.05, and we should conclude that there were significant differences. Notably, as the two aforementioned statements demonstrate, certain researchers will present findings. < or > and others will only ever give a precise p-value of 0.000001. Readers should be aware of the reporting style for p values when analyzing research. Reporting all p values for every variable in a study design is the best practice; doing otherwise is limited to reporting p values for variables that have significant findings. By including all p values, the study's validity is demonstrated, and the possibility of selective reporting or data mining is reduced. Although p values have been used by researchers historically, experts who believe that p values are problematic recommend using confidence intervals instead. P-values by themselves are insufficient to help us comprehend the magnitude of the differences or correlations. The American Statistical Association (ASA) published a statement on p values in March 2016, stating that conclusions and decision-making in science shouldn't be predicated on a set p-value threshold (e.g., 0.05). They advise concentrating on the importance of findings about the validity of the data, the quality of the measurements, and the study design. In the end, the ASA statement stated that a p-value by itself does not constitute compelling evidence. Healthcare practitioners should think about p values along with a concurrent appraisal study design validity when conceiving clinical work. A p-value from a double-blinded, randomized clinical trial, for instance, should be given more weight than one from a retrospective observational study because the former is intended to reduce bias. Since the 1950s, there has been a raging debate about p-values, and since the 1980s, there has been a suggestion to replace them with confidence intervals.

6.2.4. Confidence Intervals

Within a specified confidence interval, a range of values (e.g., 95%), as well as the precise statistical constraint value within the intended population. Most research uses a 95% CI, but investigators can set any level (e.g., 90% CI, 99% CI). A CI provides a range with the lower bound and upper bound limits of a difference or association that would be plausible for a population. Therefore, compared to p-values, confidence intervals offer more information about the precision of an estimate. For example, a CI of 95 percent means that, if a study were conducted 100 times, the range would contain the true value of 95. Taking into account the aforementioned research example, the following statement with a 95 percent confidence interval (CI) could be made: People prescribed Drug 23 showed no symptoms after three days, which was significantly faster than people prescribed Drug 22; the mean difference in days to recovery between the two groups was 4.2 days (95 percent confidence interval: 1.9 to 7.8). It is significant to remember that the standard error and sample size have an impact on the width of the CI; a smaller study sample size will result in a narrower CI (wider CI). Greater variability or a smaller sample size are indicated by a wider width. A researcher would like to see the CI's precision rise. For instance, a 95 percent confidence interval of 1.43–1.47 is far more accurate than the one given in the previous example. Confidence intervals (CIs) are useful in clinical practice and research because they indicate whether or not any clinically significant values are included in the interval.

For differences with CI, null values are occasionally used (zero for ratios and 1 for differential comparisons). CIs, however, offer more details than that. Think about the following scenario: A hospital introduces a new procedure that results in an average 25-minute (95 percent confidence interval: -2.5–41-minute) decrease in patient wait times in the emergency room. Although the range is much higher on the positive side, applying this protocol to different populations may result in longer wait times because it crosses zero.

Therefore, even though the p-value used to determine statistical significance for this may yield results that are not significant, people should still look at this range, take the study design into account, and decide if it is still worthwhile to pilot this in their place of employment. Like p-values, 95 percent confidence intervals are not able to account for researcher error (e.g., bias in the study or incorrect data analysis). When deciding which statistics to report—CIs or p-values—researchers should look into journal preferences. If in doubt, it might be helpful to report both. Here's an example: Reporting both: After three days, people who were prescribed Drug 23 did not experience any symptoms, which was a significant faster response than people who were prescribed Drug 22 ($p = 0.009$). The two groups' mean difference in days to recovery was 4.02 (95 percent confidence interval: 1.09 to 7.8).

6.2.5. Clinical Significance

Keep in mind that there are two distinct concepts: clinical significance and statistical significance. Healthcare professionals should keep in mind that while a study with a smaller sample size and statistically non-significant results may not be of interest to clinicians, one with a larger sample size and statistically significant differences may have an impact on clinical practice.

Furthermore, a non-significant finding might, as was previously mentioned, be the result of the study design rather than the relationships between the variables. When applying evidence-based medicine to clinical practice, healthcare professionals should carefully consider the design, sample size, power, probability of type I and type II errors, data analysis, and reporting of statistical findings (p values, 95 percent confidence interval, or both) to assess the practical significance of studies. It's interesting to note that some experts have demanded that work that is either statistically significant or not be included because statistical significance has never equaled clinical significance and never will. Depending on the experience of the providers and, most importantly, the severity of the disease, determining what is clinically significant can be difficult.

To assess the significance of study results, providers should conclude their knowledge and experience, as well as from the researchers' significant or insignificant findings. They should also consider the study's limitations and practical ramifications.

6.2.6. Hypothesis Testing to Improve Patient Outcomes

Similar to the detective work of statistics, hypothesis testing enables us to learn the real story behind a population. This useful tool helps us make data-driven decisions in healthcare that have the potential to save lives. Consider yourself a physician attempting to enhance the course of treatment for a particular ailment. You can test your assumptions and determine whether they still stand up to close examination by using hypothesis testing. For instance, you might predict that an innovative approach to treatment will produce better results than the conventional course of care. You can ascertain whether your hypothesis is supported or whether you need to start over by gathering data and performing statistical tests. It resembles a scientific experiment with applications to the real world. Now let's explore the intriguing field of hypothesis testing in the medical field and see how it can improve patient care. Healthcare practitioners use hypothesis testing as their statistical Swiss Army knife to determine whether their theories about a population are true or just statistical illusions. Creating a null hypothesis, which is the starting point assumption that there is no significant difference between groups or variables, and an alternative hypothesis, which is the rebellious, wild child of the null hypothesis, are the first steps in the process. Equipped with information and adept analysis, we test our theories, rejecting the null in favor of the alternative if the evidence lends credence to it. Data-driven choices that improve patient care and win over all of our data-loving colleagues are the result.

6.2.6.1. The Importance of Data in Healthcare Decision-Making

Decisions in healthcare can mean the difference between life and death. For this reason, healthcare workers must use data to guide their decisions. One statistical technique that can assist healthcare providers in making data-driven decisions is hypothesis testing. Data collection and analysis can be used to test patient care hypotheses and decide whether adjustments are necessary to get better results. In the end, both patients and healthcare providers stand to gain from this strategy's potential to improve the effectiveness and efficiency of healthcare delivery.

6.2.6.2. Identifying a Problem or Question to be Addressed

Finding an issue or query that needs to be answered is the first step in applying hypothesis testing to enhance patient care. This could take many forms, such as raising patient satisfaction levels or lowering readmissions to hospitals. After the issue or problem has been identified, we can gather information about it and create a hypothesis regarding its possible cause or potential solutions. The validity of this hypothesis and whether any adjustments are required to enhance patient care can then be ascertained by applying statistical testing techniques.

6.2.6.3. Formulating a Hypothesis and Selecting a Statistical Test

You must first develop a hypothesis regarding the issue or query you are attempting to answer before you can apply hypothesis testing to enhance patient care. This theory ought to be supported by information and observations pertaining to the problem at hand. The next stage after formulating a hypothesis is to choose a suitable statistical test to ascertain the hypothesis' validity. Depending on the type of data and the hypothesis being tested, this may entail analyzing the data using methods like t-tests, ANOVA, or regression analysis. Healthcare providers can improve patient outcomes by using data-driven decision-making and hypothesis testing in this way.

6.2.6.4. Analyzing the Results and Making Informed Decisions for Patient Care

To ascertain whether the hypothesis has been accepted or rejected, you must evaluate the data after the relevant statistical test has been completed. If the hypothesis is validated, the data indicates that there is reason to believe that the suggested course of action or intervention is successful. In the event that the hypothesis is disproved, it may be necessary to explore other options since the data do not support the intervention or suggested course of action. You can make well-informed decisions about how to enhance patient care, including changing medication dosages, introducing new treatment protocols, or giving patients more support, based on the findings of the hypothesis testing (Jones et al., 2002; Sedgwick et al., 2014).

6.3. Chi-Square (X^2) Test

A common statistical test for comparing observed data with data that would be expected based on a particular hypothesis is the chi-square test. For instance, you might be interested in learning about the goodness of fit between the observed and expected if, by Mendel's laws, you predicted that 10 of 20 offspring from a cross would be male and the actual number that was observed was 8 males. Did other factors cause the deviations or the differences between what was observed and what was expected, or were they just the product of chance? The chi-square test is always testing what scientists call the null hypothesis, which states that there is no significant difference between the expected and observed result. The question is, how much deviation can occur before you, the investigator, must conclude that something other than chance is at work, causing the observed to differ from the expected? Theoretically, we should anticipate 100 heads and 100 tails when a coin is tossed 200 times. However, these outcomes are rarely realized in real life. A Greek letter called χ^2, which is pronounced as chi-square, is used to express how much theory and observation differ from one another. The observed and expected frequencies coincide exactly if $\chi = 0$. The value of χ^2 increases with the degree of difference between the observed and expected frequencies.

Therefore, χ^2 provides an indicator of how well theory and observation match.

If O_i (i = 1, 2, ……, n) is a set of observed (experimental) frequencies and E_i (i = 1, 2, ……, n) is the corresponding set of expected (theoretical or hypothetical) frequencies, then, χ^2 is defined as

$$\chi^2 = \sum_{i=1}^{n} \left[\frac{(O_i - E_i)^2}{E_i} \right]$$

where $\Sigma O_i = \Sigma E_i$ = N (total frequency) and degrees of freedom (difference)= (n – 1).

1. If $\chi^2 = 0$, the observed and theoretical frequencies agree exactly.
2. If $\chi^2 > 0$ they do not agree exactly.

Degrees of Freedom

We must ascertain the degrees of freedom by comparing the computed value of χ2 with the table value. We can use our independent choice for any three numbers only, with the fourth being 50 minus the sum of the three numbers we choose, if we have to choose any four numbers whose sum equals 50. As a result, even though we could have chosen any four numbers, one restriction limited our options to three. Our degrees of freedom were four minus one, or three. There was only one restriction on our freedom. Our freedom of choice will be further restricted if two restrictions are placed, resulting in degrees of freedom of 4 – 2 = 2. Generally speaking, the total number of observations less the total number of independent constraints placed on the observations equals the number of degrees of freedom. The Greek letter ν, which represents "nu," is commonly used to indicate degrees of freedom or difference. Thus, for a set of data consisting of n observations, $\nu = n - k$, where k is the number of independent constraints.

Applications

χ^2 test is one of the simplest and the most general tests known. It applies to a very large number of problems in practice which can be summed up under the following heads:

1. as a test of goodness of fit.
2. as a test of independence of attributes.
3. as a test of homogeneity of independent estimates of the population variance.
4. as a test of the hypothetical value of the population variance s^2.
5. as a list to the homogeneity of independent estimates of the population correlation coefficient.

Conditions for Applying χ^2 Test

The following are the conditions that should be satisfied before the χ^2 test can be applied:

a) N, the total number of frequencies should be large. It is difficult to say what constitutes largeness, but as an arbitrary figure, we may say that N should be at least 50, however small the number of cells.

b) To determine the degrees of freedom in a statistical analysis, it is essential to evaluate the relationship between the number of observations and the constraints imposed on them. When selecting a set of values, the total number of independent choices is reduced by the constraints that govern their sum or relationship. For instance, if we are tasked with selecting five numbers that must total 100, the choice of the first four numbers inherently restricts the fifth, as it must be the difference between 100 and the sum of the first four. This leads to a calculation of degrees of freedom as the total number of observations minus the number of constraints. In this case, with five observations and one constraint, the degrees of freedom would be 5 – 1, resulting in four. If additional constraints are introduced, the degrees of freedom decrease accordingly, illustrating the fundamental principle that the flexibility in data analysis is contingent upon the number of independent choices available. The symbol ν, representing degrees of freedom, succinctly encapsulates this concept, where ν = n – k, with n denoting the total observations and k the independent constraints applied.

c) The constraints on the cell frequencies, if any, should be linear.

6.3.1. The X² Distribution

For large sample sizes, the sampling distribution of χ^2 can be closely approximated by a continuous curve known as the chi-square distribution. The probability function of χ^2 distribution is given by

$$f(\chi^2) = c(\chi^2)^{(\nu/2-1)}\, e^{-x^2/2}$$

where e = 2.71828, ν = number of degrees of freedom; c = a constant depending only on ν.

The degrees of freedom are represented symbolically by the letter ν or by difference, and they can be found using the formula ν = n – k, where k is the number of independent constraints. When fitting a Poisson distribution, the number of degrees of freedom is two less than the number of classes because the Poisson distribution's parameter is determined by using the arithmetic mean and total frequency. In general, fitting a binomial distribution results in one lower degree of freedom than the number of classes. A normal curve can have three fewer degrees of freedom than there are classes because the total frequency, mean, and standard deviation are used in the fitting process. The degrees of freedom are equal to n – 1 if the data is presented as a sequence of "n" numbers. When the distribution is Binomial, the difference is n – 1. When the distribution is Poisson, the difference is n – 2. When the distribution is Normal, the difference is n – 3.

6.3.2. X² Test As A Test of Goodness of Fit

The χ2 test allows us to determine how well theoretical distributions, like Poisson, Normal, or Binomial, perform. conform to actual distributions, i. E. distributions derived from a representative sample. Fit is deemed good if the computed χ2 value is smaller than the table value at a given level of significance (usually 5 percent), i.e., E. fluctuations in simple sampling are the cause of the discrepancy between actual and expected frequencies. A larger calculated χ2 value than the value in the table indicates a poor fit.

6.3.3. Chi-Square Test for Independence

How to perform a chi-square test for independence is covered in this section. When you have two categorical variables from a single population, you apply the test. It's employed to ascertain whether the two variables have a meaningful relationship or not. Voters may be categorized in an election survey, for instance, based on their preferred party (Democrat, Republican, or Independent) and gender (male or female). To find out if gender influences voting preference, we could perform an independence test using a chi-square test. This example is taken into consideration in the lesson's final sample problem.

6.3.3.1. When to Use Chi-Square Test for Independence

The test procedure described in this lesson is appropriate when the following conditions are met:

- The sampling method is simple random sampling.
- The variables under study are each categorical.
- If sample data are displayed in a contingency table, the expected frequency count for each cell of the table is at least 5.

This approach consists of four steps: (1) state the hypotheses, (2) formulate an analysis plan, (3) analyze sample data, and (4) interpret results.

6.3.3.2. State the Hypotheses

Suppose that Variable A has *r* levels, and Variable B has *c* levels. The null hypothesis states that knowing the level of Variable A does not help you predict the level of Variable B. That is, the variables are independent.

- H_0: Variable A and Variable B are independent.
- H_a: Variable A and Variable B are not independent.

The alternative hypothesis is that knowing the level of Variable A *can* help you predict the level of Variable B. Support for the alternative hypothesis suggests that the variables are related; but the relationship is not necessarily causal, in the sense that one variable "causes" the other.

6.3.3.3. Formulate an Analysis Plan

The analysis plan describes how to use sample data to accept or reject the null hypothesis. The plan should specify the following elements.

- **Significance level.** Often, researchers choose significance levels equal to 0.01, 0.05, or 0.10; but any value between 0 and 1 can be used.
- **Test method.** Use the chi-square test for independence to determine whether there is a significant relationship between two categorical variables.

6.3.3.4. Analyze Sample Data

Using sample data, find the degrees of freedom, expected frequencies, test statistic, and the P-value associated with the test statistic. The approach described in this section is illustrated in the sample problem at the end of this lesson.

- **Degrees of freedom.** The degrees of freedom (DF) is equal to:

  $DF = (r - 1) * (c - 1)$

  where r is the number of levels for one categorical variable, and c is the number of levels for the other categorical variable.
- **Expected frequencies.** The expected frequency counts are computed separately for each level of one categorical variable at each level of the other categorical variable. Compute r * c expected frequencies, according to the following formula.

  $E_{r,c} = (n_r * n_c) / n$

  where $E_{r,c}$ is the expected frequency count for level *r* of Variable A and level *c* of Variable B, n_r is the total number of sample observations at level r of Variable A, n_c is the total number of sample observations at level *c* of Variable B, and n is the total sample size.
- **Test statistic.** The test statistic is a chi-square random variable (X^2) defined by the following equation.

  $X^2 = \Sigma [(O_{r,c} - E_{r,c})^2 / E_{r,c}]$

where $O_{r,c}$ is the observed frequency count at level *r* of Variable A and level *c* of Variable B, and $E_{r,c}$ is the expected frequency count at level *r* of Variable A and level *c* of Variable B.

- **P-value.** The P-value is the probability of observing a sample statistic as extreme as the test statistic. Since the test statistic is a chi-square, use the Chi-Square Distribution Calculator to assess the probability associated with the test statistic. Use the degrees of freedom computed above.

6.3.3.5. Interpret Results

If the sample findings are unlikely, given the null hypothesis, the researcher rejects the null hypothesis. Typically, this involves comparing the P-value to the significance level, and rejecting the null hypothesis when the P-value is less than the significance level.

6.3.3.6. Test Your Understanding

1. Problem

A public opinion poll surveyed a simple random sample of 1000 voters. Respondents were classified by gender (male or female) and by voting preference (Republican, Democrat, or Independent). Results are shown in the contingency table below (see **Table 6.2**).

Table 6.2. *Phenomena of Voting Preferences*

	Voting Preferences			**Row total**
	Republican	**Democrat**	**Independent**	
Male	200	150	50	400
Female	250	300	50	600
Column total	450	450	100	1000

Source: https://www.transtutors.com/questions/smoking-and-grades-1266924.htm

Is there a gender gap? Do the men's voting preferences differ significantly from the women's preferences? Use a 0.05 level of significance.

2. Solution

The solution to this problem takes four steps: (1) state the hypotheses, (2) formulate an analysis plan, (3) analyze sample data, and (4) interpret results. We work through the steps below:

- **State the hypotheses.** The first step is to state the null hypothesis and an alternative hypothesis.
  - H_0: Gender and voting preferences are independent.
  - H_a: Gender and voting preferences are not independent.
- **Formulate an analysis plan**. For this analysis, the significance level is 0.05. Using sample data, we will conduct a chi-square test for independence.
- **Analyze sample data**. Applying the chi-square test for independence to sample data, we compute the degrees of freedom, the expected frequency counts, and the chi-square

test statistic. Based on the chi-square statistic and the degrees of freedom, we determine the P-value.

- $DF = (r - 1) * (c - 1) = (2 - 1) * (3 - 1) = 2$
- $E_{r,c} = (n_r * n_c) / n$
- $E_{1,1} = (400 * 450) / 1000 = 180000/1000 = 180$
- $E_{1,2} = (400 * 450) / 1000 = 180000/1000 = 180$
- $E_{1,3} = (400 * 100) / 1000 = 40000/1000 = 40$
- $E_{2,1} = (600 * 450) / 1000 = 270000/1000 = 270$
- $E_{2,2} = (600 * 450) / 1000 = 270000/1000 = 270$
- $E_{2,3} = (600 * 100) / 1000 = 60000/1000 = 60$
- $X^2 = \Sigma [(O_{r,c} - E_{r,c})^2 / E_{r,c}]$
- $X^2 = (200 - 180)^2/180 + (150 - 180)^2/180 + (50 - 40)^2/40$
- $+ (250 - 270)^2/270 + (300 - 270)^2/270 + (50 - 60)^2/60$
- $X^2 = 400/180 + 900/180 + 100/40 + 400/270 + 900/270 + 100/60$
- $X^2 = 2.22 + 5.00 + 2.50 + 1.48 + 3.33 + 1.67 = 16.2$

where DF is the degrees of freedom, r is the number of levels of gender, c is the number of levels of voting preference, n_r is the number of observations from level *r* of gender, n_c is the number of observations from level *c* of voting preference, n is the number of observations in the sample, $E_{r,c}$ is the expected frequency count when gender is level *r* and voting preference is level *c*, and $O_{r,c}$ is the observed frequency count when gender is level *r* voting preference is level *c*. The P-value is the probability that a chi-square statistic having 2 degrees of freedom is more extreme than 16.2.

- We use the Chi-Square Distribution Calculator to find $P(X^2 > 16.2) = 0.0003$.
- **Interpret results**. Since the P-value (0.0003) is less than the significance level (0.05), we cannot accept the null hypothesis. Thus, we conclude that there is a relationship between gender and voting preference.

6.4. Reliability of the Estimates

The data presented, estimates for the population as a whole although they are based on a sample survey. As such, they are prone to errors, which may be of two types.

6.4.1. Sampling Errors

Sampling errors occur because only a sample of the population is investigated. The particular sample used in this survey is one of a large number of possible samples of the same size that could have been selected using the same sampling method. Estimates based on different samples will differ from one another, and almost all of them will differ from the value obtained had a complete census has been taken – "the census value."

- The estimate X′ is the value, estimated from the specific sample of this survey, of the corresponding value X that would have been obtained had a complete census been conducted.
- The sampling error σ(X′) is a measure of the variability between the different values of the estimate that would have been obtained from all possible samples of the same size and derived by the same sampling method and the census value obtained under the same conditions of data collection.

The main aim of the sampling theory is to draw a valid conclusion about the population parameters based on the sample results. In doing this we may commit the following two types of errors:

- ***Type I Error***. When H_0 is true, we may reject it.

P(Reject H_0 when it is true) = P(Reject H_0/H_0) = α

α is called the size of the type I error also referred to as producer's risk.

- ***Type II Error***. When H_0 is wrong we may accept it P(Accept H_0 when it is wrong) = P(Accept H_0/H_1) = β . β is called the size of the type II error, also referred to as consumer risk.

For larger samples corresponding to the statistic t, the variable $z = \frac{t - E(t)}{S.E(t)}$ is normally distributed with a mean of 0 and variance of 1. The value of z given above under the null hypothesis is known as the test statistic.

The critical value of z_α of the test statistic at a level of significance α for a two-tailed test is given by

$$p(|z| > z_\alpha) = \alpha \quad (1)$$

i.e., z_α is the value of z so that the total area of the critical region on both tails is α. Since the normal curve is symmetrical, from equation (1), we get

$$p(z > z_\alpha) + p(z < -z_\alpha) = \alpha; \; i.e., \; 2p(z > z_\alpha) = \alpha; \; p(z > z_\alpha) = \alpha/2$$

i.e., the area of each tail is $\alpha/2$

The critical value $z\alpha$ is that value such that the area to the right of z_α is $\alpha/2$ and the area to the left of $-z_\alpha$ is $\alpha/2$.

In the case of the one-tailed test, $p(z > z_\alpha) = \alpha$ if it is right-tailed; $p(z < -z_\alpha) = \alpha$ if it is left-tailed.

The critical value of z for a single-tailed test (right or left) at the level of significance α is the same as the critical value of z for a two-tailed test at level of significance 2α.

Using the equation, also using the normal tables, the critical value of z at different levels of significance (α) for both single tailed and two tailed test are calculated and listed below. The equations are

$$p(|z| > z_\alpha) = \alpha; \; p(z > z_\alpha) = \alpha; \; p(z < -z_\alpha) = \alpha$$

6.4.2. Steps in Testing of Statistical Hypothesis

The steps in testing of statistical hypothesis are given below:

- ***Step 1***. Null hypothesis. Set up H_0 in clear terms.
- ***Step 2***. Alternative hypothesis. Set up H_1, so that we could decide whether we should use one-tailed test or two-tailed test.

- ***Step 3***. Level of significance. Select the appropriate level of significance in advance depending on the reliability of the estimates.
- ***Step 4***. Test statistic. Compute the test statistic $z = \dfrac{t - E(t)}{S.E(t)}$ under the null hypothesis.
- ***Step 5***. Conclusion. Compare the computed value of z with the critical value z_α at level of significance (α).

If $|z| > z_\alpha$, we reject H_0 and conclude that there is significant difference. If $|z| < z_\alpha$, we accept H_0 and conclude that there is no significant difference.

6.4.3. Non-Sampling Errors

The sampling theory generally assumes that it is possible to obtain and tabulate each population unit's true value without making any mistakes. This presumption might not hold in reality for a variety of reasons and practical limitations. As a result, there are mistakes in the tabulation and the observations. Non-sampling errors are those that result from causes other than sampling. In surveys and censuses, non-sampling errors are unavoidable. While there is no sampling error in the data gathered through full enumeration during a census, non-sampling error may still exist. Both sampling and non-sampling errors may be present in the data gathered from sample surveys. Non-sampling errors result from sources other than the inductive procedure used to extrapolate population information from a sample. While non-sampling error tends to increase with sample size, sampling errors generally decrease as sample size grows. The non-sampling errors may occasionally be significant and call for more consideration than the sampling error. It is assumed in any survey that each population unit's precise value for the characteristic to be measured has been determined. There is such a thing as a singular value. This is known as the characteristic's true value for the population value. Survey values, which are different from true values in practical applications, are data gathered on the chosen units. This discrepancy between the observed and true values is known as the response error or observational error. The primary causes of such an error are imprecise measurement methods and inconsistent investigator performance.

6.4.3.1. Sources of Non-Sampling Errors

Non-Sampling errors can occur at every stage of planning and execution of a survey or census. It occurs at planning stage, field work stage as well as at tabulation and computation stage. The main sources of the non-sampling errors are

- lack of proper specification of the domain of study and scope of investigation,
- incomplete coverage of the population or sample,
- faulty definition,
- defective methods of data collection and
- tabulation errors

More specifically, one or more of the following reasons may give rise to non-sampling errors or indicate its presence:

- The data specification may be inadequate and inconsistent with the objectives of the survey or census.
- Due to imprecise definition of the boundaries of area units, incomplete or wrong identification of units, faulty methods of enumeration, etc., the data may be duplicated or may be omitted.
- The methods of interview and observation collection may be inaccurate or inappropriate.
- The questionnaire, definitions, and instructions may be ambiguous.

- The investigators may be inexperienced or not trained properly.
- The recall errors may pose difficulty in reporting the true data.
- The scrutiny of data is not adequate.
- The coding, tabulation, etc. of the data may be erroneous.
- There can be errors in presenting and printing the tabulated results, graphs etc.
- In a sample survey, the non-sampling errors arise due to defective frames and faulty selection of sampling units.

These sources are not exhaustive but surely indicate the possible source of errors. Non-sampling errors may be broadly classified into three categories.

a. **Specification errors:** These errors occur at the planning stage due to various reasons, e.g., inadequate and inconsistent specification of data concerning the objectives of surveys/ census, omission or duplication of units due to imprecise definitions, faulty method of enumeration/interview/ ambiguous schedules etc.

b. **Ascertainment errors:** These errors occur at the field stage due to various reasons e.g., lack of trained and experienced investigations, recall errors and another type of errors in data collection, lack of adequate inspection, and lack of supervision of primary staff, etc.

c. **Tabulation errors:** These errors occur at the tabulation stage due to various reasons, e.g., inadequate scrutiny of data, errors in processing the data, errors in publishing the tabulated results, graphs, etc.

Ascertainment errors may be further sub-divided into

i. Coverage errors owing to over-enumeration or under-enumeration of the population or the sample, resulting from duplication or omission of units and the non-response.

ii. Content errors relating to the wrong entries due to the errors on the part of investigators and respondents.

The same division can be made in the case of tabulation error also. There is a possibility of missing data or repetition of data at the tabulation stage which gives rise to coverage errors and also of errors in coding, calculations, etc. which gives rise to content errors.

6.4.3.2. Treatment of Non-Sampling Errors

Some conceptual background is needed for the mathematical treatment of non-sampling errors.

1. Total error:

Difference between the sample survey estimate and the parametric true value being estimated is termed as total error.

2. Sampling error:

If complete accuracy can be ensured in the procedures such as determination, identification, and observation of sample units and the tabulation of collected data, then the total error would consist only of the error due to sampling, termed as sampling error.

The measure of sampling error is a mean squared error (MSE). The MSE is the difference between the estimator and the true value and has two components:

a. square of sampling bias.

b. sampling variance.

If the results are also subjected to the non-sampling errors, then the total error would have both sampling and non-sampling errors.

6.4.3.3. Total Bias

The difference between the expected value and the true value of the estimator is termed as total bias. This consists of sampling bias and non-sampling bias.

Non-sampling bias: For the sake of simplicity, assume that the two following steps are involved in the randomization:

i. for selecting the sample of units and
ii. for selecting the survey personnel.

Let $\hat{\bar{Y}}_{sr}$ be the estimate of the population mean $\bar{Y}$ based on s[th] sample of units supplied by the rth sample of the survey personnel. The conditional expected value of $\hat{\bar{Y}}_{sr}$ taken over the second step of randomization for a fixed sam]

$$E_r(\hat{\bar{Y}}_{sr}) = \hat{\bar{Y}}_{so},$$

which may be different from $\hat{\bar{Y}}_{sr}$ based on true values of the units in the sample. The expected value of $\hat{\bar{Y}}_{so}$ over the first step of randomization gives

$$E_s(\hat{\bar{Y}}_{so}) = \bar{Y}^*,$$

which is the value for which an unbiased estimator can be had by the specified survey process. The value $\bar{Y}^*$ maybe different from the true population mean $\bar{Y}$ and the total bias is given as

$$Bias_t(\hat{\bar{Y}}_{sr}) = \bar{Y}^* - \bar{Y}.$$

The sampling bias is given by

$$Bias(\hat{\bar{Y}}) = E_s(\hat{\bar{Y}}_s) - \bar{Y}.$$

The non-sampling bias is

$$Bias_r(\hat{\bar{Y}}_{sr}) = Bias_t(\hat{\bar{Y}}_{sr}) - Bias_s(\hat{\bar{Y}}_s)$$
$$= \bar{Y}^* - E_s(\hat{\bar{Y}}_s)$$
$$= E_s(\hat{\bar{Y}}_{so} - \hat{\bar{Y}}_s)$$

which is the expected value of the non-sampling deviation.

Complete enumeration eliminates sampling bias, leaving non-sampling bias as the only source of total bias. When it comes to sample surveys, the non-sampling bias makes up the entirety of the bias. By surveying a sample of population units with superior data collection and compilation techniques than those used in general census conditions, the non-sampling bias in a census can be estimated. This purpose may be served by the so-called post-enumeration surveys, which are typically carried out shortly after the census to assess the quality of census data. By resurveying a subsample of the original sample using improved survey techniques, the ascertainment bias in a large-scale sample survey can be estimated. Comparing the values of the units obtained from the two surveys and reconciling the disparate figures through additional investigation is another way to verify survey data. Reconciliation surveys are the term used to describe this type of checking.

6.4.3.4. Non-Sampling Variance

The MSE of $\hat{\bar{Y}}_{sr}$ based on s[th] sample of units and supplied by r[th] sample of the survey personnel is

$$MSE(\hat{\bar{Y}}_{sr}) = E_{sr}(\hat{\bar{Y}}_{sr} - \bar{Y})^2$$

where $\bar{Y}$ is the true value being estimated. This takes into account both the sampling and the non-sampling errors, i.e.,

$$MSE(\hat{\bar{Y}}_{sr}) = Var(\hat{\bar{Y}}_{sr}) + \left[Bias(\hat{\bar{Y}}_{sr}) \right]^2$$
$$= E(\hat{\bar{Y}}_{sr} - \bar{Y}^*)^2 + (\bar{Y}^* - \bar{Y})^2$$

where $\bar{Y}^*$ is the expected value of the estimator taken over both steps of randomization.

Taking the variance over the two steps of randomization, we get

$$Var_{sr}(\hat{\bar{Y}}_{sr}) = Var_s\left[E_r(\hat{\bar{Y}}_{sr}) \right] + E_s\left[Var_r(\hat{\bar{Y}}_{sr}) \right]$$
$$= \underbrace{Var_s\left[\hat{\bar{Y}}_{so} \right]}_{\text{sampling variance}} + \underbrace{E_s\left[E_r(\hat{\bar{Y}}_{sr} - \hat{\bar{Y}}_{so})^2 \right]}_{\text{non-samping variance}}.$$

Note that

$$\hat{\bar{Y}}_{sr} - \hat{\bar{Y}}_{so} = (\hat{\bar{Y}}_{sr} - \hat{\bar{Y}}_{so} - \hat{\bar{Y}}_{or} + \bar{Y}^*) + (\hat{\bar{Y}}_{or} - \hat{\bar{Y}}^*)$$

where

$$\hat{\bar{Y}}_{or} = E_s(\hat{\bar{Y}}_{sr}).$$

$$E(\hat{\bar{Y}}_{sr} - \hat{\bar{Y}}_{so})^2 = \underbrace{E_{sr}(\hat{\bar{Y}}_{sr} - \hat{\bar{Y}}_{so} - \hat{\bar{Y}}_{or} + \hat{\bar{Y}}^*)^2}_{\text{Interaction between sampling and non-sampling errors}} + \underbrace{E_r(\hat{\bar{Y}}_{or} - \hat{\bar{Y}}^*)^2}_{\text{Variance between survey personnel}}$$

The MSE of an estimator consists of,

- sampling variance,
- interaction between the sampling and the non-sampling errors,
- variance between survey personnel and
- square of the sum of sampling and non-sampling biases

In complete census, the MSE is composed of only the non-sampling variance and the square of the non-sampling bias.

6.4.3.5. Non-Response Error

The non-response error could be brought on by respondents declining to provide information or by sampling units not being reachable. This error results from the possibility that the set of units being excluded has characteristics that are so dissimilar from the set of units that are surveyed that they skew the results. Since some of the expected units in the sample or population are missing, this error is known as a non-response error. One strategy for addressing the issue of non-response is to exert every effort to gather data from a subsample of the units that did not reply on the first try.

6.4.3.6. Measurement and Control of Errors:

Some suitable methods and adequate procedures for control can be adopted before initiating the main census or sample survey. Some separate programs for estimating the different types of non-sampling errors are also required. Some such procedures are as follows:

1. Consistency checks:

   Trained and experienced personnel can perform an independent duplicate census or sample survey on a relatively smaller group. It is possible to identify non-sampling errors and determine their extent if the sample is appropriately designed and the checking procedure is executed effectively. This process is known as the "sample check method."

2. Sample check:

   Trained and experienced personnel can perform an independent duplicate census or sample survey on a relatively smaller group. It is possible to identify non-sampling errors and determine their extent if the sample is appropriately designed and the checking procedure is executed effectively. This process is known as the "sample check method."

3. Post-census and post-survey checks:

   It is a type of sample check in which a sample (or subsample) is selected of the units covered in the census (or survey) and re-enumerate or re-survey it by using better trained and more experienced survey staff than those involved in the main investigation. This procedure is called as post-survey check or post-census. The effectiveness of such check surveys can be increased by

   - re-enumerating or re-surveying immediately after the main census to avoid recall error
   - Taking steps to minimize the conditioning effect that the main survey may have on the work of the check-survey

4. External record check:

   If possible, select a sample of pertinent units from an alternative source to verify that all units have been listed in the primary inquiry and to see if there are any differences in the values when compared. It is not necessary for the list from which the check sample is taken to be exhaustive.

5. Quality control techniques:

   In large-scale surveys and censuses, the reliability of the final results can be increased by evaluating the quality of the data using statistical quality control tools like control charts and acceptance sampling techniques.

6. Study or recall error:

   Response errors can be caused by several things, including recall errors, interview techniques, respondent attitudes toward the survey, and investigator skill. The length of the reporting period and the time elapsed between the reporting period and the survey data determine the recall error. Gathering and examining information from multiple reporting periods in a sample (or sub-sample) of the units included in the survey or census is one method of researching recall errors.

7. Interpenetrating sub-samples:

   Since interpenetrating sub-samples can be used to obtain information on non-sampling errors like differences resulting from differential interviewer bias, different methods of eliciting information, etc., they aid in the assessment of the quality of the information. Following the sub-samples surveying by various teams of investigators and processing by various teams of workers during the tabulation stage, a comparison of the final estimates derived from the sub-samples offers a comprehensive assessment of the survey results' quality. (Freire et al., 2019) (Dorey et al., 2010).

A Closer Look

Parametric Tests

In the realm of health research and analysis, hypothesis testing plays a pivotal role in concluding various phenomena, treatments, or interventions. One common scenario involves assuming certain properties about the distribution of health-related data, such as employing t-tests for means and F-tests for variances. When conducting hypothesis tests for means in health-related studies, researchers often aim to assess whether there is a significant difference between the means of two groups or the mean of a sample against a known or hypothesized population mean. For instance, in clinical trials evaluating the efficacy of a new medication, researchers might employ a two-sample t-test to compare the mean improvement in health outcomes between a group receiving the medication and a control group. Similarly, in epidemiological studies comparing the average blood pressure levels between different age groups, a one-sample t-test could be utilized to determine if the mean blood pressure of a particular age group differs significantly from a population mean. The t-test assumes that the data follow a normal distribution and that the samples are independent and randomly selected, which are crucial considerations in health research to ensure the validity of the results.

On the other hand, F-tests for variances are commonly employed in health-related studies to assess whether the variability or dispersion of data differs significantly between two or more groups. Variance plays a crucial role in health research as it reflects the spread of observations around the mean and can provide insights into the consistency and stability of outcomes or measurements. For example, in assessing the effectiveness of a new surgical procedure compared to a conventional method, researchers might utilize an F-test to determine if there is a significant difference in the variability of recovery times between the two groups. Additionally, in quality control processes within healthcare settings, F-tests can be applied to evaluate whether there are significant differences in the variability of patient outcomes or treatment responses across different clinics or healthcare facilities. Similar to t-tests, F-tests assume that the data are normally distributed and that the samples are independent and randomly selected.

Summary

- Hypothesis testing procedures play a critical role in evaluating interventions, treatments, and other factors that may impact human well-being. These procedures are fundamental to clinical research, epidemiology, public health, and various other fields within the healthcare domain.
- Hypothesis testing is the method for determining the probability of an observed event that occurs only by chance. If chance were not the cause of an event, then something else must have been the cause, such as the treatment having affected the observed event (the outcome) that was measured.
- An analyst performs hypothesis testing on a statistical sample to present evidence of the plausibility of the null hypothesis. Measurements and analyses are conducted on a random sample of the population to test a theory. Analysts use a random population sample to test two hypotheses: the null and alternative hypotheses.
- Bootstrap distributions and randomization distributions are created using comparable simulation techniques. The observed sample statistic is the focal point of a bootstrap distribution, whereas the null hypothesis value is the focal point of a randomization distribution.
- A p-value is a metric that expresses the likelihood that an observed difference could have occurred by chance. As the p-value decreases the statistical significance of the observed difference increases. If the p-value is too low, you reject the null hypothesis.
- Medical providers often rely on evidence-based medicine to guide decision-making in practice. Often a research hypothesis is tested with results provided, typically with p values, confidence intervals, or both.
- P values are used in research to determine whether the sample estimate is significantly different from a hypothesized value. The p-value is the probability that the observed effect within the study would have occurred by chance if, in reality, there was no true effect.

References

1. Colquhoun, D. (2017). The reproducibility of research and the misinterpretation of p-values. *Royal Society Open Science, 4*(12), 171085.
2. Cooper, R. J., Wears, R. L., & Schriger, D. L. (2003). Reporting research results: Recommendations for improving communication. *Annals of Emergency Medicine, 41*(4), 561–564.
3. Doll, H., & Carney, S. (2007). Statistical approaches to uncertainty: P values and confidence intervals unpacked. *Equine Veterinary Journal, 39*(3), 275–276.
4. Dorey, F. (2011). Statistics in brief: Interpretation and use of p values: All p values are not equal. *Clinical Orthopaedics and Related Research, 469*(11), 3259–3261.
5. Dorey, F. J. (2010). In brief: Statistics in brief: Confidence intervals: What is the real result in the target population? *Clinical Orthopaedics and Related Research, 468*(11), 3137–3138.
6. Ferrill, M. J., Brown, D. A., & Kyle, J. A. (2010). Clinical versus statistical significance: Interpreting P values and confidence intervals related to measures of association to guide decision-making. *Journal of Pharmacy Practice, 23*(4), 344–351.

7. Fethney, J. (2010). Statistical and clinical significance, and how to use confidence intervals to help interpret both. *Australian Critical Care, 23*(2), 93–97.

8. Freire, A. P. C. F., Elkins, M. R., Ramos, E. M. C., & Moseley, A. M. (2019). Use of 95% confidence intervals in the reporting of between-group differences in randomized controlled trials: Analysis of a representative sample of 200 physical therapy trials. *Brazilian Journal of Physical Therapy, 23*(4), 302–310.

9. Gardner, M. J., & Altman, D. G. (1986). Confidence intervals rather than P values: Estimation rather than hypothesis testing. *British Medical Journal (Clinical Research Edition), 292*(6522), 746–750.

10. Hayat, M. J. (2010). Understanding statistical significance. *Nursing Research, 59*(3), 219–223.

11. Infanger, D., & Schmidt-Trucksäss, A. (2019). P value functions: An underused method to present research results and to promote quantitative reasoning. *Statistics in Medicine, 38*(21), 4189–4197.

12. Jones, M., Gebski, V., Onslow, M., & Packman, A. (2002). Statistical power in stuttering research: A tutorial. *Journal of Speech, Language, and Hearing Research, 45*(2), 243–255.

13. Liu, X. S. (2012). Implications of statistical power for confidence intervals. *British Journal of Mathematical and Statistical Psychology, 65*(3), 427–437.

14. Porcher, R. (2009). Reporting results of orthopaedic research: Confidence intervals and p values. *Clinical Orthopaedics and Related Research, 467*(10), 2736–2737.

15. Sedgwick, P. (2014). Pitfalls of statistical hypothesis testing: Type I and type II errors. *BMJ, 349*, g4287.

16. Spanos, A. (2014). Recurring controversies about P values and confidence intervals revisited. *Ecology, 95*(3), 645–651.

17. Tijssen, J. G., & Kolm, P. (2016). Demystifying the new statistical recommendations: The use and reporting of p values. *Journal of the American College of Cardiology, 68*(2), 231–233.

Chapter 7

POWER AND SAMPLE SIZE DETERMINATION

Contents

Introduction 194
7.1. Issues in Estimating Sample Size for Confidence Intervals Estimates 196
7.2. Issues in Estimating Sample Size for Hypothesis Testing 204
Summary 215
References 215

Introduction

Deciding on the right sample size to address the research question is a crucial step in any investigation. This module will concentrate on formulas that can be used to determine the sample size required to generate a confidence interval estimate with a given precision margin or to guarantee that a test of hypothesis has a high likelihood of identifying a significant parameter difference. Research questions should be sufficiently addressed by the number of participants in the studies, which should be planned accordingly. Both an insufficient number of participants and an excessive number of participants in a study waste time and resources for the investigators, participants, assessment tools, analysis, and other purposes. These circumstances can also be seen as unethical since it's possible that participants were put in danger as a result of a study that was unable to provide a crucial answer.

Based on statistical criteria, the formulas presented here provide estimates of the required sample size or sizes. However, budgetary or logistical limitations frequently dictate the sample size in research projects. Let's take an example where a study to assess a novel Down syndrome screening tool is suggested. Assume that the screening procedure is based on the examination of a blood sample obtained from expectant mothers. To assess the screening test's characteristics (eg., sensitivity and specificity), every expectant mother will be required to give a blood sample and have an amniocentesis performed. The goal is to compare the outcomes of the screening test and the amniocentesis, which is considered the gold standard. Assume that each participant will pay $250 for the collection and processing of their blood sample and $900 for their amniocentesis. Just these budgetary limitations may significantly reduce the total number of women who are eligible for enrolment. Analyzing the results of a statistical analysis requires taking into account both statistical and clinical significance; similarly, choosing the appropriate sample size for a study requires taking into account both logistical and statistical considerations.

Orientation and Directional Terms:

Terms	Definition	Illustration
Hypothesis	A hypothesis is a proposed explanation for a phenomenon. For a hypothesis to be a scientific hypothesis, the scientific method requires that one can test it.	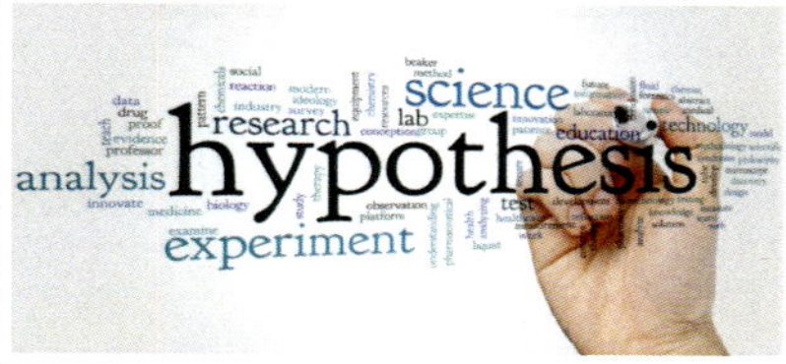
Margin of error	The margin of error is a statistic expressing the amount of random sampling error in the results of a survey.	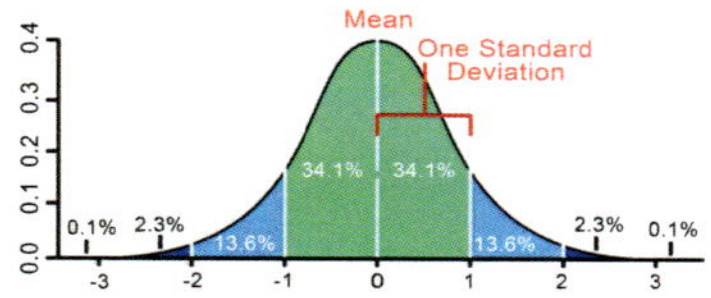
Blood pressure	Blood pressure is measured using two numbers: The first number, called systolic blood pressure, measures the pressure in your arteries when your heart beats.	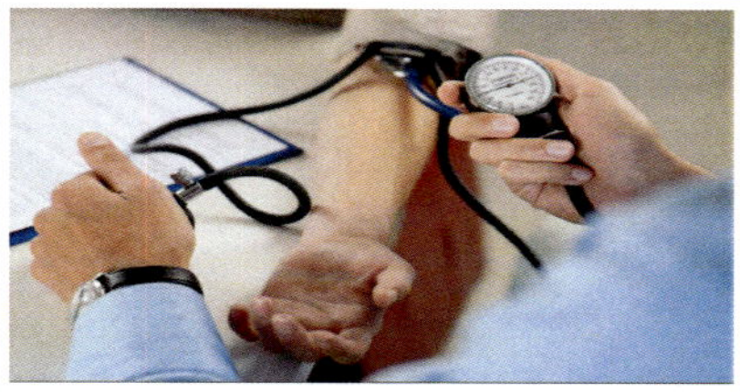
Confidence interval	A confidence interval is the mean of your estimate plus and minus the variation in that estimate.	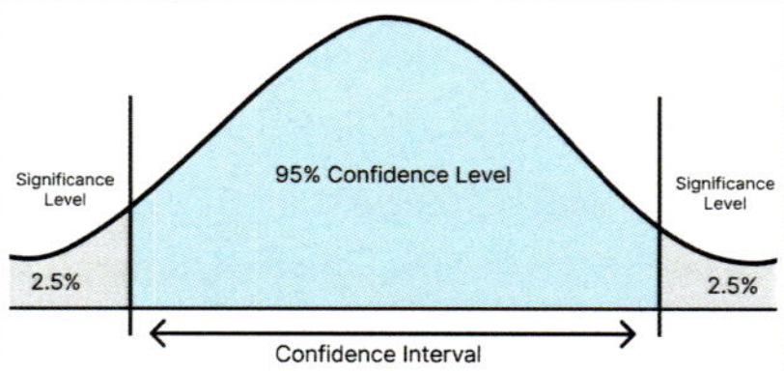
Hypothesis Testing	Hypothesis testing is a tool for making statistical inferences about the population data.	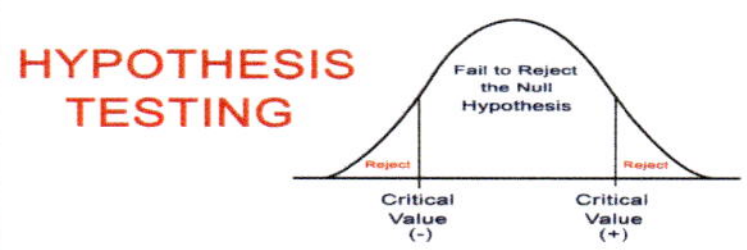

7.1. Issues in Estimating Sample Size for Confidence Intervals Estimates

The module on confidence intervals provided methods for estimating confidence intervals for various parameters (e.g., μ, p, (μ_1- μ_2), μ_d, (p_1-p_2)). Confidence intervals for every parameter take the following general form:

Point Estimate ± Margin of Error

In the module on confidence intervals, we derived the formula for the confidence interval for μ as

$$\overline{X} \pm z\frac{\sigma}{\sqrt{n}}.$$

In actuality, the population standard deviation is estimated using the sample standard deviation. It should be noted that when the sample size is small (n<30), a different formula is used to estimate the mean of a continuous outcome in a single population. To reflect the desired level of confidence, a value from the t distribution is used instead of one from the conventional normal distribution. We utilize the large sample formula displayed here when calculating sample sizes.

Note: The final sample size may be small, and the right confidence interval formula needs to be applied during the analysis phase. The point estimate for the population mean is the sample mean and the margin of error is $z\frac{\sigma}{\sqrt{n}}$. When designing studies, we want to know how big of a sample size is required to guarantee that the margin of error is small enough to be useful. Assume, for instance, that we wish to determine the average weight of female college students. After conducting research, we arrive at the following 95 percent confidence interval: 125 + 40 pounds, or 85 to 165 pounds. The confidence interval is meaningless because of the enormous margin of error. If the margin of error is 5 or 10 pounds, the 95 percent confidence interval would have a width (lower limit to upper limit) of 10 or 20 pounds, which would be instructive for the investigator. The desired margin of error must be specified by the investigator in order to calculate the required sample size. It is crucial to remember that this is a clinical or practical problem rather than a statistical one. Assume, for instance, that we wish to determine the average birth weight of children born to pregnant women who smoke. It is evident that the birth weight range of infants is considerably narrower than that of female college students. As a result, it makes sense to produce a confidence interval for the mean birth weight with a margin of error of no more than one or two pounds.

The margin of error in the one-sample confidence interval for μ can be written as follows:

$$E = z\frac{\sigma}{\sqrt{n}}.$$

Finding the sample size, n, that guarantees the margin of error, "E," stays below a given value is our aim. With a little algebra, we can solve for n using the formula above: multiply both sides of the equation by the square root of n. Then, since any number divided by itself equals 1, eliminate the square root of n from the denominator and numerator on the right side of the equation.

This leaves:

$$\sqrt{n}\,E = Z\sigma$$

Now divide both sides by "E" and cancel out "E" from the numerator and denominator on the left side. This leaves:

$$\sqrt{n} = \frac{Z\sigma}{E}$$

Finally, square both sides of the equation to get:

$$n = \left(\frac{z\sigma}{E}\right)^2.$$

This formula generates the sample size, **n**, required to ensure that the margin of error, **E**, does not exceed a specified value. To solve for **n**, we must input "**Z**," "**σ**," and "**E**."

- **Z** is the value from the table of probabilities of the standard normal distribution for the desired confidence level (e.g., Z = 1.96 for 95% confidence)
- **E** is the margin of error that the investigator specifies as important from a clinical or practical standpoint.
- **σ** is the standard deviation of the outcome of interest.

It can be challenging to estimate σ at times. We are organizing a study to estimate the unknown mean of a specific outcome variable in a population when we apply the sample size formula above. We are unlikely to be aware of that variable's standard deviation. Researchers frequently utilize the standard deviation from a prior study or a study conducted in a different but comparable population when calculating sample sizes. It is reasonable to use an appropriate estimate for the standard deviation because the computation of sample size does not involve statistical inference. The estimate can be obtained from an alternative study that was published in the literature; some researchers estimate the standard deviation by conducting a small pilot study. Typically, a pilot study has a small participant count (e.g., n=10) who are chosen at random, as opposed to by convenience. The sample standard deviation, which can be calculated using information from the pilot study participants, is a useful approximation for σ in the sample size formula. No matter how the estimate of the outcome's variability is calculated, it should always be conservative (i.e., as big as is appropriate), to ensure that the final sample size is not excessively small.

The formula $n = \left(\frac{z\sigma}{E}\right)^2$ produces the minimum sample size to ensure that the margin of error in a confidence interval will not exceed **E**. Investigators should take attrition or loss to follow-up into account when planning studies. The number of participants with complete data required to guarantee that the confidence interval's margin of error does not exceed E is provided by the formula above.

7.1.1. Sample Size for One Sample, Continuous Outcome

In studies where the plan is to estimate the mean of a continuous outcome variable in a single population, the formula for determining sample size is given below:

$$n = \left(\frac{z\sigma}{E}\right)^2$$

where **Z** is the value from the standard normal distribution reflecting the confidence level that will be used (e.g., Z = 1.96 for 95%), **σ** is the standard deviation of the outcome variable and **E** is the desired margin of error. The formula above generates the minimum number of subjects required to ensure that the margin of error in the confidence interval for μ does not exceed **E**.

Example 7.1.

Between the ages of three and five, children with congenital heart disease have a mean systolic blood pressure that an investigator wants to determine. With a margin of error of five units and a 95 percent confidence interval (so Z=1.96), how many children should be enrolled in the study? The investigators conducted a literature search and discovered that children with other cardiac defects have a systolic blood pressure standard deviation of between 15 and

20, although the exact value is unknown. To get the most conservative (largest) sample size, we take into account the larger standard deviation when estimating the sample size.

$$n = \left(\frac{z\sigma}{E}\right)^2 = \left(\frac{1.96 \times 20}{5}\right)^2 = 61.5.$$

A sample size of 62 is required to guarantee that the mean systolic blood pressure in children with congenital heart disease between the ages of 3 and 5 is within 5 units of the true mean, according to the 95 % confidence interval estimate.

Note: The sample size formulas always produce the bare minimum of subjects required to guarantee the desired precision, so we always round up. If we had taken a 15 standard deviation assumption, then n=35 would have been the sample size. It would be wise to use the larger standard deviation and schedule a study with 62 children because the estimates of the standard deviation were obtained from studies of children with other cardiac defects. Choosing the smaller sample size might result in an estimate of the confidence interval with a higher margin of error.

Example 7.2.

The mean birth weight of infants born to mothers who are 19 years of age or younger at full term (about 40 weeks gestation) is to be estimated by an investigator. For mothers who are 20 years of age or older, the mean birth weight of their full-term babies is 3510 g, with a standard deviation of 385 g. To guarantee that a 95 % confidence interval estimate of the mean birth weight of their infants has a margin of error not exceeding 100 g, how many women, aged 19 or younger, must be enrolled in the study?

$$n = \left(\frac{z\sigma}{E}\right)^2 = \left(\frac{1.96 \times 385}{100}\right)^2 = 56.9.$$

A sample of size 57 is required to guarantee that the 95 percent confidence interval estimate of the mean birth weight is within 100 grams of the true mean. The possibility that some women may deliver babies early must be taken into account by the researcher when designing the study. If women are recruited for the study while they are pregnant, then more than 57 women must be recruited in order to have 57 full-term deliveries available for analysis, after removing those who deliver prematurely. For instance, if five percent of the pregnant women are anticipated to give birth early (i.e., 95 % of the women will give birth at full term), then 60 women must sign up to make sure that 57 of them do.

The number of women who must be enrolled, N, is computed as

N (number to enrol) × (% retained) = Desired sample size,

$$N \times 0.95 = 57,$$

$$N = \frac{57}{0.95} = 60.$$

7.1.2. Sample Size for One Sample, Dichotomous Outcome

The formula for calculating sample size is used in research where the goal is to estimate the percentage of successes in a dichotomous outcome variable in a single population.

$$n = p(1-p)\left(\frac{z}{E}\right)^2.$$

where Z is the value, representing the confidence level to be used, from the standard normal distribution (e.g., where E is the intended margin of error and Z is 1.96 for the 95 percentiles. P is the population's success percentage. The study's goal is to produce a 95% confidence interval for the p, or unknown population proportion. The formula for calculating the sample size needed to determine p appears to require knowledge of p; however, this is a circular argument, as we would not need a study if we knew the population's success percentage! What we actually need is an estimated or predicted value for p. Since p has a range of 0 to 1, p(1-p) also has a range of 0 to 1. P=0.5 is the value of p that maximizes p(1-p). Therefore, the most conservative, or largest, sample size can be obtained using p=0.5, if there is no information available to approximate p.

Example 7.3.

An investigator wishes to calculate the percentage of first-year students at his university who smoke cigarettes at the moment (i.e., the rate of smoking among people). To guarantee that a 95% confidence interval estimate of the percentage of freshmen who smoke is within five percent of the actual percentage, how many freshmen should be included in the study?

Because we have no information on the proportion of freshmen who smoke, we use 0.5 to estimate the sample size as follows:

$$n = p(1-p)\left(\frac{z}{E}\right)^2 = 0.5(1-0.5)\left(\frac{1.96}{0.05}\right)^2 = 384.2.$$

To ensure that the 95% confidence interval estimate of the proportion of freshmen who smoke is within 5% of the true proportion, a sample of size 385 is needed.

Assume that two years ago, a similar study was carried out and it was discovered that 27% of freshmen smoked. It can be used to plan the study if the researcher thinks this is a realistic estimate of prevalence today.

$$n = p(1-p)\left(\frac{z}{E}\right)^2 = 0.27(1-0.27)\left(\frac{1.96}{0.05}\right)^2 = 302.9.$$

A sample of size 303 is required to guarantee that the 95% confidence interval estimate of the percentage of freshmen who smoke is within 5% of the true proportion. You will note that this sample size is significantly lower than the one that was previously estimated. A sample size based on a population proportion of 0.5 is always less than or equal to the one produced when the magnitude of the proportion in the population is known.

Example 7.4.

The goal of the study is to determine how common breast cancer is in Boston among women in their 40s and 45s. According to national data, one in 235 women will receive a breast cancer diagnosis by the age of 40. Given this, how many women must be included in the study to guarantee that the estimate is accurate? This corresponds to a prevalence of 43 per 10,000 women or a proportion of 0.0043 (0.43 %). Let's say the researcher wants the estimate to have a 95% confidence level and fall between 10 and 10,000 women.

The sample size is computed as follows:

$$n = p(1-p)\left(\frac{z}{E}\right)^2 =$$

$$0.0043(1-0.0043)\left(\frac{1.96}{0.0010}\right)^2 = 16,447.8.$$

A sample size of n=16,448 will guarantee that the prevalence of breast cancer is within 0.10, or 10 women per 10,000, of its true value, according to a 95% confidence interval estimate. Investigators may conclude that a sample of this size is not practical. Assume that, in terms of practicality, the investigators believed a sample size of five thousand would be appropriate. How precisely can we estimate the prevalence with a sample of size n=5,000? Recall that the confidence interval formula to estimate prevalence is:

$$\hat{p} \pm z\sqrt{\frac{\hat{p}(1-\hat{p})}{n}}.$$

Assuming that the prevalence of breast cancer in the sample is close to that based on national data, we would expect the margin of error to be approximately equal to

$$z\sqrt{\frac{\hat{p}(1-\hat{p})}{n}} = 1.96\sqrt{\frac{0.0043(1-0.0043)}{5000}} = 0.0018.$$

A 95 % confidence interval with n = 55000 women should have a margin of error of 0.0018, or 18 per 10,000. Whether this is accurate enough to address the research question is up to the investigators to determine. Please take note that the underlying assumption of this calculation is that Boston's breast cancer prevalence is comparable to the country as a whole. This could be a reasonable assumption or it might not be. The current study's goal is to determine the prevalence in Boston. The research team will need to carefully consider the implications of choosing a sample size of n = 5000, n = 16,448, or any other size in between, with input from clinical investigators and biostatisticians.

7.1.3. Sample Sizes for Two Independent Samples, Continuous Outcome

In studies where the plan is to estimate the difference in means between two independent populations, the formula for determining the sample sizes required in each comparison group is given below:

$$n_i = 2\left(\frac{z\sigma}{E}\right)^2$$

where Z is the value from the standard normal distribution indicating the confidence level that will be used, E is the intended margin of error, and n_i is the sample size needed in each group (i=1,2). Once more, the outcome variable's standard deviation is reflected by σ. Remember from the confidence intervals module that we used Sp, the pooled estimate of the common standard deviation, as a measure of outcome variability (based on pooling the data) when generating a confidence interval estimate for the difference in means, where Sp is computed as follows:

$$S_p = \sqrt{\frac{(n_1-1)s_1^2 + (n_2-1)s_2^2}{n_1+n_2-2}}$$

S_p can be calculated and applied to the sample size formula if information on the variability of the outcome in each comparison group is available. Nonetheless, it frequently happens that information about the variability of the result is limited to one group—typically the untreated (e.g., placebo control) or group that was not exposed. When organizing a clinical trial to examine a novel medication or method, information from previous trials involving a placebo or an active control group (i.e., a customary drug or course of therapy administered for the ailment being researched). To plan a future trial, one can use the standard deviation of the outcome variable measured in patients assigned to the placebo, control, or unexposed group.

Keep in mind that sample size estimates are produced by the sample size formula for samples of equal size. Alternative formulas can be utilized if a study is planned in which varying numbers of patients will be assigned, or varying numbers of patients will make up the comparison groups.

Example 7.5.

A clinical trial to assess a novel medication intended to raise HDL cholesterol (the "good" cholesterol) is being planned by an investigator. Participants will be recruited and randomly assigned to receive either a placebo or the new medication. Following 12 weeks of the prescribed treatment, each participant's HDL cholesterol will be assessed. The investigator anticipates that 10% of all participants will either drop out of the study or be lost to follow-up, based on experience with similar trials. The difference in mean HDL levels between patients receiving the new medication and those receiving a placebo will be measured, and a 95% confidence interval will be estimated. The maximum margin of error that the investigator would like to see is three units.

The sample sizes (i.e., the number of participants who must receive the new drug and the number who must receive a placebo) are computed as

$$n_i = 2\left(\frac{z\sigma}{E}\right)^2.$$

Determining the variability in the outcome of interest, in this case the HDL cholesterol standard deviation (σ), is a crucial task. We can use information from the Framingham Heart Study to plan this investigation. The standard deviation of HDL cholesterol is 17.1 among participants in the Framingham Offspring Study who were not receiving treatment for high cholesterol at the time of the seventh examination. We use this value and the other inputs to compute the sample sizes:

$$n_i = 2\left(\frac{z\sigma}{E}\right)^2 = 2\left(\frac{1.96 \times 17.1}{3}\right)^2 = 249.6.$$

The 95 % confidence interval for the difference in mean HDL levels will have a margin of error of no more than three units if samples of sizes $n_1 = 250$ and $n_2 = 250$ are used. Once more, the number of participants with complete data is indicated by these sample sizes. Ten percent attrition, or dropout, was the hypothesised rate by the investigators for both groups. To ensure that a total sample size of 500 is available at 12 weeks, the investigator needs to recruit more participants to allow for attrition.

N (number to enrol) × (% retained) = Desired sample size

$$N \times 0.90 = 500.$$

$$N = \frac{500}{0.90} = 556.$$

The investigator must enrol 556 participants. Each patient will be randomly assigned to receive either the new drug or a placebo; assuming that 10% are lost to follow-up, 500 will be available for analysis.

Example 7.6.

An investigator wishes to compare two diet plans for obese children. There are two types of diets: one low in fat and the other low in carbohydrates. At the beginning of the study, children are supposed to be weighed and enrolled. The low-fat or low-carb diet will then be assigned to each child at random. Every child will adhere to the prescribed diet for eight weeks, after which he or she will be weighed once more. We'll figure out how many pounds each child lost. According to data from adult diet trials, the researcher anticipates that 20% of all children will not finish the study. The investigator would like the margin of error to be no more than 3 pounds. The difference in weight loss between the two diets will be quantified using an estimated 95% confidence interval. How many kids ought to be enlisted for the research?

The sample sizes (i.e., the number of children who must follow the low-fat diet and the number of children who must follow the low-carbohydrate diet) are computed as

$$n_i = 2\left(\frac{z\sigma}{E}\right)^2.$$

Once more, the problem is figuring out how variable the outcome of interest is—in this case, the standard deviation (σ) of pounds lost over 8 weeks. Investigators used information from adult studies to plan this investigation. Assume that one such study had 100 participants in each diet group and compared the same diets for adults. According to the study, the average amount of weight lost over the course of eight weeks on a low-fat diet was 8.4 pounds, and the average amount of weight lost over the course of eight weeks on a low-carb diet was 7.7 pounds. These data can be used to estimate the common standard deviation in weight lost as

$$S_p = \sqrt{\frac{(n_1-1)s_1^2+(n_2-1)s_2^2}{n_1+n_2-2}} =$$

$$\sqrt{\frac{(100-1)(8.4)^2+(100-1)(7.7)^2}{100+100-2}} = 8.1.$$

We now use this value and the other inputs to compute the sample sizes:

$$n_i = 2\left(\frac{z\sigma}{E}\right)^2 = 2\left(\frac{1.96\times 8.1}{3}\right)^2 = 56.0.$$

The 95% confidence interval for the difference in weight lost between diets will have a margin of error of no more than 3 pounds if samples of sizes n_1 = 56 and n_2 = 56 are used. Once more, the number of children with complete data is indicated by these sample sizes. The researchers calculated an attrition rate of 20 percent. To guarantee that the entire sample size of 112 will be accessible after 8 weeks, the researcher must enlist additional participants to account for participant attrition.

N (number to enrol) × (% retained) = Desired sample size.

$$N \times 0.80 = 112.$$

$$N = \frac{112}{0.80} = 140.$$

The investigator must enrol 140 children. Each child will be randomly assigned to either the low-fat or low-carbohydrate diet; assuming that 20% are lost to follow-up, 112 will be available for analysis.

7.1.4. Sample Size for Matched Samples, Continuous Outcome

In studies where the plan is to estimate the mean difference of a continuous outcome based on matched data, the formula for determining sample size is given below:

$$n = \left(\frac{z\sigma_d}{E}\right)^2$$

where Z is the value, representing the confidence level to be used, from the standard normal distribution (e.g., E is the intended margin of error, σd is the standard deviation of the difference scores and Z = 1.96 for 95%). It's critical that the difference scores' standard deviation (e.g., Here, the sample size is suitably estimated using the difference between matched pairs or the difference based on measurements over time.

Example 7.7.

Let's say the researcher is thinking of using a crossover trial as an alternative design. Every child in the crossover trial adheres to one diet for eight weeks. Every eight weeks, the amount of weight lost is measured after the period. Youngsters will be grouped at random into the first diet (i.e., some people will start with a low-fat diet, while others will start with a low-carb diet. Over the 16-week study, 30% of the participants are expected to drop out, according to the investigators. Each child's weight loss on the low-fat and low-carb diets will be compared, and a confidence interval for the mean weight loss difference will be calculated. To guarantee a margin of error of no more than 3 pounds for a 95% confidence interval estimate of the mean difference in weight lost, how many kids are needed?

We require an estimate of the variability in the difference in weight loss between diets, rather than the variability in weight loss within either diet program, to calculate the sample size. Assume, from an adult crossover trial, that the standard deviation of the weight loss difference between a low-fat and a low-carb diet is roughly 9.1 lbs.

The sample size is computed as

$$n = \left(\frac{z\sigma_d}{E}\right)^2 = \left(\frac{1.96 \times 9.1}{3}\right)^2 = 35.3.$$

A sample size of 36 children with complete data is required to guarantee that the 95% confidence interval estimate of the mean difference in weight loss between diets is within 3 pounds of the true mean. The researchers calculated an attrition rate of thirty percent. To ensure that the total sample size of 36 is available at 16 weeks, the investigator needs to recruit 52 participants to allow for attrition:

N (number to enrol) × (% retained) = Desired sample size.

$$N \times 0.70 = 36.$$

$$N = \frac{36}{0.70} = 52.$$

As you can see, the crossover trial requires fewer patients than the trial that takes into account two parallel or concurrent comparison groups. Every child in the crossover trial receives every treatment (diet). Crossover trials have the potential to yield efficient sample sizes. In other ways though, the crossover can be difficult. When there is a loss to follow-up, the crossover trial presents challenges. Since every participant provides data for every treatment, if a participant disappears after finishing the first treatment, the data from that participant are useless without knowledge of the second treatment. When it comes to participant loss during follow-up, diet studies present unique challenges. Occasionally, individuals lose weight and decide they don't need to continue with the study, which leads to their withdrawal. Some participants give up because they are dissatisfied and fail to lose weight. When choosing the best study design, these and other factors need to be carefully taken into account.

7.1.5. Sample Sizes for Two Independent Samples, Dichotomous Outcome

In research where the goal is to calculate the variance in proportions between two separate populations (to estimate the difference in risk), the formula for determining the sample sizes required in each comparison group is:

$$n_i = \left[p_1(1-p_1) + p_2(1-p_2)\right]\left(\frac{z}{E}\right)^2$$

where n_i is the sample size required in each group (i=1,2), Z is the value from the standard normal distribution reflecting the confidence level that will be used (e.g., Z = 1.96 for 95%), and E is the desired margin of error. p_1 and p_2 are the proportions of successes in each comparison group. Again, here we are planning a study to generate a 95% confidence interval for the difference in unknown proportions, and the formula to estimate the sample sizes needed requires p_1 and p_2. To estimate the sample size, we need approximate values of p_1 and p_2. The values of p_1 and p_2 that maximize the sample size are p_1=p_2=0.5. Thus, if there is no information available to approximate p_1 and p_2, then 0.5 can be used to generate the most conservative, or largest, sample sizes.

As with the scenario involving two independent samples and a continuous outcome at the top of this page, it is possible that information about the percentage of successes in one group—typically the untreated (e.g., placebo control) or group that was not exposed. If so, the above formula can be applied to both p_1 and p_2 using the known proportion. For samples of the same size, the formula above yields sample size estimates. Alternative formulas can be utilized if a study is planned in which varying numbers of patients will be assigned, or varying numbers of patients will make up the comparison groups.

Example 7.8.

The goal of the investigation is to calculate the risk of preterm birth from smoking during pregnancy. Premature deliveries occur before 37 weeks of pregnancy; a normal pregnancy lasts about 40 weeks. In the United States, about 12 % of infants are born prematurely, according to the 2005 National Vital Statistics report. The researcher intends to gather information by reviewing medical records and to produce a 95 percent confidence interval for the difference between the percentages of babies born prematurely to pregnant women who smoked and those who did not. To guarantee that the 95 % confidence interval for the proportional difference has a margin of error of no more than 4 %, how many women should be enrolled in the study?

The numbers of the samples (i.e., the number of pregnant women who smoked and did not smoke) can be calculated using the above formula. According to national data, 12 % of babies are born before their due date. In calculating the sample size, we will utilize that estimate for both groups.

$$n_i = \left[p_1(1-p_1)+p_2(1-p_2)\right]\left(\frac{z}{E}\right)^2 =$$

$$\left[0.12(1-0.12)+0.12(1-0.12)\right]\left(\frac{1.96}{0.04}\right)^2 = 507.1.$$

The 95% confidence interval for the variation in the proportions of preterm deliveries will have a margin of error of no more than 4 percent if samples of size n_1=508 pregnant smokers and n_2=508 pregnant non-smokers are used.

7.2. Issues in Estimating Sample Size for Hypothesis Testing

In the module on hypothesis testing for means and proportions, we introduced techniques for means, proportions, differences in means, and differences in proportions. While each test involved details that were specific to the outcome of interest (e.g., continuous or dichotomous) and to the number of comparison groups (one, two, more than two), there were common elements to each test. For example, in each test of hypothesis, two errors can be committed. The first is called a Type I error and refers to the situation where we incorrectly reject H_0 when in fact it is true. In the first step of any test of hypothesis, we select a level of significance, α, and α = P(Type I error) = P(Reject H_0 | H_0 is true). Because we purposely select a small value for α, we control the probability of committing a Type I error. The second type of error is called a Type II error and it is defined as the probability we do not reject H_0 when it is false. The probability of a Type II error is denoted β, and β =P(Type II error) = P(Do not Reject H_0 | H_0 is false). In hypothesis testing, we usually focus on power, which is defined as the probability that we reject H_0 when it is false, i.e., power = 1- β = P(Reject H_0 | H_0 is false). Power is the probability that a test correctly rejects a false null hypothesis. A good test is one with a low probability of committing a Type I error (i.e., small α) and high power (i.e., small β, high power). Here are some formulas to help you figure out how big of a sample you need to guarantee a high power test. The computation of sample size is contingent upon several factors, including the effect size, variability of the outcome, desired test power (which is equivalent to 1-β), and the level of significance, aα. The difference in the parameter of interest that indicates a difference with clinical significance is called the effect size. Like the margin of error in applications involving confidence intervals, the effect size is established using practical or clinical standards rather than statistical standards.

It can be challenging to understand statistical power. We will first go over power conceptually before presenting the formulas to find the sample sizes needed to guarantee high power in a test.

Suppose we want to test the following hypotheses at aα=0.05:

H_0: μ = 90

versus

H_1: μ ≠ 90.

Let us assume that we choose a sample size of n = 100 to test the hypotheses. Assume for this example that the outcome's standard deviation is σ = 20. After calculating the sample mean, we must determine whether or not the sample mean supports the alternative hypothesis. To accomplish this, compute a test statistic and compare it to the relevant critical value. We will probably choose a sample whose mean is near to 90 if the null hypothesis (μ=90) is correct. It is also feasible, though, to choose a sample with a mean that is significantly different from 90.

Recall from the Central Limit Theorem, that for large n (here n=100 is sufficiently large), the distribution of the sample means is approximately normal with a mean of

$$\mu\bar{X} = \mu = 90$$

and

$$\text{Standard deviation} = \sigma\bar{X} = \frac{\sigma}{\sqrt{n}} = \frac{20}{\sqrt{100}} = 2.0$$

If the null hypothesis is true, it is possible to observe any sample mean shown in the figure below; all are possible under H_0: μ = 90 (see **Figure 7.1**).

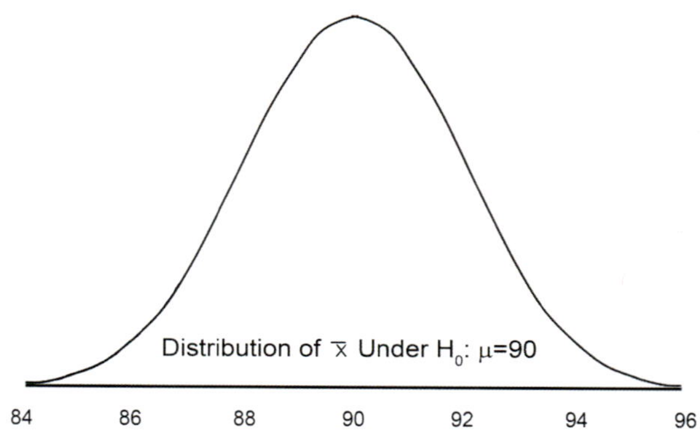

Figure 7.1. *Distribution of $\bar{X}$ Under H0: μ = 90.*

Source: *https://sphweb.bumc.bu.edu/otlt/mph-modules/bs/bs704_power/Distribution%20of%20x-bar.png.*

When we set up the decision rule for our test of hypothesis, we determine critical values based on α=0.05 and a two-sided test. When we run tests of hypotheses, we usually standardize the data (e.g., convert to Z or t) and the critical values are appropriate values from the probability distribution used in the test. To facilitate interpretation, we will continue this discussion with x- as opposed to Z. The critical values for a two-sided test with α=0.05 are 86.06 and 93.92 (these values correspond to -1.96 and 1.96, respectively, on the Z scale), so the decision rule is as follows: (see **Figure 7.2**).

Reject H_0 if x- ≤ 86.06 or if x- ≥ 93.92.

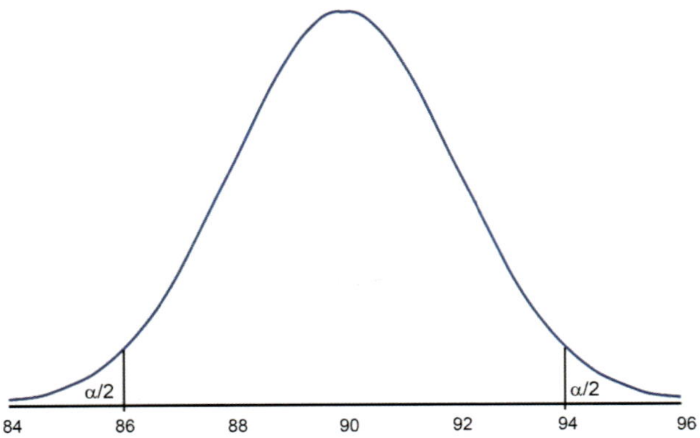

Figure 7.2. *Rejection Region for Test H0: μ = 90 versus H1: μ ≠ 90 at α =0.05.*

Source: https://sphweb.bumc.bu.edu/otlt/mph-modules/bs/bs704_power/Rejection%20Region.png.

The areas in the two tails of the curve represent the probability of a Type I Error, α= 0.05. This concept was discussed in the module on Hypothesis Testing.

Now, suppose that the alternative hypothesis, H_1, is true (i.e., μ ≠ 90) and that the true mean is 94. The figure below shows the distributions of the sample mean under the null and alternative hypotheses. The values of the sample mean are shown along the horizontal axis (see **Figure 7.3**).

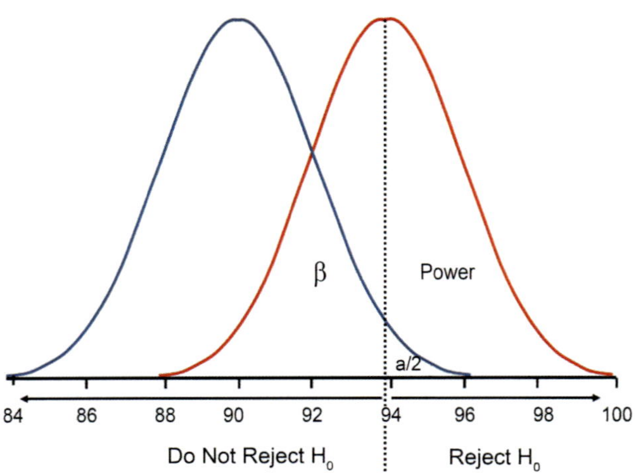

Figure 7.3. *Distribution of* $\overline{X}$ *Under H0: μ = 90 and Under H1: μ = 94.*

Source: https://sphweb.bumc.bu.edu/otlt/mph-modules/bs/bs704_power/Rejection%20Region2.png.

If the true mean is 94, then the alternative hypothesis is true. In our test, we selected α = 0.05 and rejected H_0 if the observed sample mean exceeds 93.92 (focusing on the upper tail of the rejection region for now). The critical value (93.92) is indicated by the vertical line. The probability of a Type II error is denoted β, and β = P(Do not Reject H_0 | H_0 is false), i.e., the probability of not rejecting the null hypothesis if the null hypothesis were true. β is shown in the figure above as the area under the rightmost curve (H_1) to the left of the vertical line (where we do not reject H_0). Power is defined as 1- β = P (Reject H_0 | H_0 is false) and is shown in the figure as the area under the rightmost curve (H_1) to the right of the vertical line (where we reject H_0).

Note that β and power are related to α, the variability of the outcome, and the effect size. From the figure above we can see what happens to β and power if we increase α. Suppose, for example, we increase α to α=0.10. The upper critical value would be 92.56 instead of 93.92. The vertical line would shift to the left, increasing α, decreasing β, and increasing power. While a better test is one with higher power, it is not advisable to increase α as a means to increase power. Nonetheless, there is a direct relationship between α and power (as α increases, so does power).

β and power are also related to the variability of the outcome and to the effect size. The effect size is the difference in the parameter of interest (e.g., μ) that represents a clinically meaningful difference. The figure above graphically displays α, β, and power when the difference in the mean under the null as compared to the alternative hypothesis is 4 units (i.e., 90 versus 94). The figure below shows the same components for the situation where the mean under the alternative hypothesis is 98 (see **Figure 7.4**).

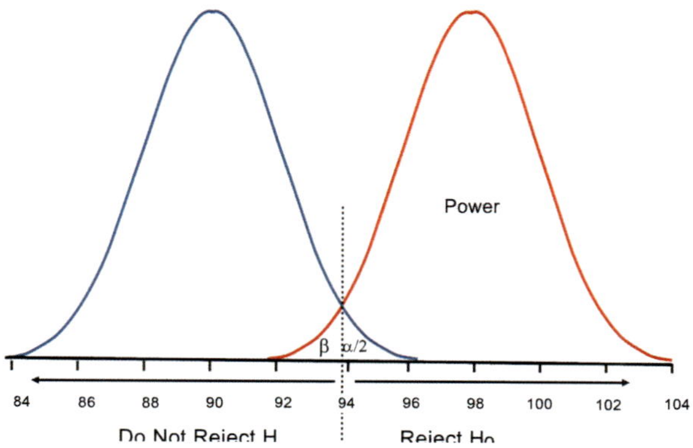

Figure 7.4. *Distribution of* $\bar{X}$ *Under H0:* $\mu = 90$ *and Under H1:* $\mu = 98$.

Source: https://sphweb.bumc.bu.edu/otlt/mph-modules/bs/bs704_power/Rejection%20Region3.png.

Notice that there is much higher power when there is a larger difference between the mean under H_0 as compared to H_1 (i.e., 90 versus 98). A statistical test is much more likely to reject the null hypothesis in favor of the alternative if the true mean is 98 than if the true mean is 94. Notice also in this case that there is little overlap in the distributions under the null and alternative hypotheses. If a sample mean of 97 or higher is observed it is very unlikely that it came from a distribution whose mean is 90. In the previous figure for H_0: $\mu = 90$ and H_1: $\mu = 94$, if we observed a sample mean of 93, for example, it would not be as clear as to whether it came from a distribution whose mean is 90 or one whose mean is 94.

7.2.1. Ensuring That a Test Has High Power

Most people think about 80 or 90 % power when designing studies (just as we typically use 95% as the confidence level for confidence interval estimates). The required power, the degree of significance, and the effect size are the inputs used in the sample size calculations. The effect size is chosen to reflect a change in the parameter of interest that is significant either practically or clinically. The following formulas yield the smallest sample size necessary to guarantee that the test of the hypothesis will have a given probability of rejecting the null hypothesis in the event that it is false (i.e., a designated power). Researchers must once more take attrition or loss to follow-up into consideration when designing studies. The following formulas yield the required number of participants based on complete data.

7.2.2. Sample Size for One Sample, Continuous Outcome

In studies where the plan is to perform a test of hypothesis comparing the mean of a continuous outcome variable in a single population to a known mean, the hypotheses of interest are:

$$H_0: \mu = \mu_0 \text{ and } H_1: \mu \neq \mu_0$$

where μ_0 is the known mean (e.g., a historical control). The formula for determining sample size to ensure that the test has a specified power is given below:

$$n = \left(\frac{z_{1-\alpha/2} + z_{1-\beta}}{\text{ES}} \right)^2$$

where α is the selected level of significance and $Z_{1-\alpha/2}$ is the value from the standard normal distribution holding $1-\alpha/2$ below it. For example, if $\alpha=0.05$, then $1-\alpha/2 = 0.975$ and $Z=1.960$. $1-\beta$ is the selected power, and $Z_{1-\beta}$ is the value from the standard normal distribution holding $1-\beta$ below it. Sample size estimates for hypothesis testing are often based on achieving 80% or 90% power. The $Z_{1-\beta}$ values for these popular scenarios are given below:

- For 80% power $Z_{0.80} = 0.84$

- For 90% power $Z_{0.90}$ =1.282

ES is the *effect size*, defined as follows:

$$ES = \frac{|\mu_1 - \mu_0|}{\sigma},$$

where μ_0 is the mean under H_0, μ_1 is the mean under H_1 and σ is the standard deviation of the outcome of interest. The numerator of the effect size, the absolute value of the difference in means $|\mu_1 - \mu_0|$, represents what is considered a clinically meaningful or practically important difference in means.

It can occasionally be challenging to estimate the standard deviation, which is comparable to the problem we encountered when organizing research to estimate confidence intervals. Researchers frequently utilize the standard deviation from a prior study or a study conducted in a different but similar population when calculating sample sizes. No matter how the estimate of the outcome's variability is calculated, it should always be conservative (i.e., as big as is appropriate), to ensure that the final sample size is not excessively small.

Example 7.9.

An investigator is testing the hypothesis that individuals without diabetes who consume at least two cups of coffee per day have higher fasting blood glucose levels, which is a risk factor for coronary heart disease. In a cross-sectional study, they plan to compare the mean fasting blood glucose levels in this group. The mean fasting blood glucose level in individuals without diabetes is 95.0 mg/dL with a standard deviation of 9.8 mg/dL. If the mean blood glucose level in individuals who drink at least two cups of coffee per day is found to be 100 mg/dL, this would have clinical significance. To ensure the test has 80% power to detect this difference with a two-sided test at a 5% level of significance, the study should enrol a certain number of patients.

The effect size is computed as:

$$ES = \frac{|\mu_1 - \mu_0|}{\sigma} = \frac{|100-95|}{9.8} = 0.51.$$

The population mean difference that is meaningful is represented by the effect size, which in this case is 95 versus 100, or 0.51 standard deviation units different. To compute the sample size, we now substitute the effect size and the appropriate Z values for the chosen α and power.

$$n = \left(\frac{z_{1-\alpha/2} + z_{1-\beta}}{ES}\right)^2 = \left(\frac{1.96+0.84}{0.51}\right)^2 = 30.1.$$

Therefore, a sample of size n=31 will ensure that a two-sided test with α =0.05 has 80% power to detect a 5 mg/dL difference in mean fasting blood glucose levels.

Participants in the study will be required to fast for the entire night and give a blood sample so that the glucose levels can be measured. The researchers predict that 10% of participants won't fast or won't adhere to the study's protocol based on experience. To guarantee that 31 of the participants are available for analysis, a total of 35 will be enrolled in the study.

N (number to enrol) * (% following protocol) = desired sample size

Therefore N (number to enrol) = desired sample size/(% retained)

N = 31/0.90 = 35.

7.2.3. Sample Size for One Sample, Dichotomous Outcome

In studies where the plan is to perform a test of hypothesis comparing the proportion of successes in a dichotomous outcome variable in a single population to a known proportion, the hypotheses of interest are:

$$H_0: p = p_0,$$
$$H_1: p \neq p_0$$

where p_0 is the known proportion (e.g., a historical control). The formula for determining the sample size to ensure that the test has a specified power is given below:

$$n = \left(\frac{z_{1-\alpha/2} + z_{1-\beta}}{\text{ES}} \right)^2$$

where α is the selected level of significance and $Z_{1-\alpha/2}$ is the value from the standard normal distribution holding 1- α/2 below it. 1- β is the selected power and $Z_{1-\beta}$ is the value from the standard normal distribution holding 1- β below it , and ES is the effect size, defined as follows:

$$\text{ES} = \frac{|p_1 - p_0|}{\sqrt{p_0(1-p_0)}},$$

where p_0 is the proportion under H_0 and p_1 is the proportion under H_1. The numerator of the effect size, the absolute value of the difference in proportions $|p_1 - p_0|$, again represents what is considered a clinically meaningful or practically important difference in proportions.

Example 7.10.

According to a recent Framingham Heart Study report, 26% of individuals without cardiovascular disease had elevated LDL cholesterol levels, which are measured as LDL > 159 mg/dL. An elevated LDL cholesterol is expected to be present in a greater proportion of patients with a history of cardiovascular disease, according to an investigator's hypothesis. A two-sided test with a five percent level of significance will be employed. How many patients should be studied to guarantee that the power of the test is ninety percent to detect a five percent difference in the proportion with elevated LDL cholesterol?

We first compute the effect size:

$$\text{ES} = \frac{|p_1 - p_0|}{\sqrt{p_0(1-p_0)}} = \frac{0.05}{\sqrt{0.26(1-0.26)}} = 0.11.$$

We now substitute the effect size and the appropriate Z values for the selected α and power to compute the sample size.

$$n = \left(\frac{z_{1-\alpha/2} + z_{1-\beta}}{\text{ES}} \right)^2 = \left(\frac{1.96 + 1.282}{0.11} \right)^2 = 868.6.$$

A sample of size n=869 will ensure that a two-sided test with α =0.05 has 90% power to detect a 5% difference in the proportion of patients with a history of cardiovascular disease who have an elevated LDL cholesterol level.

Implantable stents are made by a manufacturer of medical devices. Approximately 10 percent of the stents are considered defective during the manufacturing process. The goal of the manufacturer's test is to determine if more than 10% of stents are defective. Corrective action is required if the process yields more than 15% of defective stents. As a result, the manufacturer requires that the test have 90% power to identify a variation in proportions this significant. For your computations, use a two-sided test with a five percent significance level for the number of stents that need to be evaluated.

7.2.4. Sample Sizes for Two Independent Samples, Continuous Outcome

In studies where the plan is to perform a test of hypothesis comparing the means of a continuous outcome variable in two independent populations, the hypotheses of interest are:

$$H_0: \mu_1 = \mu_2$$
$$H_1: \mu_1 \neq \mu_2,$$

where μ_1 and μ_2 are the means in the two comparison populations. The formula for determining the sample sizes to ensure that the test has a specified power is:

$$n_i = 2\left(\frac{z_{1-\alpha/2} + z_{1-\beta}}{\text{ES}}\right)^2$$

where n_i is the sample size required in each group (i=1,2), α is the selected level of significance and $Z_{1-\alpha/2}$ is the value from the standard normal distribution holding 1- α /2 below it, and 1- β is the selected power and $Z_{1-\beta}$ is the value from the standard normal distribution holding 1- β below it. ES is the effect size, defined as:

$$\text{ES} = \frac{|\mu_1 - \mu_2|}{\sigma},$$

where the absolute value of the mean difference between the two groups predicted by the alternative hypothesis, H1, is represented by the expression |μ1 - μ2|. The standard deviation of the desired outcome is denoted by σ. Remember from the Hypothesis Testing module that we used S_p, the pooled estimate of the common standard deviation, as a measure of outcome variability when we conducted tests of hypothesis comparing the means of two independent groups.

S_p is computed as follows:

$$S_p = \sqrt{\frac{(n_1 - 1)s_1^2 + (n2 - 1)s_2^2}{(n_1 + n_2 - 2)}}$$

If information on the variability of the result in every comparison group is available, Sp can be calculated and utilized to produce sample sizes. In clinical research, it is common for the variability of results to be primarily documented for a single group, often the untreated or placebo control group. When designing a clinical trial to evaluate a new medication or treatment, insights from prior studies that included a placebo or active control group can be invaluable. The standard deviation of the outcome variable from patients in the placebo or control group can serve as a critical reference for planning future trials. It is important to recognize that the sample size estimates for equal-sized groups are derived from established formulas. However, if a study involves unequal patient assignments or varying sizes in comparison groups, alternative formulas should be employed to ensure accurate planning and analysis.

Example 7.11.

A clinical trial is being planned by an investigator to assess the effectiveness of a novel medication intended to lower systolic blood pressure. Participants will be recruited and randomly assigned to receive either a placebo or the new medication. After each participant has received the prescribed treatment for 12 weeks, their systolic blood pressure will be measured. The investigator projects that 10% of all participants will either drop out of the study or be lost to follow-up, based on experience with similar trials. A 5-unit drop in mean systolic blood pressure would indicate a clinically significant drop in blood pressure with the new medication. A two-sided test with a 5% level of significance will be used; how many patients should be enrolled in the trial to guarantee that the test's power is 80% to detect this difference?

An estimate of the variability in systolic blood pressure is required in order to calculate the effect size. The Framingham Heart Study's data analysis revealed that the systolic blood pressure's standard deviation was 19 points. The trial can be planned using this value.

The effect size is:

$$\text{ES} = \frac{|\mu_1 - \mu_2|}{\sigma} = \frac{5}{19.0} = 0.26.$$

We now substitute the effect size and the appropriate Z values for the selected α and power to compute the sample size.

$$n_i = 2\left(\frac{z_{1-\alpha/2} + z_{1-\beta}}{\text{ES}}\right)^2 = 2\left(\frac{1.96+0.84}{0.26}\right)^2 = 232.0.$$

Samples of size n_1=232 and n_2= 232 will ensure that the test of hypothesis will have 80% power to detect a 5-unit difference in mean systolic blood pressures in patients receiving the new drug as compared to patients receiving the placebo. However, the investigators hypothesized a 10% attrition rate (in both groups), and to ensure a total sample size of 232 they need to allow for attrition.

N (number to enrol) * (% retained) = desired sample size

Therefore N (number to enrol) = desired sample size/(% retained)

N = 232/0.90 = 258.

The investigator must enrol 258 participants to be randomly assigned to receive either the new drug or placebo.

A researcher is organizing an investigation to evaluate the correlation between alcohol intake and senior college grade point average. The idea is to classify students as heavy drinkers or not using the standard criterion of five or more drinks consumed on a typical drinking day. A two independent samples test of means will be used to compare the mean grade point averages of students who are classified as heavy drinkers versus those who are not. A significant difference in grade point averages (concerning drinking status) is 0.25 units, and the standard deviation of grade point averages is assumed to be 0.42. Use a two-sided test with a 5% level of significance to determine how many college seniors should be enrolled in the study in order to guarantee that the test's power is 80% to detect a 0.25 unit difference in mean grade point averages.

7.2.5. Sample Size for Matched Samples, Continuous Outcome

In studies where the plan is to perform a test of hypothesis on the mean difference in a continuous outcome variable based on matched data, the hypotheses of interest are:

$$H_0: \mu_d = 0,$$

$$H_1: \mu_d \neq 0,$$

where μ_d is the mean difference in the population. The formula for determining the sample size to ensure that the test has a specified power is given below:

$$n = \left(\frac{z_{1-\alpha/2} + z_{1-\beta}}{\text{ES}}\right)^2,$$

where α is the selected level of significance and $Z_{1-\alpha/2}$ is the value from the standard normal distribution holding 1- α/2 below it, 1- β is the selected power and $Z_{1-\beta}$ is the value from the standard normal distribution holding 1- β below it and ES is the effect size, defined as follows:

$$\text{ES} = \frac{\mu_d}{\sigma_d},$$

where μ_d is the mean difference expected under the alternative hypothesis, H_1, and σ_d is the standard deviation of the difference in the outcome (e.g., the difference based on measurements over time or the difference between matched pairs).

Example 7.12.

An investigator wishes to assess whether treating patients with chronic migraine headaches with acupuncture can effectively reduce their pain. Enrolling patients with migraine headaches is the plan. Before receiving any treatment, each patient will be asked to rate the intensity of the pain they feel from their next migraine. A pain score between 1 and 100 will be used to record the pain, with higher scores denoting more severe pain. After that, each patient will receive an acupuncture treatment. Every patient will be asked to rate the intensity of their migraine once more (post-treatment). For every patient, the difference in pain will be calculated. To determine whether there is a statistically significant difference in pain scores before and after treatment, a two-sided test of the hypothesis will be performed at $\alpha = 0.05$. Assuming that the standard deviation of the difference scores is roughly 20 units, how many patients should be included in the study to guarantee that the test has 80% power to detect a difference of 10 units on the pain scale?

First, compute the effect size:

$$\mathrm{ES} = \frac{\mu_d}{\sigma_d} = \frac{10}{20} = 0.50.$$

Then substitute the effect size and the appropriate Z values for the selected α and power to compute the sample size.

$$n = \left(\frac{z_{1-\alpha/2} + z_{1-\beta}}{\mathrm{ES}}\right)^2 = \left(\frac{1.96 + 0.84}{0.50}\right)^2 = 31.4.$$

A sample of size n=32 patients with migraine will ensure that a two-sided test with α =0.05 has 80% power to detect a mean difference of 10 points in pain before and after treatment, assuming that all 32 patients complete the treatment.

7.2.6. Sample Sizes for Two Independent Samples, Dichotomous Outcomes

In studies where the plan is to perform a test of hypothesis comparing the proportions of successes in two independent populations, the hypotheses of interest are:

$$H_0: p_1 = p_2$$

versus

$$H_1: p_1 \neq p_2$$

where p_1 and p_2 are the proportions in the two comparison populations. The formula for determining the sample sizes to ensure that the test has a specified power is given below:

$$n_i = 2\left(\frac{z_{1-\alpha/2} + z_{1-\beta}}{\mathrm{ES}}\right)^2$$

where n_i is the sample size required in each group (i=1,2), α is the selected level of significance and $Z_{1-\alpha/2}$ is the value from the standard normal distribution holding 1- α/2 below it, and 1- β is the selected power and $Z_{1-\beta}$ is the value from the standard normal distribution holding 1- β below it. ES is the effect size, defined as follows:

$$\mathrm{ES} = \frac{|p_1 - p_2|}{\sqrt{p(1-p)}},$$

where $|p_1 - p_2|$ is the absolute value of the difference in proportions between the two groups expected under the alternative hypothesis, H_1, and p is the overall proportion, based on pooling the data from the two comparison groups (p can be computed by taking the mean of the proportions in the two comparison groups, assuming that the groups will be of approximately equal size).

Example 7.13.

According to an investigator's hypothesis, students who regularly use their athletic facility have a higher incidence of flu than their non-user peers. The research will take place in the spring. Every student will be questioned about whether they have had the flu and whether they have utilized the sports facilities frequently over the previous six months. To compare the percentage of students who regularly used the athletic facility and contracted the flu with the percentage of students who did not and contracted the illness, a hypothesis test will be carried out. About thirty-five percent of the students get the flu in a typical year. A clinically significant rise in flu cases among individuals who frequently used the sports facility would be thirty percent. We will use a two-sided test with a 5% level of significance; how many students should be enrolled in the study to ensure that the test's power is 80% to detect this difference in the proportions?

We first compute the effect size by substituting the proportions of students in each group who are expected to develop flu, $p_1=0.46$ (i.e., 0.35*1.30=0.46) and $p_2=0.35$ and the overall proportion, p=0.41 (i.e., (0.46+0.35)/2):

$$\text{ES} = \frac{|p_1 - p_2|}{\sqrt{p(1-p)}} = \frac{|0.46-0.35|}{\sqrt{0.41(1-0.41)}} = 0.22.$$

We now substitute the effect size and the appropriate Z values for the selected α and power to compute the sample size.

$$n_i = 2\left(\frac{z_{1-\alpha/2}+z_{1-\beta}}{\text{ES}}\right)^2 = 2\left(\frac{1.96+0.84}{0.22}\right)^2 = 324.0.$$

Samples of size $n_1=324$ and $n_2=324$ will ensure that the test of hypothesis will have 80% power to detect a 30% difference in the proportions of students who develop flu between those who do and do not use the athletic facilities regularly. (Buschman et al., 2001) (Plaskon et al., 2003).

A Closer Look

Hypothesis Testing

Hypothesis testing is a statistical method used to determine if there is enough evidence to support a specific claim about a population parameter. The process begins with formulating two competing hypotheses: the null hypothesis (H0), which represents a baseline or default position, and the alternative hypothesis (H1 or Ha), which reflects the claim being tested. Data is collected through experimentation or observation, and a test statistic is calculated. This statistic is then compared to a critical value derived from the chosen significance level (alpha), usually set at 0.05. If the test statistic falls within the critical region, the null hypothesis is rejected in favor of the alternative. Conversely, if it falls outside, there isn't enough evidence to reject the null hypothesis. This process helps in making informed decisions based on empirical evidence, ensuring that conclusions drawn are statistically significant rather than due to random chance.

Summary

- The formulas presented here generate estimates of the necessary sample size(s) required based on statistical criteria. However, in many studies, the sample size is determined by financial or logistical constraints.
- It involves a value from the t distribution, as opposed to one from the standard normal distribution, to reflect the desired level of confidence.
- An investigator wants to estimate the mean systolic blood pressure in children with congenital heart disease who are between the ages of 3 and 5.
- It is extremely important that the standard deviation of the *difference* scores (e.g., the difference based on measurements over time or the difference between matched pairs) is used here to appropriately estimate the sample size.
- Similar to the situation for two independent samples and a continuous outcome at the top of this page, it may be the case that data are available on the proportion of successes in one group, usually the untreated (e.g., placebo control) or unexposed group.
- In the module on hypothesis testing for means and proportions, we introduced techniques for means, proportions, differences in means, and differences in proportions.
- An investigator is planning a clinical trial to evaluate the efficacy of a new drug designed to reduce systolic blood pressure.
- An investigator wants to evaluate the efficacy of an acupuncture treatment for reducing pain in patients with chronic migraine headaches. The plan is to enroll patients who suffer from migraine headaches.

References

1. Buschman, N. A., Foster, G., & Vickers, P. (2001). Adolescent girls and their babies: Achieving optimal birth weight. Gestational weight gain and pregnancy outcome in terms of gestation at delivery and infant birth weight: A comparison between adolescents under 16 and adult women. *Child: Care, Health and Development, 27*(2), 163–171.
2. National Center for Health Statistics. (2005). *Health, United States, 2005 with Chartbook on Trends in the Health of Americans*. Hyattsville, MD: US Government Printing Office.
3. Plaskon, L. A., Penson, D. F., Vaughan, T. L., & Stanford, J. L. (2003). Cigarette smoking and risk of prostate cancer in middle-aged men. *Cancer Epidemiology, Biomarkers & Prevention, 12*, 604–609.
4. Ramachandran, V., Sullivan, L. M., Wilson, P. W., Sempos, C. T., Sundstrom, J., Kannel, W. B., Levy, D., & D'Agostino, R. B. (2005). Relative importance of borderline and elevated levels of coronary heart disease risk factors. *Annals of Internal Medicine, 142*, 393–402.
5. Rutter, M. K., Meigs, J. B., Sullivan, L. M., D'Agostino, R. B., & Wilson, P. W. (2004). C-reactive protein, the metabolic syndrome, and prediction of cardiovascular events in the Framingham Offspring Study. *Circulation, 110*, 380–385.
6. Wechsler, H., Lee, J. E., Kuo, M., & Lee, H. (2000). College binge drinking in the 1990s: A continuing problem results of the Harvard School of Public Health. *College Health, 48*, 199–210.

Chapter 8

MULTIVARIABLE METHODS

Contents

Introduction 217
8.1. Correlation and Regression 219
8.2. Sensitivity to Outliers, Outlier Rejection, and Robust Regression 228
8.3. Multiple Linear Regression 234
8.4. Logistic Regression 236
Summary 241
References 241

Introduction

Multivariable methods in statistics are powerful analytical techniques used to understand complex relationships between multiple variables simultaneously. Unlike univariable analysis, which focuses on the relationship between one variable and an outcome, multivariable methods allow researchers to consider the influence of several variables on an outcome of interest. These methods are essential for gaining deeper insights into the multifaceted nature of real-world phenomena, where multiple factors often interact to shape outcomes. One fundamental concept in multivariable methods is multivariable regression analysis, which extends the principles of simple linear regression to incorporate multiple predictor variables. In multivariable regression, researchers examine how a dependent variable (or outcome) is influenced by two or more independent variables (or predictors), while accounting for the interplay between them. This enables researchers to assess the unique contribution of each predictor variable to the outcome, controlling for the effects of other variables.

Orientation and Directional Terms

Term	Definition	Illustration
Correlation	It is a statistical measure that expresses the extent to which two variables are linearly related (meaning they change together at a constant rate). It's a common tool for describing simple relationships without making a statement about cause and effect.	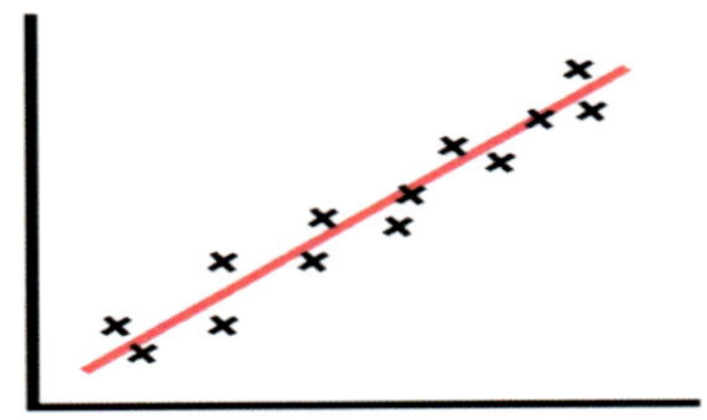
Regression Analysis	Regression analysis is a set of statistical methods used for the estimation of relationships between a dependent variable and one or more independent variables.	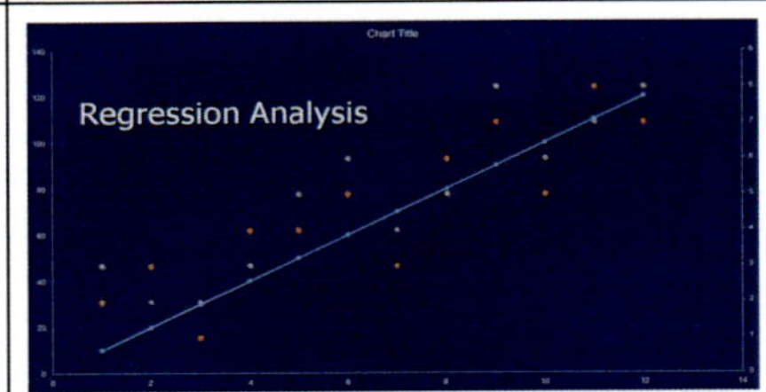
Qualitative Variable	A qualitative variable, also called categorical, is one in which the variable categories are not described as numbers but instead by verbal groupings. There are two classifications of categorical data: nominal and ordinal	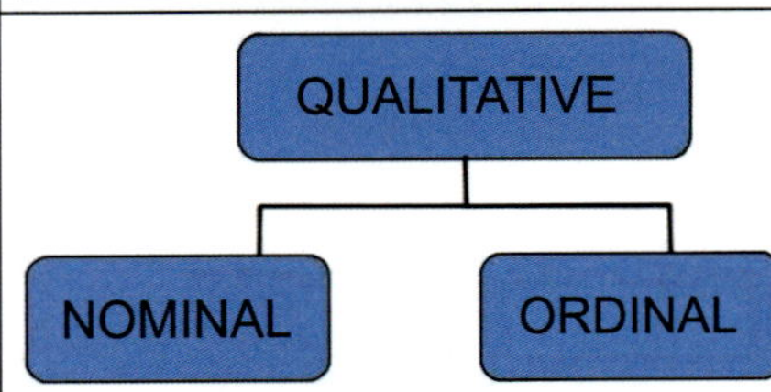
Scatter Diagram	It is a type of plot or mathematical diagram using Cartesian coordinates to display values for typically two variables for a set of data. If the points are coded, one additional variable can be displayed.	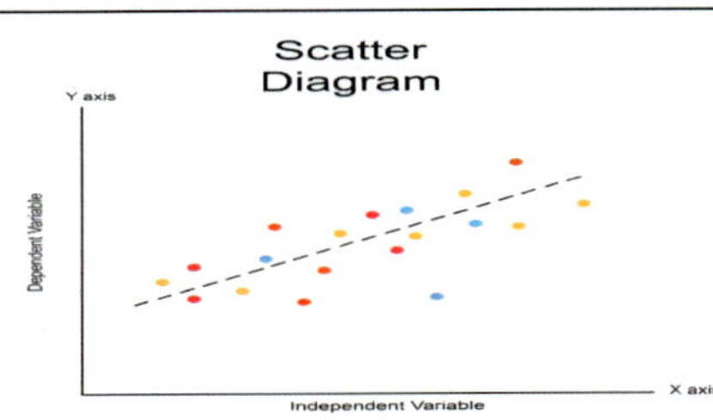
Normal Distribution	It is a continuous probability distribution wherein values lie in a symmetrical fashion mostly situated around the mean.	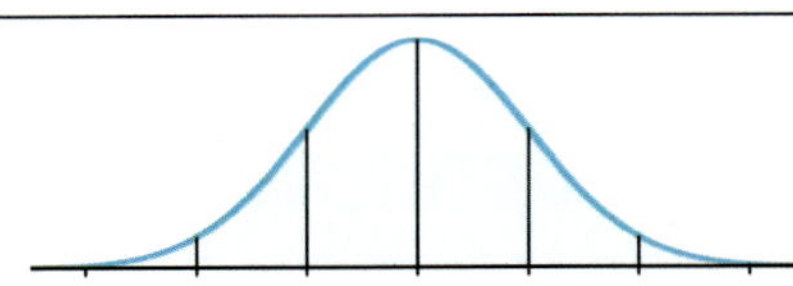

8.1. Correlation and Regression

Correlation and linear regression are the methods most frequently used to look into the relationship between two quantitative variables. Regression expresses the relationship as an equation, whereas correlation quantifies the strength of the linear relationship between two variables. For example, in patients attending an accident and emergency unit (A&E), we could use correlation and regression to determine whether there is a relationship between age and urea level and whether the level of urea can be predicted for a given age.

8.1.1. Scatter Diagram

The first step in examining a relationship between two variables is to visually represent the data values using a scatter diagram. Examine the information provided in Table 8.1. The logarithmically transformed admission serum urea (natural logarithm [ln] urea) and ages (years) of 20 patients attending an A&E are listed below. To achieve a more Normal distribution, the urea levels were transformed. The scatter plot for age and ln urea (Figure 8.1) indicates that these variables have a positive linear relationship with one another.

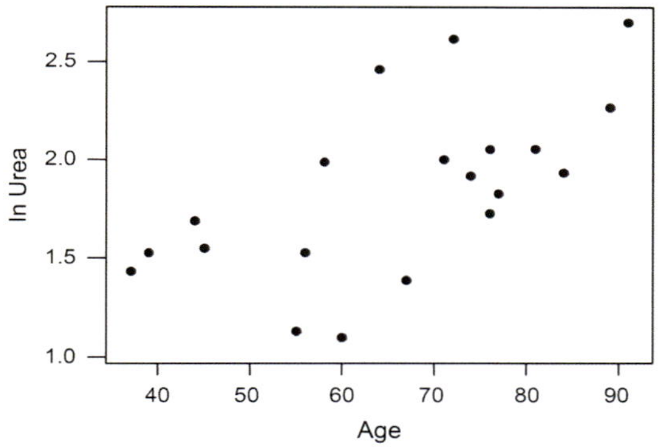

Figure 8.1. *Scatter diagram for ln Urea and age.*

Source: Viv Bewick, Liz Cheek and Jonathan Ball: Correlation and regression: ISSN 1364-8535.

Table 8.1. *Age and Ln Urea for 20 Patients Attending an Accident and Emergency Unit*

Subject	Age (years)	ln urea
1	60	1.099
2	76	1.723
3	81	2.054
4	89	2.262
5	44	1.686
6	58	1.988
7	55	1.131
8	74	1.917
9	45	1.548
10	67	1.386
11	72	2.617
12	91	2.701
13	76	2.054
14	39	1.526
15	71	2.002
16	56	1.526
17	77	1.825
18	37	1.435
19	64	2.460
20	84	1.932

Source: Viv Bewick, Liz Cheek and Jonathan Ball: Correlation and regression: ISSN 1364-8535.

8.1.2. Correlation

On a scatter diagram, the closer the points lie to a straight line, the stronger the linear relationship between two variables. To quantify the strength of the relationship, we can calculate the correlation coefficient. In algebraic notation, if we have two variables x and y, and the data take the form of n pairs (i.e., $[x_1, y_1]$, $[x_2, y_2]$, $[x_3, y_3]$ ... $[x_n, y_n]$), then the correlation coefficient is given by the following equation:

$$r = \frac{\sum_{i=1}^{n}(x_i - \bar{x})(y_i - \bar{y})}{\sqrt{\sum_{i=1}^{n}(x_i - \bar{x})^2 \sum_{i=1}^{n}(y_i - \bar{y})^2}}$$

where $\bar{X}$ is the mean of the x values, and $\bar{Y}$ is the mean of the y values.

This is the Pearson correlation coefficient, also known as the product-moment correlation coefficient. R is always between -1 and +1 in value. Strong positive linear relationships are indicated by a correlation coefficient value near +1 (i.e., one variable rises in proportion to the other; **Figure 8.2**). When the value is near to -1, a strong negative linear relationship (i.e., As one variable rises, the other falls; see **Figure 8.3**). There is no linear relationship when the value is near to 0 (**Figure 8.4**), but a nonlinear relationship between the variables is possible (**Figure 8.5**).

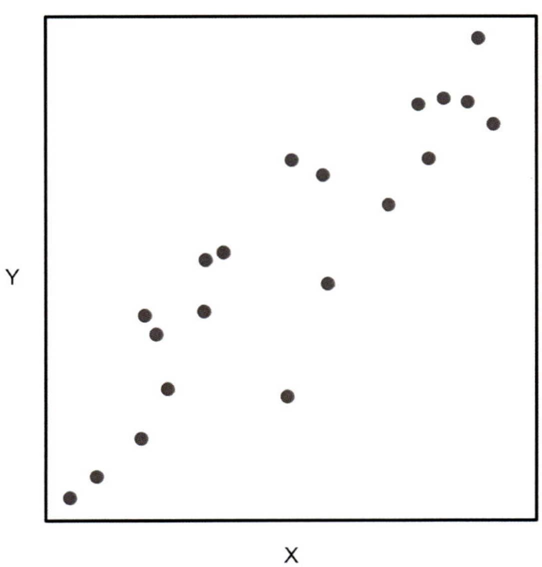

Figure 8.2. *Correlation coefficient (r) = +0.9. positive linear relationship.*

Source: Viv Bewick, Liz Cheek and Jonathan Ball: Correlation and regression: ISSN 1364-8535.

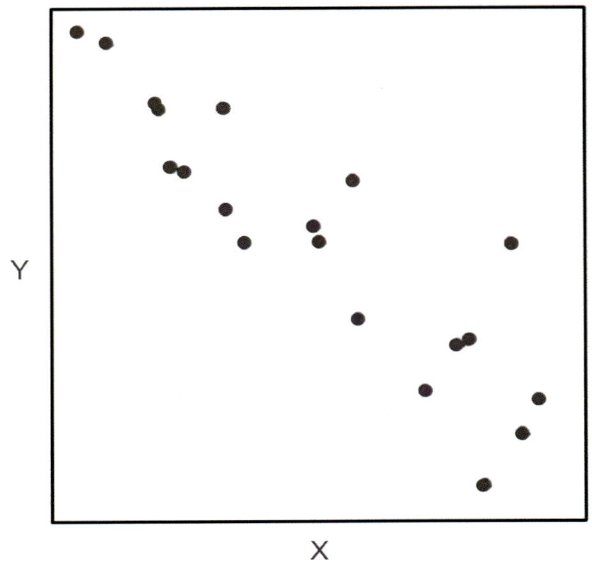

Figure 8.3. *Correlation coefficient (r) = –0.9. negative linear relationship.*

Source: https://www.ncbi.nlm.nih.gov/pmc/articles/PMC374386/pdf/cc2401.pdf.

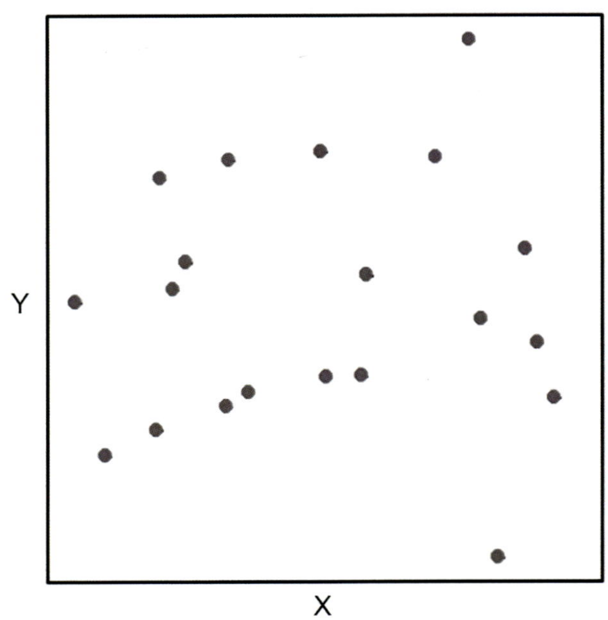

Figure 8.4. *Correlation coefficient (r) = 0.04. no relationship.*

Source: https://www.ncbi.nlm.nih.gov/pmc/articles/PMC374386/pdf/cc2401.pdf.

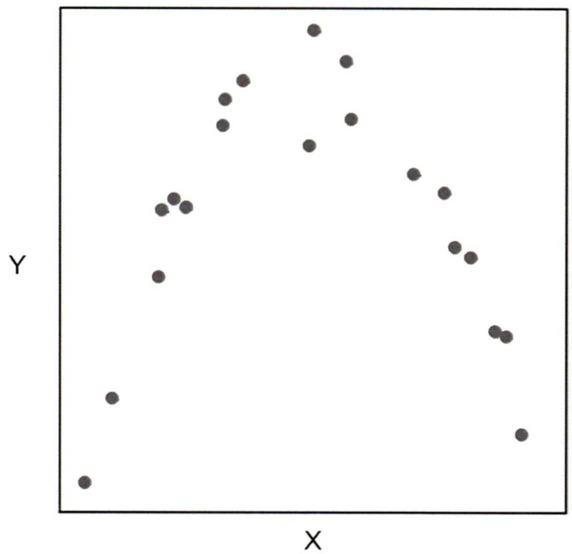

Figure 8.5. *Correlation coefficient (r) = −0.03. nonlinear relationship.*

Source: https://www.ncbi.nlm.nih.gov/pmc/articles/PMC374386/pdf/cc2401.pdf.

For the A&E data, the correlation coefficient is 0.62, indicating a moderate positive linear relationship between the two variables.

8.1.2.1. Hypothesis Test of Correlation

To determine whether there is a linear relationship between the variables in the population as a whole, we can use the correlation coefficient. The population correlation coefficient of zero is the null hypothesis. You can compare the value of r with those in Table 8.2, or you can use most statistical packages to get exact P values. P-value is less than 0.01 for the A&E data, as shown by r = 0.62 with a sample size of 20, which is greater than the value bolded in Table 8.2 for P = 0.01. Consequently, there is enough data to infer that ln urea and age have a linear relationship and that the true population correlation coefficient is not 0.

Table 8.2. *5% and 1% Points for the Distribution of the Correlation Coefficient Under the Null Hypothesis that the Population Correlation is 0 in a Two-Tailed Test*

	r values for two-tailed probabilities (*P*)			Two-tailed probabilities (*P*)	
Sample size	0.05	0.01	Sample size	0.05	0.01
3	1.00	1.00	23	0.41	0.53
4	0.95	0.99	24	0.40	0.52
5	0.88	0.96	25	0.40	0.51
6	0.81	0.92	26	0.39	0.50
7	0.75	0.87	27	0.38	0.49
8	0.71	0.83	28	0.37	0.48
9	0.67	0.80	29	0.37	0.47
10	0.63	0.76	30	0.36	0.46
11	0.60	0.73	40	0.31	0.40
12	0.58	0.71	50	0.28	0.36
13	0.55	0.68	60	0.25	0.33
14	0.53	0.66	70	0.24	0.31
15	0.51	0.64	80	0.22	0.29
16	0.50	0.62	90	0.21	0.27
17	0.48	0.61	100	0.20	0.26

18	0.47	0.59	110	0.19	0.24
19	0.46	0.58	120	0.18	0.23
20	0.44	**0.56**	130	0.17	0.23
21	0.43	0.55	140	0.17	0.22
22	0.42	0.54	150	0.16	0.21

Source: Viv Bewick, Liz Cheek and Jonathan Ball: Correlation and regression: ISSN 1364-8535.

8.1.2.2. Confidence Interval for the Population Correlation Coefficient

The hypothesis test does not indicate the strength of the linear relationship, even though it does show whether one exists. A confidence interval for the population correlation coefficient can provide this extra information.

To calculate a confidence interval, r must be transformed to give a normal distribution making use of Fisher's z transformation:

$$z_r = \frac{1}{2}\log_e\left(\frac{1+r}{1-r}\right)$$

The standard error of z_r is approximately:

$$\frac{1}{\sqrt{n-3}}$$

and hence a 95% confidence interval for the true population value for the transformed correlation coefficient z_r is given by z_r - (1.96 × standard error) to z_r + (1.96 × standard error). Because z_r is Normally distributed, 1.96 deviations from the statistic will give a 95% confidence interval.

For the A&E data the transformed correlation coefficient z_r between ln urea and age is:

$$\frac{1}{2}\log_e\left(\frac{1+0.62}{1-0.62}\right)=0.725$$

The standard error of z_r is:

$$\frac{1}{\sqrt{20-3}}=0.242$$

The 95% confidence interval for z_r is therefore 0.725 – (1.96 × 0.242) to 0.725 + (1.96 × 0.242), giving 0.251 to 1.199.

We must use the inverse of Fisher's transformation on the lower and upper limits of this confidence interval to obtain the 95% confidence interval for the correlation coefficient. The lower limit is:

$$\frac{e^{2\times0.251}-1}{e^{2\times0.251}+1}$$

giving 0.25 and the upper limit is:

$$\frac{e^{2\times1.199}-1}{e^{2\times1.199}+1}$$

giving 0.83. Therefore, we are 95% confident that the population correlation coefficient is between 0.25 and 0.83.

The width of the confidence interval depends on the sample size, and therefore it is possible to calculate the sample size required for a given level of accuracy.

8.1.2.3. Misuse of Correlation

There are several common situations in which the correlation coefficient can be misinterpreted.

One of the most frequent mistakes made when interpreting the correlation coefficient is not taking into account the possibility that the apparent correlation is caused by a third variable that is connected to both of the variables under investigation. Correlation is not the same as causality. Other potential underlying variables and whether the relationship holds in different populations must be taken into account in order to bolster the case for causality.

It is possible for two variables to have a nonlinear relationship that the correlation coefficient would not be able to adequately describe, or possibly even identify. There are situations when a data set includes different subgroups, like men and women. Clusters of points could emerge from this, inflating the correlation coefficient (**Figure 8.6**). An isolated outlier could have the same kind of impact.

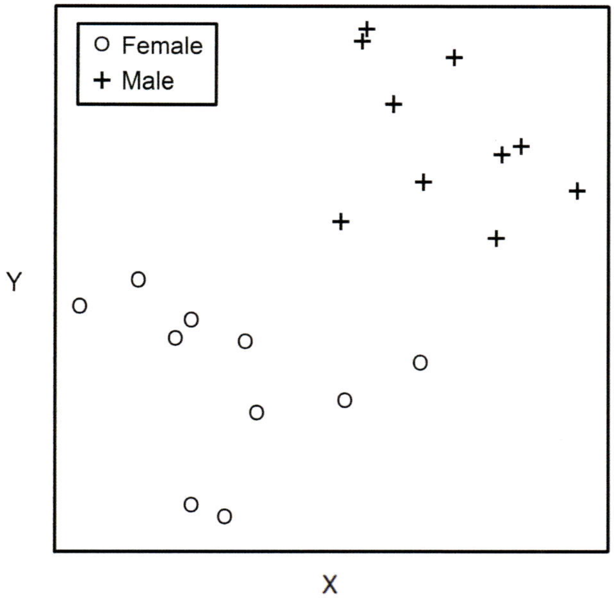

Figure 8.6. *Subgroups in the data resulting in a misleading correlation. All data: r = 0.57; males: r = -0.41; females: r = -0.26.*

Source: Viv Bewick, Liz Cheek, and Jonathan Ball: Correlation and regression: ISSN 1364-8535.

One variable's values must be neither predetermined nor limited to a specific range. As a result of the subjects' non-random sampling, the true correlation coefficient may be estimated incorrectly.

When comparing two measurement techniques, a correlation coefficient can also occasionally be interpreted incorrectly. One may mistakenly assume that a high correlation indicates agreement between the two approaches. A more suitable analysis would look into the variations between observation pairs, like the one developed by Bland and Altman.

8.1.3. Regression

We are interested in how age (the predictor, or x variable) affects ln urea (the response, or y variable) in the A&E example. To forecast ln urea and, consequently, urea for a specific age, we need to estimate the underlying linear relationship. It is possible to determine this line's equation via regression. The regression line is the common name for this line.

Note that in a scatter diagram the response variable is always plotted on the vertical (y) axis.

8.1.3.1. Equation of a Straight Line

The equation of a straight line is given by y = a + bx, where the coefficients a and b are the intercept of the line on the y-axis and the gradient, respectively. The equation of the regression line for the A&E data (**Figure 8.7**) is as follows: ln urea = 0.72 + (0.017 × age) (calculated using the method of least squares, which is described below). The gradient of this line is 0.017, which indicates that for an increase of 1 year in age the expected increase in ln urea is 0.017 units (and hence the expected increase in urea is 1.02 mmol/l). The predicted ln urea of a patient aged 60 years, for example, is 0.72 + (0.017 × 60) = 1.74 units. This transforms to a urea level of $e^{1.74}$ = 5.70 mmol/l. The y intercept is 0.72, meaning that if the line were projected back to age = 0, then the ln urea value would be 0.72. However, this is not a meaningful value because age = 0 is a long way outside the range of the data and therefore there is no reason to believe that the straight line would still be appropriate.

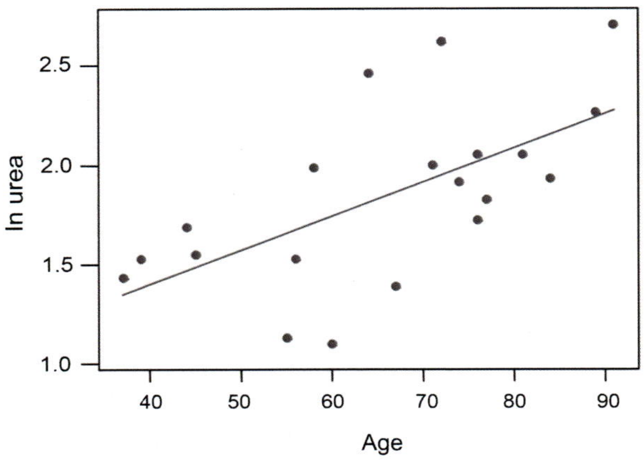

Figure 8.7. *Regression line for ln urea and age: ln urea = 0.72 + (0.017 × age).*

Source: Viv Bewick, Liz Cheek and Jonathan Ball: Correlation and regression: ISSN 1364-8535.

8.1.3.2. Method of Least Squares

The least squares method is used to obtain the regression line. For every value of x in the data set, the line y = a + bx that we draw through the points provides a predicted or fitted value of y. The deviation, also known as the residual, is the vertical difference, for a given value of x, between the observed and fitted values of y (**Figure 8.8**). The values of a and b that minimize the sum of the squares of all the deviations are found using the least squares method. This gives the following formulae for calculating a and b:

$$a = \bar{y} - b\bar{x} \qquad b = \frac{\sum_{i=1}^{n}(x_i - \bar{x})(y_i - \bar{y})}{\sum_{i=1}^{n}(x_i - \bar{x})^2}$$

Usually, these values would be calculated using a statistical package or the statistical functions on a calculator.

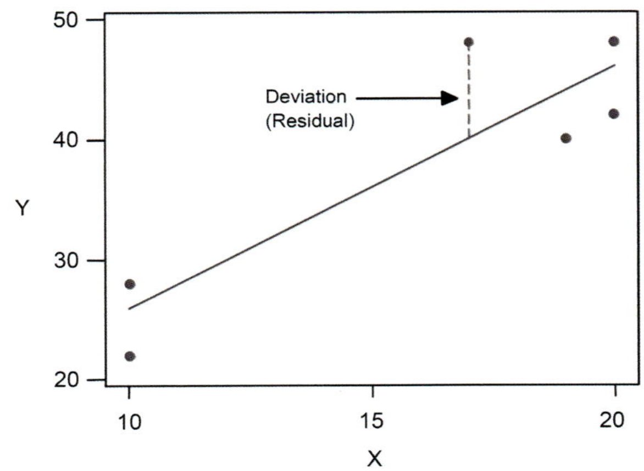

Figure 8.8. *Regression line obtained by minimizing the sums of squares of all of the deviations.*

Source: Viv Bewick, Liz Cheek and Jonathan Ball: Correlation and regression: ISSN 1364-8535.

8.1.3.3. Hypothesis Tests and Confidence Intervals

The population intercept and gradient are each equal to 0, and we can test this null hypothesis using test statistics obtained from dividing the estimate of the coefficient by its standard error.

$$\text{The standard error of the intercept} = s\sqrt{\left[\frac{1}{n} + \frac{\bar{x}^2}{\sum_{i=1}^{n}(x_i - \bar{x})^2}\right]}$$

$$\text{and for the gradient} = \frac{s}{\sqrt{\sum_{i=1}^{n}(x_i - \bar{x})^2}}$$

$$\text{where } s = \sqrt{\frac{\sum_{i=1}^{n}(y_i - \bar{y})^2 - b\sum_{i=1}^{n}(x_i - \bar{x})^2}{(n-2)}}$$

The test statistics are compared with the t distribution on n − 2 (sample size − number of regression coefficients) degrees of freedom.

The 95% confidence interval for each of the population coefficients are calculated as follows: coefficient ± (t_{n-2} × the standard error), where t_{n-2} is the 5% point for a t distribution with n – 2 degrees of freedom.

For the A&E data, the output (Table 8.3) was obtained from a statistical package. The *P* value for the coefficient of ln urea (0.004) gives strong evidence against the null hypothesis, indicating that the population coefficient is not 0 and that there is a linear relationship between ln urea and age. The coefficient of ln urea is the gradient of the regression line and its hypothesis test is equivalent to the test of the population correlation coefficient discussed above. The *P* value for the constant of 0.054 provides insufficient evidence to indicate that the population coefficient is different from 0. Although the intercept is not significant, it is still appropriate to keep it in the equation. There are some situations in which a straight line passing through the origin is known to be appropriate for the data, and in this case, a special regression analysis can be carried out that omits the constant.

Table 8.3. *Regression Parameter Estimates, P Values, and Confidence Intervals for the Accident and Emergency Unit Data*

	Coefficient	Standard error of the coefficient	t	*P*	Confidence interval
Constant, or intercept	0.72	0.346	2.07	0.054	-0.01 to +1.45
ln urea	0.017	0.005	3.35	0.004	0.006 to 0.028

Source: Viv Bewick, Liz Cheek, and Jonathan Ball: Correlation and regression: ISSN 1364-8535.

8.1.3.4. Analysis of Variance

The least squares approach reduces the sum of squares of the point deviations around the regression line. Examine the small sample of data shown in Figure 8.9. This figure demonstrates that, for a given value of x, the total deviation, or the distance of y from the mean of y, is equal to the sum of the distances between y and the line (the deviation not explained by the regression) and the fitted y value from the mean (the deviation explained by the regression).

The regression line for these data is given by y = 6 + 2x. The observed, fitted values and deviations are given in Table 8.4. The sum of squared deviations can be compared with the total variation in y, which is measured by the sum of squares of the deviations of y from the mean of y. Table 8.4 illustrates the relationship between the sums of squares. Total sum of squares = sum of squares explained by the regression line + sum of squares not explained by the regression line. The explained sum of squares is referred to as the 'regression sum of squares' and the unexplained sum of squares is referred to as the 'residual sum of squares.'

This partitioning of the total sum of squares can be presented in an analysis of variance table (Table 8.5). The total degrees of freedom = n – 1, the regression degrees of freedom = 1, and the residual degrees of freedom = n – 2 (total – regression degrees of freedom). The mean squares are the sums of squares divided by their degrees of freedom.

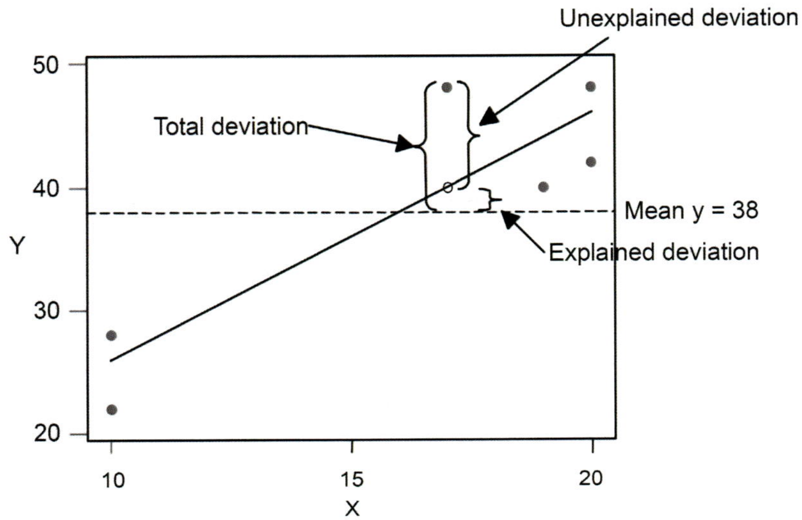

Figure 8.9. *Total, explained and unexplained deviations for a point.*

Source: Viv Bewick, Liz Cheek and Jonathan Ball: Correlation and regression: ISSN 1364-8535.

Table 8.4. *Small Data Set with the Fitted Values from the Regression, the Deviations, and their Sums of Squares*

x (mean x = 16)	y (mean y = 38)	Fitted y = 6 + 2x	Unexplained Deviation = y – Fitted y	Explained Deviation = Fitted y – mean y	Total Deviation = y – Mean y
10	22	26	-4	-12	-16
10	28	26	2	-12	-10
20	42	46	-4	8	4
20	48	46	2	8	10
19	40	44	-4	6	2
17	48	40	8	2	10
		Sum of squares	120	456	576

Source: Viv Bewick, Liz Cheek, and Jonathan Ball: Correlation and regression: ISSN 1364-8535.

Table 8.5. *Analysis of Variance for a Small Data Set*

Source of variation	Degrees of freedom	Sum of squares	Mean square	F	*P*
Regression	1	456	456	15.2	0.018
Residual	4	120	30		
Total	5	576			

Source: Viv Bewick, Liz Cheek, and Jonathan Ball: Correlation and regression: ISSN 1364-8535.

The regression mean squares and residual mean squares would roughly match if there was no linear relationship between the variables. An F test can be used to evaluate the null hypothesis, which states that there is no linear relationship. The test statistic can be obtained by comparing it to the F distribution with 1 and n – 2 degrees of freedom. The test statistic is computed as the regression mean square divided by the residual mean square. Usually, a statistical program that can generate an exact P-value is used to conduct this analysis. Actually, for regression with a single predictor, the t test of the gradient and the F test from the analysis of variance are identical. With multiple predictors, this isn't the case, but we'll look into this more in a later review. The gradient test and the correlation test are equivalent, resulting in three tests with the same P-values. Therefore, it makes no difference which of these tests is used when there is only one predictor variable.

The analysis of variance for the A&E data (Table 8.6) gives a *P* value of 0.006 (the same *P* value as obtained previously), again indicating a linear relationship between ln urea and age.

Table 8.6. *Analysis of Variance for the Accident and Emergency Unit Data*

Source of Variation	Degrees of Freedom	Sum of Squares	Mean Square	F	*P*
Regression	1	1.462	1.462	11.24	0.004
Residual	18	2.342	0.130		
Total	19	3.804			

Source: Viv Bewick, Liz Cheek and Jonathan Ball: Correlation and regression: ISSN 1364-8535.

8.1.3.5. Coefficient of Determination

Another useful quantity that can be obtained from the analysis of variance is the coefficient of determination (R^2).

$$R^2 = \frac{\text{Regression sum of squares}}{\text{Total sum of squares}}$$

It is the proportion of the total variation in y accounted for by the regression model. Values of R^2 close to 1 imply that most of the variability in y is explained by the regression model. R^2 is the same as r^2 in regression when there is only one predictor variable.

For the A&E data, $R^2 = 1.462/3.804 = 0.38$ (i.e., the same as 0.62^2), and therefore age accounts for 38% of the total variation in ln urea. This means that 62% of the variation in ln urea is not accounted for by age differences. This may be due to inherent variability in ln urea or to other unknown factors that affect the level of ln urea.

8.1.3.6. Prediction

An approximation of the population mean of y for a specific value of x is the fitted value of y. As a result, it can be applied to supply a population mean confidence interval. The confidence intervals will fluctuate in tandem with the fitted values as x changes.

The 95% confidence interval for the fitted value of y for a particular value of x, say x_p, is again calculated as fitted y ± (t_{n-2} × the standard error). The standard error is given by:

$$s\sqrt{\left[\frac{1}{n}+\frac{(x_p-\bar{x})^2}{\sum_{i=1}^{n}(x_i-\bar{x})^2}\right]}$$

Fig 8.10 shows the range of confidence intervals for the A&E data. For example, the 95% confidence interval for the population mean ln urea for a patient aged 60 years is 1.56 to 1.92 units. This transforms to urea values of 4.76 to 6.82 mmol/l.

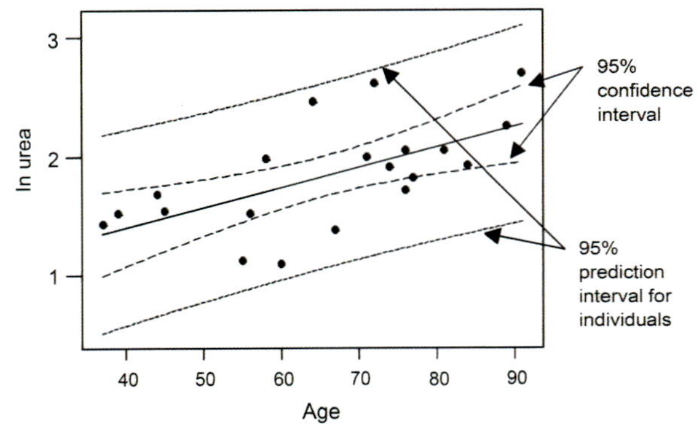

Figure 8.10. *Regression line, its 95% confidence interval and the 95% prediction interval for individual patients.*

Source: Viv Bewick, Liz Cheek and Jonathan Ball: Correlation and regression: ISSN 1364-8535.

A predicted value for an individual can also be obtained from the fitted value for y, and a prediction interval or reference range can be obtained (**Figure 8.10**). The standard error is provided by: however the prediction interval is computed similarly to the confidence interval.

$$s\sqrt{\left[\frac{1}{n}+\frac{(x_p-\bar{x})^2}{\sum_{i=1}^{n}(x_i-\bar{x})^2}\right]}$$

For example, the 95% prediction interval for the ln urea for a patient aged 60 years is 0.97 to 2.52 units. This transforms to urea values of 2.64 to 12.43 mmol/l. Both confidence intervals and prediction intervals become wider for values of the predictor variable further from the mean.

8.2. Sensitivity to Outliers, Outlier Rejection, and Robust Regression

Unusual or extreme values within a data set are referred to as outliers. Many human characteristics and biochemical parameters should be normally distributed, with most cases falling between ±2 standard deviations. Nonetheless, extreme values could appear in a big data set. These extreme values could result from coding, measurement, or data entry errors, or they could be the result of real rare events. A scatter diagram, like the one in **Figure 8.11**, can be used to visualize outliers.

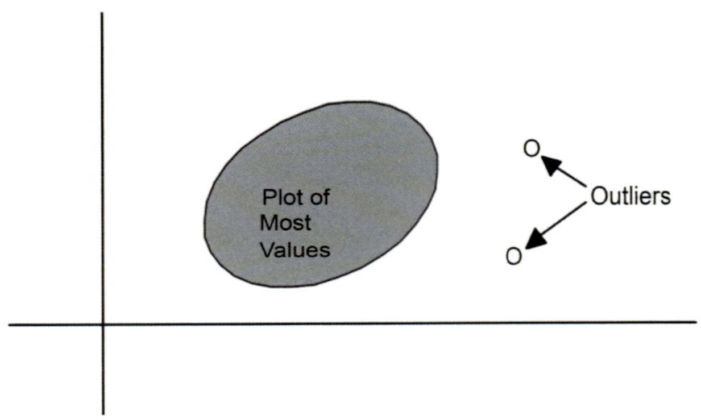

Figure 8.11. *Scatter diagram with outliers.*

Source: Michael r. Chernick, Robert h. Friis: Introductory Biostatistics for the Health Sciences: ISBN 0-471-41137-X.

The least squares method of regression calculates "b" (the regression slope) and "a" (the intercept) by minimizing the sum of squares $[\Sigma(Y-\hat{Y})^2]$ about the regression line. Outliers cause distortions in the estimates obtained by the least squares method. Robust regression techniques are used to detect outliers and minimize their influence in regression analyses.

A regression line's intercept and slope can both be affected by a small number of outliers. The square of the residual is the penalty for deviating from the line of best fit, which explains the significant effect of outliers. As a result, the slope and intercept must be set so that these outliers have smaller deviations than many of the more "normal" observations.

The position of outliers within the space delineated by the measurement distribution for X (the independent variable) also affects their impact. Leverage points are observations for extremely high or low values of X that, even in the absence of outliers, have a significant impact on the line's slope. Robust regression is an alternative to least squares regression because it is less susceptible to outliers than the least squares model. A sort of quantile regression known as a minimum absolute deviation model, or median regression, is an illustration of robust regression.

In the now-famous 2000 presidential election, the vote total for Patrick Buchanan in Florida's Palm Beach County was a very dramatic example of a significant outlier. Many people think that a sizable portion of the votes that were meant for Gore were cast for Buchanan. The so-called butterfly ballot's confusing design may have contributed to this outcome.

In any case, a consistent pattern that allows one to predict the number of votes for Buchanan based on the number of votes for Bush or Gore can be seen upon closely examining two scatter plots (**Figure 8.12**, which shows the vote totals by county for Buchanan versus Bush, and **Figure 8.13**, which shows the vote totals by county for Buchanan versus Gore). All counties except Palm Beach, where Buchanan's vote total significantly exceeded expectations, would benefit greatly from this prediction model. Palm Beach stood out conspicuously. Let's examine the information that is readily available and posted online.

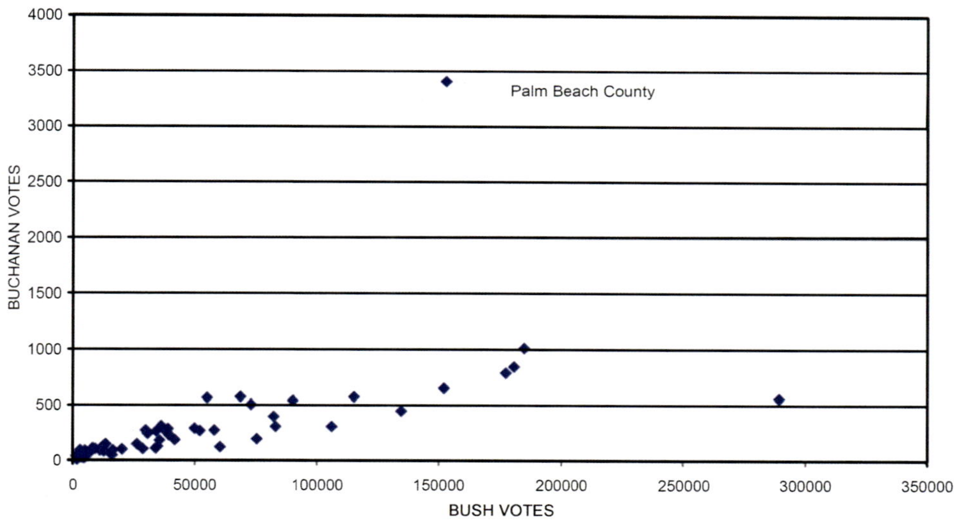

Figure 8.12. *A scatterplot of the votes for Bush versus the votes for*

Buchanan. Florida presidential votes (all counties).

Source: Michael r. Chernick, Robert h. Friis: Introductory Biostatistics for the Health Sciences: ISBN 0-471-41137-X.

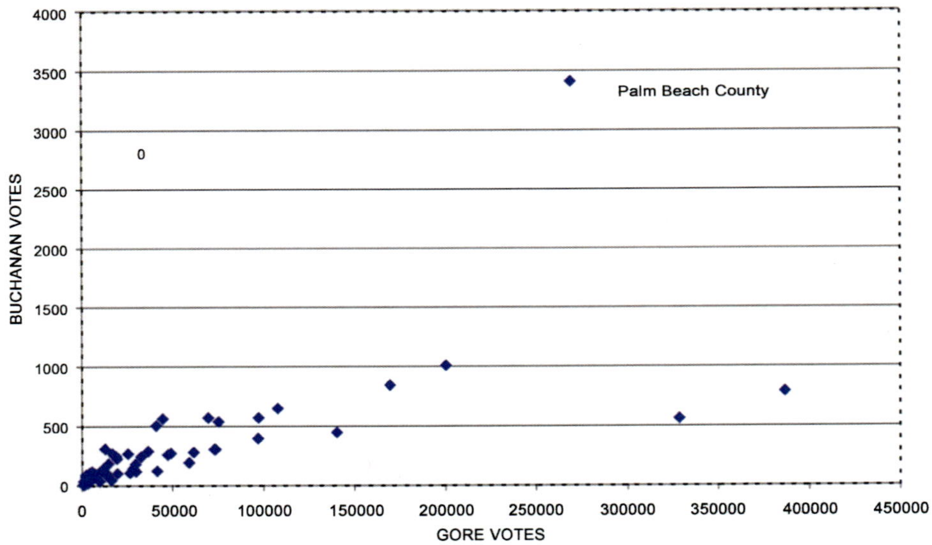

Figure 8.13. *Votes for Gore to votes for Buchanan. Florida presidential votes (all counties).*

Source: Michael r. Chernick, Robert h. Friis: Introductory Biostatistics for the Health Sciences: ISBN 0-471-41137-X.

The counties and the total number of votes that Bush, Gore, and Buchanan received in each county are displayed in **Table 8.7**. The size of the county had a major impact on the distribution of votes; nevertheless, a scatter plot shows a fairly linear relationship, for example, between the total votes cast for Bush and Buchanan. Given that the total number of votes cast for Bush is known, a regression equation could be created to predict the total number of votes cast for Buchanan. Palm Beach County is a notable outlier to this trend. This instance contains an outlier that provides valuable insight into the butterfly ballot issue.

The highest number of votes (3407 votes) went to Buchanan from Palm Beach County. Pinellas County received only 1010 votes for Buchanan, making it the county with the next highest number of votes cast. Though larger counties than Palm Beach are Broward and Dade, Buchanan received only 789 and 561 votes in those two counties, respectively. The votes cast for Bush and Buchanan are plotted against each other in **Figure 8.12**. Palm Beach County is clearly an outlier based on this figure.

Next, comparing votes for Gore to votes for Buchanan in **Figure 8.12**, and votes for Nader to votes for Buchanan in **Figure 8.14**, we observe the same pattern. With the exception of Palm Beach County, each scatter plot shows the number of votes received by each candidate in relation to the size of each county. It will be observed that the votes cast for Nader and Buchanan have a slightly higher correlation than the votes cast for Bush or Gore, and that the votes cast for Bush and Buchanan have a slightly higher correlation than the votes cast for Gore. We can use this regression function to predict Buchanan's vote totals if we take Palm Beach County out of the scatter plot and fit a regression function with or without an intercept term.

Table 8.7. *2000 Presidential Vote by County in Florida*

County	Gore	Bush	Buchanan
Alachua	47,300	34,062	262
Baker	2,392	5,610	73
Bay	18,850	38,637	248
Bradford	3,072	5,413	65
Brevard	97,318	115,185	570
Broward	386,518	177,279	789
Calhoun	2,155	2,873	90
Charlotte	29,641	35,419	182
Citrus	25,501	29,744	270
Clay	14,630	41,745	186
Collier	29,905	60,426	122
Columbia	7,047	10,964	89
Dade	328,702	289,456	561
De Soto	3,322	4,256	36
Dixie	1,825	2,698	29
Duval	107,680	152,082	650
Escambia	40,958	73,029	504
Flagler	13,891	12,608	83
Franklin	2,042	2,448	33
Gadsden	9,565	4,750	39
Gilchrist	1,910	3,300	29
Glades	1,420	1,840	9
Gulf	2,389	3,546	71
Hamilton	1,718	2,153	24
Hardee	2,341	3,764	30
Hendry	3,239	4,743	22
Hernando	32,644	30,646	242
Highlands	14,152	20,196	99
Hillsborough	169,529	180,713	845
Holmes	2,154	4,985	76
Indian River	19,769	28,627	105
Jackson	6,868	9,138	102
Jefferson	3,038	2,481	29
Lafayette	788	1,669	10
Lake	36,555	49,965	289
Lee	73,530	106,123	306
Leon	61,425	39,053	282
Levy	5,403	6,860	67
Liberty	1,011	1,316	39
Madison	3,011	3,038	29
Manatee	49,169	57,948	272
Marion	44,648	55,135	563
Martin	26,619	33,864	108
Monroe	16,483	16,059	47
Nassau	6,952	16,404	90
Okaloosa	16,924	52,043	267

County	Gore	Bush	Buchanan
Okeechobee	4,588	5,058	43
Orange	140,115	134,476	446
Osceola	28,177	26,216	145
Palm Beach	268,945	152,846	3,407
Pasco	69,550	68,581	570
Pinellas	200,212	184,884	1,010
Polk	74,977	90,101	538
Putnam	12,091	13,439	147
Santa Rosa	12,795	36,248	311
Sarasota	72,854	83,100	305
Seminole	58,888	75,293	194
St. Johns	19,482	39,497	229
St. Lucie	41,559	34,705	124
Sumter	9,634	12,126	114
Suwannee	4,084	8,014	108
Taylor	2,647	4,051	27
Union	1,399	2,326	26
Volusia	97,063	82,214	396
Wakulla	3,835	4,511	46
Walton	5,637	12,176	120
Washington	2,796	4,983	88

Source: *Michael r. Chernick, Robert h. Friis: Introductory Biostatistics for the Health Sciences: ISBN 0-471-41137-X.*

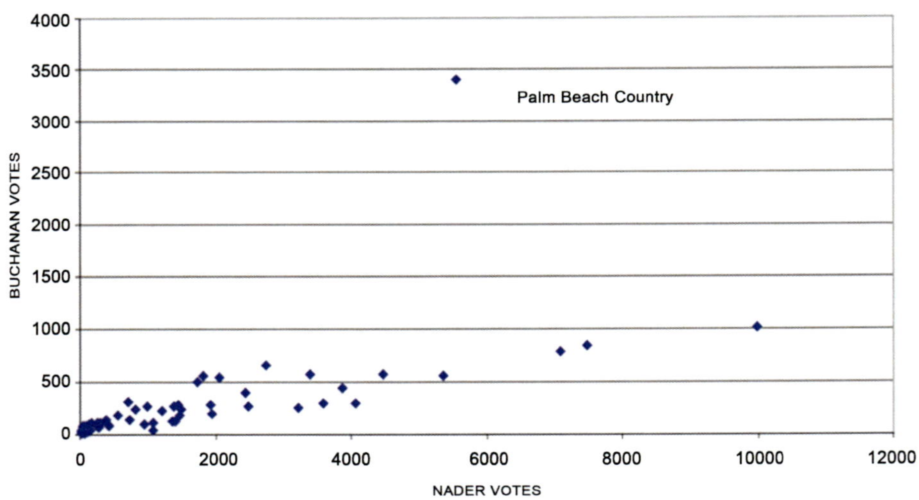

Figure 8.14. *Votes for Nader to*

votes for Buchanan. Florida presidential votes (all counties).

Source: Michael r. Chernick, Robert h. Friis: Introductory Biostatistics for the Health Sciences: ISBN 0-471-41137-X.

For instance, Figures 8.15 and 8.16 display regression equations with and without intercepts for forecasting Buchanan's votes based on votes for Nader in all counties except Palm Beach. These equations are then applied to predict the election outcome in Palm Beach. Subsequently, the predicted results are compared to the actual 3407 votes recorded for Buchanan in Palm Beach County.

Since Nader received 5564 votes in Palm Beach County, we derive, using the equation in Figure 8.15, the prediction of Y for Buchanan: $\hat{Y}$ = 0.1028(5564) + 68.93 = 640.9092. Or, if we use the zero intercept formula, we have $\hat{Y}$ = 0.1194 (5564) = 664.3416.

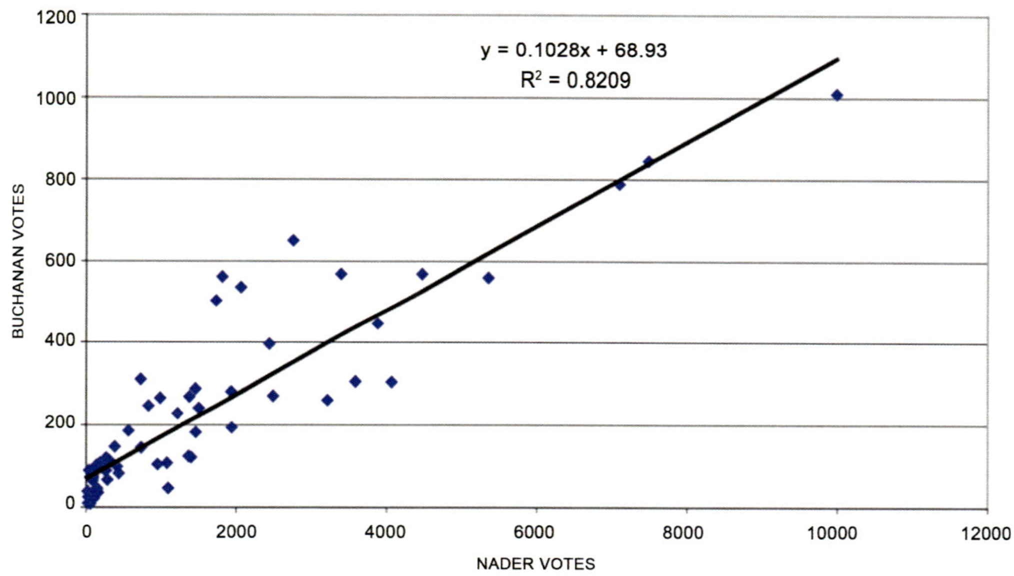

Figure 8.15. *The prediction of Y for Buchanan: Y^ = 0.1028(5564) + 68.93 = 640.9092. Florida presidential vote (palm beach county omitted).*

Source: Michael r. Chernick, Robert h. Friis: Introductory Biostatistics for the Health Sciences: ISBN 0-471-41137-X.

Similar predictions for the votes for Buchanan using the votes for Bush as the covariate X give the equations $\hat{Y}$ = 0.0035 X + 65.51 = 600.471 and $\hat{Y}$ = 0.004 X = 611.384 (zero intercept formula), since Bush reaped 152,846 votes in Palm Beach County. Votes for Gore also could be used to predict the votes for Buchanan, although the correlation is lower (r = 0.7940 for the equation with intercept, and r = 0.6704 for the equation without the intercept).

Using the votes for Gore, the regression equations are $\hat{Y}$ = 0.0025 X + 109.24 and $\hat{Y}$ = 0.0032 X, respectively, for the fit with and without the intercept. Gore's 268,945 votes in Palm Beach County lead to predictions of 781.6025 and 1075.78 using the intercept and non-intercept equations, respectively (see Figure 8.16).

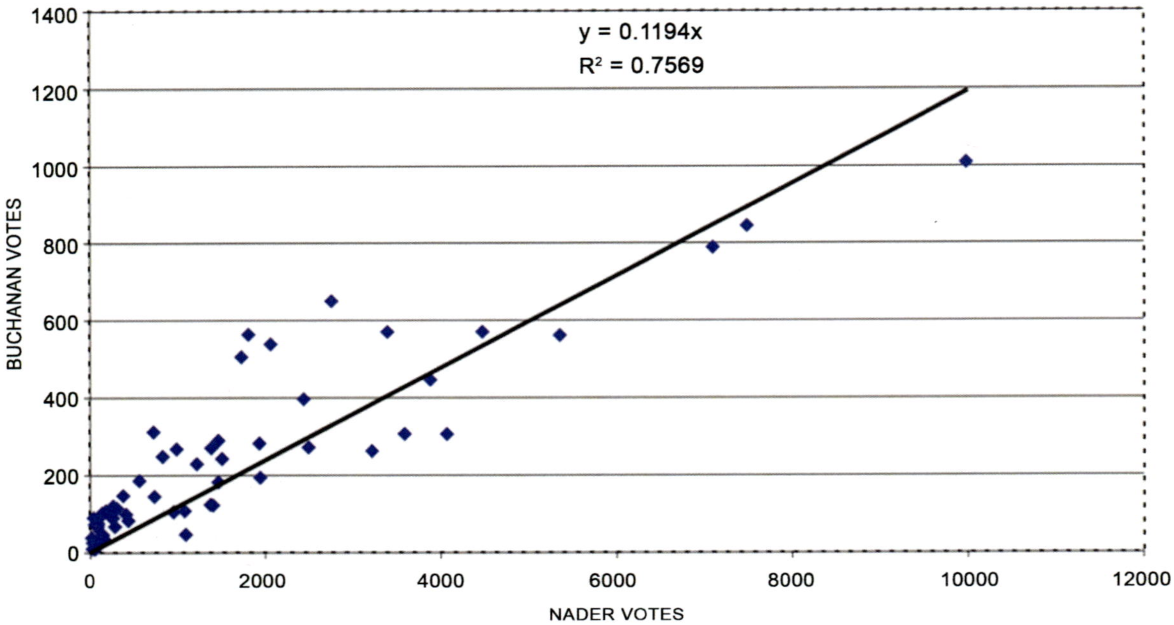

Figure 8.16. *The prediction of Y for Buchanan: Y^ = 0.1194 (5564) = 664.3416. Florida presidential vote (palm beach county omitted).*

Source: Michael r. Chernick, Robert h. Friis: Introductory Biostatistics for the Health Sciences: ISBN 0-471-41137-X.

In every instance, the estimated number of votes for Buchanan varied from about 600 to approximately 1076 votes, significantly lower than the 3407 votes he ultimately received. This difference in predicted and actual votes strongly suggests that up to 2000 of the votes attributed to Buchanan might have been meant for Gore.

Increasing the votes for Gore would remove the outlier in the number of votes cast for Buchanan in Palm Beach County. This adjustment addresses the concerns of voters who were confused by the butterfly ballot. An analysis of the ballot suggests that the hole punched for Buchanan could easily be mistaken for Gore's, but not for any other candidate. Using multiple regression could provide a more accurate prediction of the votes for Buchanan. (Aggarwal et al., 2017) (Altman et al., 1991).

8.3. Multiple Linear Regression

Multiple linear regression is a statistical method for predicting the value of a variable by using two or more other variables. It is also called multiple regression and is an expansion of linear regression. The variable we are trying to predict is called the dependent variable, while the variables used to make this prediction are called independent or explanatory variables (see **Figure 8.17**).

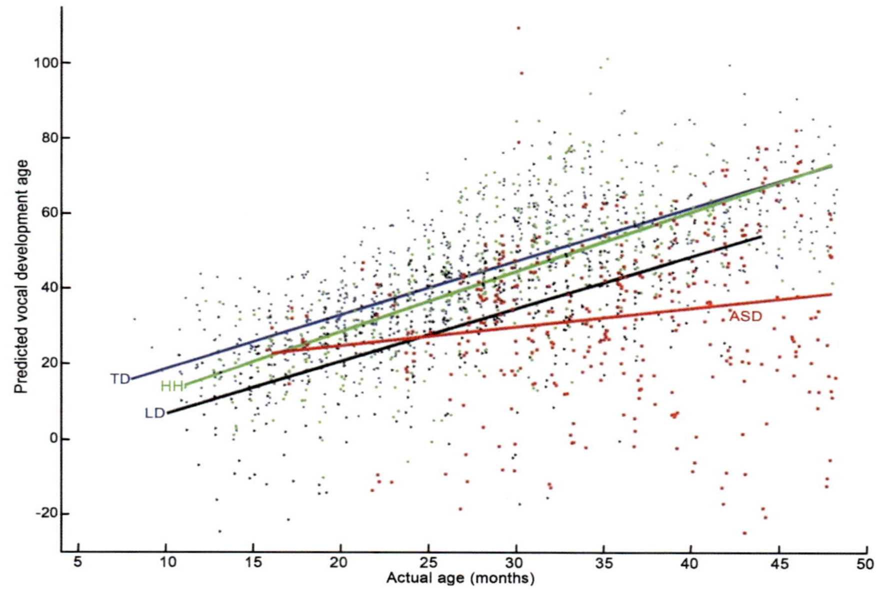

Figure 8.17. *Multiple linear regression model predictions for individual observations.*

Source: https://corporatefinanceinstitute.com/resources/data-science/multiple-linear-regression/.

8.3.1. Multiple Linear Regression Formula

$$yi = \beta 0 + \beta 1xi1 + \beta 2xi2 + ... + \beta pxip + \epsilon$$

Where:

- **yi** is the dependent or predicted variable
- **β0** is the y-intercept, i.e., the value of y when both xi and x2 are 0.
- **β1** and **β2** are the regression coefficients representing the change in y relative to a one-unit change in **xi1** and **xi2**, respectively.
- **βp** is the slope coefficient for each independent variable
- ϵ is the model's random error (residual) term.

Simple linear regression allows statisticians to make predictions about one variable using information about another variable. It works to determine the relationship between the two variables on a straight line.

Multiple regression is a statistical method used to analyze the relationship between a dependent variable and two or more independent variables. This relationship can be linear, meaning it follows a straight line, or non-linear, where the variables do not follow a straight line. Both linear and non-linear regression aim to predict a specific response using multiple variables. However, non-linear regression is often more challenging to implement as it involves making assumptions based on trial and error.

8.3.2. Assumptions of Multiple Linear Regression

Multiple linear regression is based on the following assumptions:

8.3.2.1. A Linear Relationship between the Dependent and Independent Variables

One of the main assumptions in multiple linear regression is that a linear relationship exists between the dependent variable and each of the independent variables. To verify this relationship, it is recommended to create scatterplots and visually examine them for linearity. If the scatterplot does not show a linear relationship, the analyst may need to consider running a non-linear regression or transforming the data using statistical software such as SPSS.

8.3.2.2. The Independent Variables are not Highly Correlated with Each Other

Multi-collinearity should not be present in the data, which occurs when the independent variables are highly correlated with each other. When multicollinearity is present, it becomes difficult to determine which specific independent variable is contributing to the variance in the dependent variable. The most effective method to test for multi-collinearity is the Variance Inflation Factor (VIF) method.

8.3.2.3. The variance of the Residuals is Constant

Multiple linear regression assumes that the residuals have consistent variance throughout the linear model, a concept known as homoscedasticity. To test this assumption, analysts should plot the standardized residuals against the predicted values to check for even distribution across all independent variable values. This can be done through a scatterplot or using statistical software to visualize the entire model.

8.3.2.4. Independence of Observation

The observations are supposed to be independent of each other, according to the model. In other words, the model assumes that the residual values are independent. The Durbin-Watson statistic is used to verify this assumption. The test will display values between 0 and 4, with values between 0 and 2 indicating positive autocorrelation and values between 2 and 4 indicating negative autocorrelation. The middle point, i.e., a value of two indicates the absence of autocorrelation.

8.3.2.5. Multivariate Normality

Multivariate normality is present when residuals show a normal distribution. To assess this assumption, examine the distribution of residual values. Two common methods to test for this are by using a histogram with a normal curve overlay or by using the Normal Probability Plot method.

8.4. Logistic Regression

The process of estimating the relationship between continuous predictor (independent) variables and an outcome (dependent) variable on a continuous scale is known as linear regression analysis. Specifically, we examine the relationship between a binary (or dichotomous) outcome (e.g., yes/no, success/failure, alive/dead) with one or more continuous or categorical predictors.

Let us examine a hypothetical study that compares two treatments for patients with oesophageal varices: sclerotherapy and variceal ligation [Table 8.8a]. The odds ratio (OR) for death in the sclerotherapy arm of 2.05 relative to the ligation arm is revealed by a straightforward (univariate) analysis. This indicates that a patient undergoing sclerotherapy has a nearly twofold higher chance of dying than a patient undergoing ligation.

Table 8.8. *Relation of Death (a Dichotomous Outcome) with (a) Treatment Given (Variceal Ligation Versus Sclerotherapy), (b) Prior Beta-Blocker Therapy, and (c) Both Treatment Given and Prior Beta-Blocker Therapy*

(a) Treatment given (variceal ligation versus sclerotherapy)

Treatment given	Outcome		Row totals
	Dead	Survived	
Variceal ligation	18	46	64
Variceal sclerotherapy	29	36	65
Total	47	82	129

(b) Prior beta-blocker therapy

Concurrent treatment	Outcome		Row totals
	Dead	Survived	
Beta-blocker	12	48	60
No beta-blocker	35	34	69
Total	47	82	129

(c) Both treatment given and prior beta-blocker therapy

Type of treatment	Dead	Survived	Total	Odds ratio for death in "ligation" arm versus "sclerotherapy" arm
Beta-blocker				
Ligation	8	20	28	2.8
Sclerotherapy	4	28	32	
No beta-blocker				
Ligation	10	26	36	0.12
Sclerotherapy	25	8	33	

Source: *https://www.ncbi.nlm.nih.gov/pmc/articles/PMC5543767/.*

However, we are aware that a person's risk of dying can be influenced by several factors besides their treatment preference. These could include, but are not limited to, age, gender, the presence of other illnesses, and the use of beta-blockers concurrently. To examine how beta-blocker therapy affects death, we can create a 2 × 2 table [Table 8.8b]. This shows the OR for death in the 4.1 "no beta-blocker" arm compared to the "beta-blocker" arm. Similarly, we can ascertain how death is related to other predictors, like gender, age, and the existence of additional illnesses. These analyses, which are referred to as univariate analyses and provide us with unadjusted ORs, evaluate the relationship between one predictor factor and the dichotomous outcome variable, which is death.

But frequently, our interest lies in determining whether different predictors are confounded; for instance, did a similar percentage of patients in the ligation and sclerotherapy arms receive beta-blockers? This can be achieved by stratifying the data and creating distinct tables for two levels of the most likely confounder, such as beta-blocker and no beta-blocker [Table 8.8c]. This analysis makes it clear that ligation raised the risk of death for people taking beta-blockers while lowering the risk for people not taking beta-blockers. Consequently, we should not compare the effects of ligation and sclerotherapy without considering beta-blocker administration. In a similar vein, we might be interested in finding out if patients' ages, a continuous variable, differed between the two treatment groups and whether this variation might have had an impact on the relationship between treatment and death. In actuality, our goal is to evaluate the combined impact of multiple predictor variables (continuous and categorical) on a single binary result. This is accomplished through the use of "multivariable logistic regression," a method that enables us to examine the impact of several variables on a dichotomous outcome at the same time.

8.4.1. How Does Multiple Logistic Regression Work?

The statistical program first determines, in the absence of any predictor, the baseline odds of having the outcome versus not having the outcome. We now have the constant, also referred to as the intercept. Following the selection of the independent (input/predictor) variables, the regression coefficient (also referred to as "beta") and P value are computed for each of the variables in the model. The software thus provides the results in a format that resembles [Table 8.9a]. The "P" value indicates whether or not a given variable significantly influences the outcome's likelihood of occurring. An equation [Table 8.9b] that includes the constant term and the regression coefficient for each variable that has been determined to be significant (often using $P < 0.05$) can also be used to express these results. Given a person's profile of predictor factors, the equation offers a model that can be used to predict the likelihood that an event will occur for that person.

Table 8.9. *Different Methods of Representing Results of a Multivariate Logistic Analysis: (A) as a Table Showing Regression Coefficients and Significance Levels, (B) as an Equation for Log (Odds) Containing Regression Coefficients for Each Variable, and (C) as an Equation for Odds Using Coefficients (Or Anti-Loge) of Regression Coefficients (which Represents Adjusted Odds Ratios) for Each Variable*

(a) Regression coefficients and significance levels

Predictor factor	Regression coefficient (β)*	Significance level (*P*)	aOR=Exp(β) (exponential or anti-log$_e$ of the regression coefficient)
Constant	−3.06	0.001	0.05
Treatment (sclerotherapy vs. ligation)	0.34	0.023	1.40
Gender (female vs. male)	−1.76	0.006	0.17
Age	0.06	0.008	1.06
Presence of other illnesses (yes vs. no)	1.26	0.310	3.53

*Positive values of β imply aOR >1.0, or a positive association, negative values imply aOR <1.0, or a protective association (and of 0 would imply aOR=1.0, or no association). aOR=adjusted odds ratio

(b) Equation for log (odds) containing regression coefficients for each variable

$\log_e$ (odds of death)= −3.06 + 0.34 (sclerotherapy) − 1.76 (gender) + 0.061 (age)
(i) The sign for the gender term is negative in keeping with the negative sign of its coefficient (as shown in section "a" above), and (ii) the variable "presence of other illnesses" has been left out since it was not significant (had a $P>0.05$)

(c) Equation for odds using coefficients (or anti-log$_e$) of regression coefficients (which represents aORs) for each variable

Odds of death=0.047 × $(1.4^{[1 \text{ if sclerotherapy}, 0 \text{ if ligation}]})$ × $(0.17^{[1 \text{ if female}, 0 \text{ if male}]})$ × $([1.06]^{age})$

The equation in (b) above is additive, and that in (c) above is multiplicative. aOR=adjusted odds ratio

Source: https://www.ncbi.nlm.nih.gov/pmc/articles/PMC5543767/

The coefficients, which are a little challenging to understand on their own, show the odds associated with each factor in logarithmic form (using the natural base, denoted by "e"). As can be seen in the final column of Table 8.9a, the software tools frequently also automatically compute antilogs (exponentials) of the coefficients. These provide adjusted ORs (aOR) for having the desired outcome if a specific exposure is present, while controlling for the impact of other predictor factors. An alternate model representation can be created using these aORs [Table 8.9c].

For categorical predictors, the aOR is concerning a reference category (exposure absent). For example, the aOR for treatment gives the chance of death in the sclerotherapy group as compared to the ligation group, i.e., patients receiving sclerotherapy are 1.4 times more likely to die than those receiving ligation, after adjusting for age, gender, and presence of other illnesses. For gender, it refers to the odds of death in women versus men (i.e., women are 0.25 times [one-fourth] as likely to die as males, after adjusting for type of treatment, age, and presence of other illnesses). Most software tools allow the user to choose the reference category. For example, for gender, one could choose "female" as the reference category – in that case, the result would provide the odds of death in men as compared to women. The results would be different in that case – with software returning the aOR for gender of 4 (= 1/0.25), i.e., men are four times more likely to die than women after adjusting for other factors. If a factor has more than two categories (e.g., non-smoker, ex-smoker, current smoker), then separate ORs are calculated for each of the other categories relative to a particular reference category (ex-smoker vs. nonsmoker; current smoker vs. nonsmoker).

If predictors are continuous (e.g., age), the aOR shows how the odds of the desired outcome rise for each unit increase in the input variable. In the aforementioned example, the odds of dying increase by 6% (OR of 1.06) for every year of age increase. This increase is multiplicative; for example, a three-year increase in age would result in a $1.06 \times 1.06 \times 1.06$ (or $[1.06]^3$) increase in the odds of dying. (Antwi et al., 2017) (Atkinson et al., 1985).

A Closer Look

Multivariable Regression

Multivariable regression analysis is a statistical technique used to understand the relationship between multiple independent variables and a single dependent variable. It's an extension of simple linear regression, where only one independent variable is considered. In multivariable regression, the aim is to model the relationship between the dependent variable and two or more independent variables while controlling for the potential effects of other variables.

The process of conducting a multivariable regression analysis typically involves several steps. First, researchers select a dependent variable they want to predict or explain and identify multiple independent variables they believe may influence it. These independent variables can be continuous, categorical, or binary.

Next, researchers gather data on these variables from their sample or population of interest. It's essential to ensure the data is reliable, valid, and representative of the population being studied.

Once the data is collected, researchers use statistical software to run the regression analysis. The output of the analysis includes coefficients for each independent variable, which represent the strength and direction of their relationship with the dependent variable. These coefficients indicate how much the dependent variable is expected to change when the independent variable changes, holding all other variables constant.

In addition to coefficients, the output typically includes other statistics such as p-values, R-squared values, and standard errors, which help assess the overall fit of the model and the significance of individual predictors.

Interpreting the results of a multivariable regression analysis requires careful consideration of several factors. Researchers need to assess the magnitude and direction of the coefficients, as well as their statistical significance. They also need to consider potential confounding variables and interactions between independent variables.

Overall, multivariable regression analysis is a powerful tool for examining complex relationships between variables and can provide valuable insights in various fields, including epidemiology, economics, social sciences, and healthcare research. However, it's essential to use this technique appropriately and interpret the results with caution, taking into account the limitations and assumptions of the analysis.

Summary

- Correlation and regression are statistical methods used to explore the relationship between variables and make predictions based on data. While both techniques are related and often used together, they serve different purposes and provide distinct insights into the data.
- A data set may sometimes comprise distinct subgroups, for example, males and females. This could result in clusters of points leading to an inflated correlation coefficient. A single outlier may produce the same sort of effect.
- The regression line is obtained using the method of least squares. Any line $y = a + bx$ that we draw through the points gives a predicted or fitted value of y for each value of x in the data set. For a particular value of x the vertical difference between the observed and fitted value of y is known as the deviation, or residual.
- The fitted value of y for a given value of x is an estimate of the population mean of y for that particular value of x. As such it can be used to provide a confidence interval for the population mean. The fitted values change as x changes, and therefore the confidence intervals will also change.
- Multiple linear regression refers to a statistical technique that is used to predict the outcome of a variable based on the value of two or more variables. It is sometimes known simply as multiple regression, and it is an extension of linear regression. The variable that we want to predict is known as the dependent variable, while the variables we use to predict the value of the dependent variable are known as independent or explanatory variables.
- Linear regression analysis which estimates the relationship of an outcome (dependent) variable on a continuous scale with continuous predictor (independent) variables.

References

1. Aggarwal, R., & Ranganathan, P. (2017). Common pitfalls in statistical analysis: Linear regression analysis. *Perspectives in Clinical Research, 8*, 100–102.
2. Altman, D. G. (1991). *Practical Statistics for Medical Research*. London: Chapman & Hall.
3. Antwi, E., Groenwold, R. H., Browne, J. L., Franx, A., Agyepong, I. A., & Koram, K. A., et al. (2017). Development and validation of a prediction model for gestational hypertension in a Ghanaian cohort. *BMJ Open, 7*, e012670.
4. Atkinson, A. C. (1985). *Plots, Transformations, and Regression*. New York: Oxford University Press.
5. Belsley, D. A., Kuh, E., & Welsch, R. E. (1980). *Regression Diagnostics*. New York: Wiley.
6. Bland, M. (2001). *An Introduction to Medical Statistics* (3rd ed.). Oxford: Oxford University Press.
7. Bland, M., & Altman, D. G. (1986). Statistical methods for assessing agreement between two methods of clinical measurement. *The Lancet, 1*, 307–310.
8. Bloomfield, P., & Steiger, W. (1983). *Least Absolute Deviations*. Boston: Birkhauser.

9. Campbell, M. J., & Machin, D. (1999). *Medical Statistics: A Commonsense Approach* (3rd ed.). Chichester, England: Wiley.
10. Carroll, R. J., & Ruppert, D. (1988). *Transformation and Weighting in Regression*. New York: Chapman and Hall.
11. Chatterjee, S., & Hadi, A. S. (1988). *Sensitivity Analysis in Linear Regression*. New York: Wiley.
12. Chatterjee, S., Price, B., & Hadi, A. S. (1999). *Regression Analysis by Example* (3rd ed.). New York: Wiley.
13. Cook, R. D. (1998). *Regression Graphics*. New York: Wiley.
14. Cook, R. D., & Weisberg, S. (1982). *Residuals and Influence in Regression*. London: Chapman and Hall.
15. Draper, N. R., & Smith, H. (1998). *Applied Regression Analysis* (3rd ed.). New York: Wiley.
16. Hosmer, D. W., & Lemeshow, S. (2000). *Applied Logistic Regression* (2nd ed.). New York: Wiley.
17. Jaske, D. R. (1994). Illustrating the Gauss–Markov theorem. *The American Statistician, 48*, 237–238.
18. McCullagh, P., & Nelder, J. A. (1989). *Generalized Linear Models* (2nd ed.). London: Chapman and Hall.
19. Montgomery, D. C., & Peck, E. A. (1992). *Introduction to Linear Regression Analysis* (2nd ed.). New York: Wiley.
20. Myers, R. H. (1990). *Classical and Modern Regression with Applications* (2nd ed.). North Scituate, MA: PWS-Kent.
21. Peduzzi, P., Concato, J., Kemper, E., Holford, T. R., & Feinstein, A. R. (1996). A simulation study of the number of events per variable in logistic regression analysis. *Journal of Clinical Epidemiology, 49*, 1373–1379.
22. Ranganathan, P., Aggarwal, R., & Pramesh, C. S. (2015). Common pitfalls in statistical analysis: Odds versus risk. *Perspectives in Clinical Research, 6*, 222–224.
23. Rousseeuw, P. J., & Leroy, A. M. (1987). *Robust Regression and Outlier Detection*. New York: Wiley.
24. Ryan, T. P. (1997). *Modern Regression Methods*. New York: Wiley.
25. Staudte, R. G., & Sheather, S. J. (1990). *Robust Estimation and Testing*. New York: Wiley.
26. Vittinghoff, E., & McCulloch, C. E. (2007). Relaxing the rule of ten events per variable in logistic and Cox regression. *American Journal of Epidemiology, 165*, 710–718.
27. Weisberg, S. (1985). *Applied Linear Regression* (2nd ed.). New York: Wiley.
28. Whitley, E., & Ball, J. (2002). Statistics review 2: Samples and populations. *Critical Care, 6*, 143–148. https://doi.org/10.1186/cc1473
29. Zar, J. H. (1999). *Biostatistical Analysis* (4th ed.). New Jersey: Prentice Hall.

Chapter

NONPARAMETRIC TESTS

9

Contents

Introduction 244

9.1. Parametric and Nonparametric Tests 246

9.2. Nonparametric Testing 249

9.3. Tests with Two Independent Samples 251

9.4. Tests with Matched Samples 257

9.5. Tests with More than Two Independent Samples 268

Summary 275

References 275

Introduction

Nonparametric tests in biostatistics play a vital role in public health research by providing robust statistical methods for analyzing data when certain assumptions of traditional parametric tests are not met or when dealing with non-normal distributions. Unlike parametric tests, which make assumptions about the underlying distribution of the data, nonparametric tests offer flexibility and can be applied to a wide range of data types, including ordinal, nominal, and continuous variables.

Nonparametric tests are statistical methods that do not rely on specific population parameters, such as means and variances. Instead, they focus on the ranks or frequencies of data points, making them particularly useful when the data do not follow a normal distribution or when sample sizes are small. In public health research, where data may be inherently skewed or have outliers, nonparametric tests offer reliable alternatives to parametric tests. One commonly used nonparametric test is the Wilcoxon rank-sum test (also known as the Mann-Whitney U test), which compares two independent groups to determine if there is a significant difference between them. This test is valuable when the assumptions of the independent samples t-test are violated, such as non-normality or unequal variances.

Another widely used nonparametric test is the Kruskal-Wallis test, which extends the idea of the rank-sum test to compare more than two independent groups. It is particularly useful for analyzing differences among multiple groups when the assumptions of the analysis of variance (ANOVA) cannot be met.

In addition to comparing groups, nonparametric tests can also assess relationships between variables. The Spearman rank correlation coefficient, for example, measures the strength and direction of association between two variables based on their ranks rather than their actual values. This makes it suitable for analyzing monotonic relationships, even when the data do not meet the assumptions of Pearson's correlation coefficient.

Overall, nonparametric tests offer valuable tools for analyzing data in public health research, especially when dealing with non-normal distributions, small sample sizes, or ordinal data. By providing robust statistical methods that do not rely on stringent assumptions, nonparametric tests contribute to the rigor and validity of statistical analyses in biostatistics and public health.

Orientation and Directional Terms

Term	Definition	Illustration
Hypothesis	A hypothesis is an assumption or idea that is proposed for argument so that it can be tested to see if it might be true. In statistics, a hypothesis is a formal statement that explains the relationship between two or more variables in a specified population.	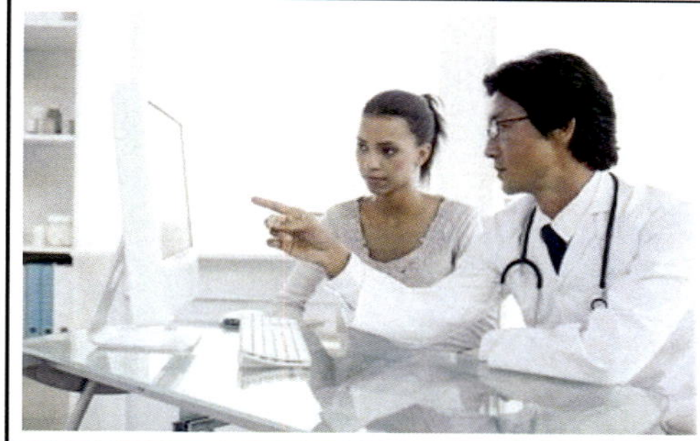
Parametric tests	Parametric tests are statistical tests that assume data follows a normal distribution, or "bell-shaped curve." They are used in biostatistics when samples are randomly drawn from a population and observations within a group are independent.	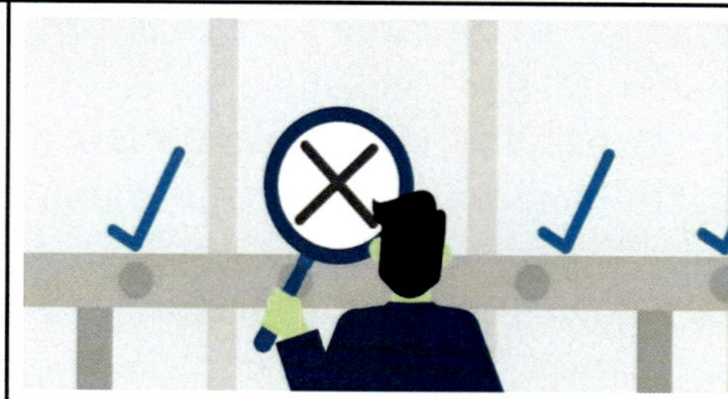
Ordinal-scale data	Ordinal data is quantitative data that has a natural order, but the difference between the data is unknown. In medicine, ordinal variables are often used to describe patient characteristics, attitudes, behaviours, or status.	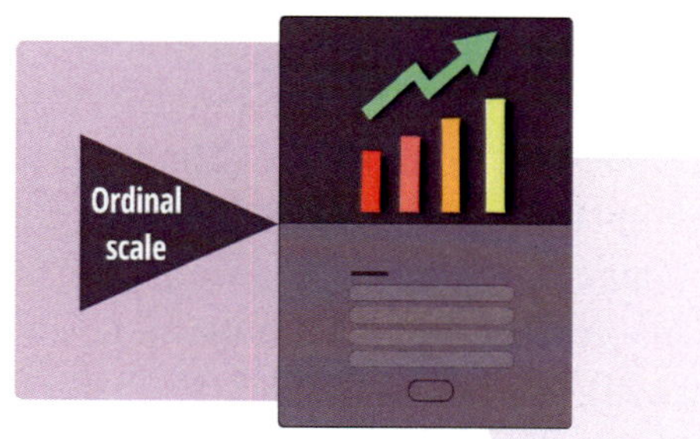
Test statistic	Test statistic is a numerical value that summarizes a data set and is used in statistical hypothesis testing	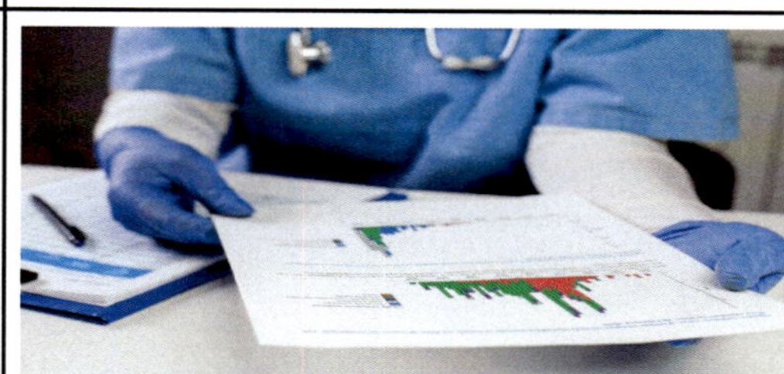
Mann–Whitney U test	The Mann-Whitney U test, also known as the Wilcoxon Rank Sum Test or Mann Whitney Wilcoxon Test, is a non-parametric statistical test that compares two sample means from the same population to determine if they are equal.	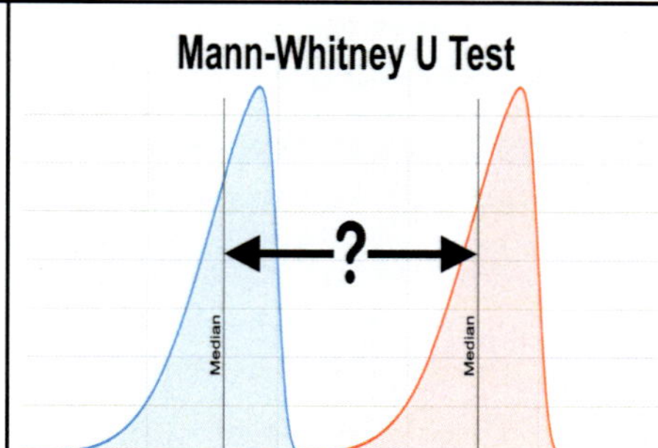

9.1. Parametric and Nonparametric Tests

Several hypothesis tests for outcomes that are ordinal, continuous, dichotomous, and categorical. Whereas tests for dichotomous, categorical, and ordinal outcomes concentrated on comparing proportions, tests for continuous outcomes compared means.

For their proper application, parametric tests and their assumptions are predicated. For instance, all parametric tests rely on the assumption that the outcome is roughly normally distributed in the population when conducting hypothesis tests for means of continuous outcomes. This indicates that the outcome follows a normal distribution in the entire population, which is not observed, rather than that the data in the observed sample follow a normal distribution. In numerous cases, investigators feel at ease using the normalcy assumption (i.e., fewer observations are at either extreme and the majority are in the middle of the distribution). It also turns out that a lot of statistical tests are robust, meaning that even in the case where some or all of the assumptions are not met, the tests retain their statistical properties. Based on the Central Limit Theorem, tests are robust if the normalcy assumption is broken when the sample size is large.

Nonparametric tests are appropriate alternative tests when the sample size is small and the outcome distribution is unknown and cannot be assumed to be approximately normally distributed.

Due to their lower assumption base, nonparametric tests are also referred to as distribution-free tests (e.g., they don't assume that the result will be roughly normally distributed. Parametric tests involve specific probability distributions (e. g., the normal distribution), and the tests entail estimating the distribution's essential parameters (e.g., the sample data's mean (or difference in means). Fewer assumptions come at the expense of nonparametric tests' typically lower power compared to parametric counterparts (i.e., when the alternative is accurate, they might be less inclined to dismiss H_0.

Determining whether a continuous outcome has a normal distribution and, therefore, whether a parametric or nonparametric test is appropriate, can be challenging at times. Some statistical tests can be employed to evaluate the likelihood that data originate from a normal distribution. The most widely used ones are the Shapiro-Wilk, Anderson-Darling, and Kolmogorov-Smirnov tests. Every test compares observed data to quantiles of the normal (or another specified) distribution, effectively serving as a goodness-of-fit test. For every test, the null hypothesis is H_0: The data are normally distributed, as opposed to H_1: The data are not normally distributed. Should the test be noteworthy (e.g., $p < 0.05$), then a nonparametric test is necessary because the data do not fit into a normal distribution. It should be mentioned that low power may affect these normal tests. In particular, if the data do not follow a normal distribution, the tests may fail to reject H_0: Data follow a normal distribution. Unfortunately, low power is a significant problem when the sample size is small, which is frequently the case when we want to use these tests. The most useful method for determining normality is to use a histogram to examine the distributional form of the outcome in the sample and supplement it with information from other studies, if any, that could help determine how the outcome is distributed in the population.

In certain cases, it is evident that the result does not fit into a normal distribution. These scenarios include those in which the result has distinct limits of detection, is an ordinal variable or a rank or has definite outliers. The following are some examples of these kinds of results. Imagine a clinical trial in which participants are asked to rate the severity of their symptoms after receiving the prescribed treatment for six weeks. The following response options can be used to rate the severity of symptoms on a 5-point ordinal scale: symptoms got much worse, symptoms got slightly worse, no change, symptoms improved slightly, or symptoms are much improved. Assume the trial has n = 20 participants in total, who are randomized to receive either a placebo or the experimental treatment. The distribution of the outcome data is depicted in Figure 9.1. There is a discrepancy in the outcome distribution (symptom severity); more participants report improved symptoms than worsening symptoms.

In certain investigations, a rank is the result. For instance, the health of a newborn is frequently evaluated using the APGAR score in obstetrical research. The APGAR score, which describes a baby's condition at birth, is named after Dr. Virginia Apgar. The five factors that make up the APGAR score are skin appearance, respiration, activity (or muscle tone), grimace (reflex or response to stimulation), and pulse rate. Based on particular clinical criteria, each of the five criteria is rated as 0 (very unhealthy), 1 (healthy), or 2 (well). The five component scores add up to the APGAR score, which is a number between 0 and 10. Infants scoring seven or above are regarded as normal; those scoring four to six are regarded as low; and those scoring zero to three are deemed critically low. The APGAR scores are sometimes recalculated and then examined, for instance, one minute, five minutes, and ten minutes after delivery. Most newborns have APGAR scores of 7 or higher, which is within the normal range, but the scores do not typically follow a normal distribution.

The results of certain studies are continuous, but they can contain extreme values or outliers. One outcome that is prone to anomalies is the length of stay in the hospital after a specific surgical procedure. Let's say researchers want to determine if patients in for-profit versus nonprofit hospitals stay longer in the hospital after receiving a liver transplant in an observational study. Assume that the number of days spent in the hospital after a transplant is calculated for n = 100 participants, with 50 coming from nonprofit and 50 from for-profit hospitals. The results are displayed in Figure 9.2.

Note that 75% of the participants stay at most 16 days in the hospital following a transplant, while at least one patient stays 35 days, which would be considered an outlier. We use $Q_1 - 1.5(Q_3 - Q_1)$ as a lower limit and $Q_3 + 1.5(Q_3 - Q1)$ as an upper limit to detect outliers. In Figure 9.2, $Q_1 = 12$ and $Q_3 = 16$; thus outliers are values below 12 − 1.5(16 − 12) = 6 or above 16 + 1.5(16 − 12) = 22.

In certain investigations, the result is a continuous variable that is measured somewhat imprecisely (e.g., with distinct detection bounds). Certain assays or instruments are unable to detect the presence of particular quantities above or below predetermined thresholds. For instance, the number of copies of the virus in a specific volume of blood is known as the viral load, which indicates the quantity of virus present in the body.

It can have hundreds of millions of copies or be "not detected" or "below the limit of detection." As a result, measurements for some sample members maybe 1,254,000 copies or 874,050 copies, while measurements for other participants may be marked as "not detected.." In cases where a significant proportion of participants exhibit undetectable viral load, the viral load distribution is not normally distributed.

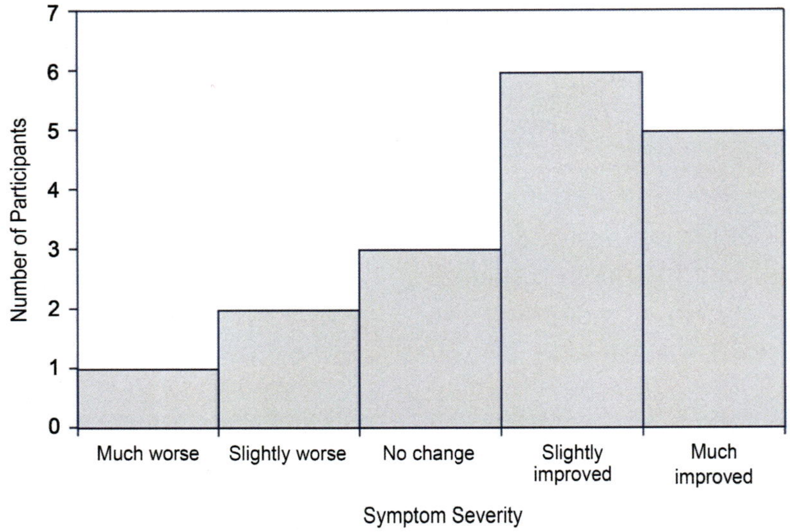

Figure 9.1. *Distribution of symptom severity in total sample.*

Source: Lisa M. Sullivan, Essentials of Biostatistics in Public Health Third Edition, ISBN 9781284108194.

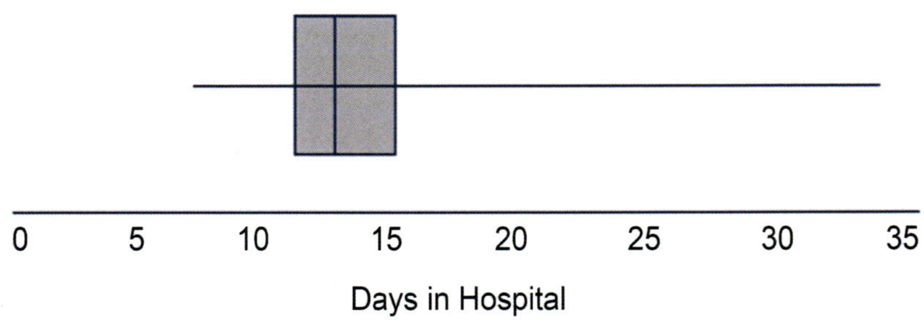

Figure 9.2. *Distribution of days in the hospital following transplant.*

Source: Lisa M. Sullivan, Essentials of Biostatistics in Public Health Third Edition, ISBN 9781284108194.

The hypotheses in nonparametric tests do not concern population parameters (e.g., $m_1 = m_2$ or m = 50. The null hypothesis, on the other hand, is more broad. For instance, in a parametric test, the null hypothesis is H_0: $m_1 = m_2$. when comparing two independent groups in terms of a continuous outcome. In a nonparametric test, on the other hand, the null hypothesis is that the two populations are equal, which is frequently taken to mean that they are equal about their central tendency.

There are several clear benefits to using nonparametric tests. Nonparametric tests might be the only method available for analyzing the data when the results are as described above. It is challenging to use parametric methods for analysis of outcomes that are ordinal, ranked, susceptible to outliers, or imprecisely measured without making significant assumptions about their distributions and choices regarding how to code certain values (e.g., "not detected.." Nonparametric tests can also be reasonably easy to perform, as we explain here.

Here, we outline a few well-liked nonparametric tests for continuous results. If readers are interested in a more thorough explanation of nonparametric tests, they should consult Conover. It is important to reiterate before moving further that parametric tests are more appropriate if the data are approximately normally distributed. In general, parametric tests are more potent and capable of testing a larger variety of alternative hypotheses. Nonetheless, there are circumstances where a nonparametric test is preferable because the assumptions underlying a parametric test are broken.

9.2. Nonparametric Testing

Techniques for summarizing data gathered in a sample are presented, and we made distinctions between different kinds of variables or results. We specifically covered the following outcomes: ordinal and categorical (which have more than two response options and are ordered and unordered, respectively); continuous variables (also referred to as quantitative or measurement variables); and dichotomous outcomes (which have only two possible response options, typically coded as "yes" and "no"). Theoretically, there are an infinite number of possible responses for continuous variables.

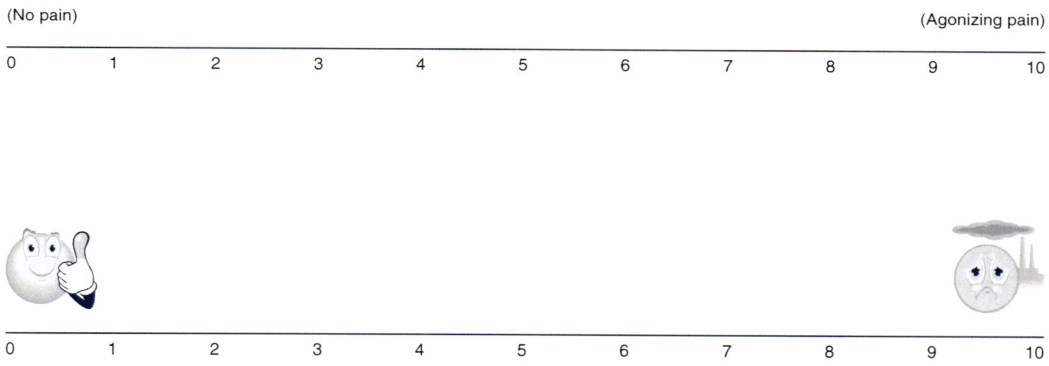

Figure 9.3. *Visual pain scales.*

Source: Lisa M. Sullivan, Essentials of Biostatistics in Public Health Third Edition, ISBN 9781284108194.

The methods we outline here can be used with non-normally distributed ordinal, ranked, or continuous outcomes. Remember that quantitative measures of continuous outcomes are determined by a particular measurement scale (e.g., height in inches, or weight in pounds). Some researchers distinguish between data on an ordinal, interval, and continuous scale. Similar to continuous data, interval data are measured on a fixed scale (i.e., the disparity between neighbouring scale scores is constant throughout the whole range of scores). Ratios cannot be interpreted, but differences between interval scores can. An example of an interval-scale result is temperature, expressed in either Celsius or Fahrenheit. Though 80° is not twice as warm as 40°, the difference between 70° and 80° is the same as the difference between 30° and 40°. The ordered categories don't need to be equally spaced, and ordinal results may be less specific. An example of an ordinal outcome is the severity of the symptoms; it is unclear if the distinction between "much worse" and "slightly worse" and "no change" and "slightly improved" is the same. In certain research, participants' self-reported signs and symptoms are evaluated using visual scales. This is how pain is commonly measured. On a visual scale, like the one in the upper part of Figure 9.3, participants are occasionally shown. They are asked to select the number that most accurately describes their level of pain (0 being no pain and 10 being excruciating pain). As seen in the bottom section of Figure 9.3, visual anchors are occasionally used with pain scales.

Even though 10 is worse than 9 which is worse than 8, the difference between adjacent scores in the upper part of Figure 9.3 may not always be the same. To draw valid conclusions from statistical analysis and, in particular, to avoid inflating precision, it is critical to comprehend how results are measured.

The general procedure is the same for the nonparametric procedures that we describe here. Whether the outcome variable is continuous, interval, or ordinal, it is ranked from lowest to highest, and the ranks—rather than the measured or raw values—are what is analyzed. Let's take an example where we take a sample of n = 6 participants and record their self-reported pain using a visual analog scale with anchors at 0 (no pain) and 10 (agonizing pain).

7 5 9 3 0 2

The following is the assignment of the ranks, which are used to run a nonparametric test: First, the data are sorted from smallest to largest. Next, a rank of 1 is given to the lowest-value score, a rank of 2 to the next lowest, and so on. A rank of n (in this case, n = 6) is given to the largest value. Below are the observed data and corresponding ranks:

Ordered Observed Data:	0	2	3	5	7
Ranks:	1	2	3	4	5

An additional complicating factor occurs when the sample contains ties (i.e., when two or more participants measure the same value). Assume, for instance, that our sample of n = 6 includes the following data:

Observed Data:	7	7	9	3	0	2

The 4th and 5th ordered values are both equal to 7. When assigning ranks, the recommended procedure is to assign the mean rank of 4.5 to each (i.e., the mean of 4 and 5), as follows:

Ordered Observed Data:	0	2	3	7	7	9
Ranks:	1	2	3	4.5	4.5	6

Using the same approach, suppose that there are three values of 7. In this case, we assign a rank of 5 (the mean of 4, 5, and 6) to the 4th, 5th, and 6th ordered values, as follows:

Ordered Observed Data:	0	2	3	7	7	7
Ranks:	1	2	3	5	5	5

Assigning the mean rank when there are ties ensures that the sum of the ranks is the same in each sample (1 + 2 + 3 + 4 + 5 + 6 = 21, 1 + 2 + 3 + 4.5 + 4.5 + 6 = 21, and 1 + 2 + 3 + 5 + 5 + 5 = 21).

The sum of the ranks will always equal n(n + 1)/2 when using this method. Prior to beginning the analysis, it is helpful to verify the sum of the ranks when performing nonparametric tests.

To conduct nonparametric tests, we again follow the five-step approach outlined for hypothesis testing.

- ***Step 1. Set up hypotheses and select the level of significance a.***

  The research hypothesis can be one- or two-sided (one- or two-tailed), similar to parametric testing, depending on the relevant research question.

- ***Step 2. Select the appropriate test statistic.***

A single figure that condenses the sample data is the test statistic. The observed data are transformed into ranks in nonparametric tests, and the ranks are then condensed into a test statistic.

- ***Step 3. Set up the decision rule.***

  The decision rule is a statement that specifies when the null hypothesis should be rejected. If the test statistic is large in some nonparametric tests, we reject H0; if the test statistic is small in other tests, we reject H_0. As we go over the various tests, these are differentiated.

- ***Step 4. Compute the test statistic.***

  Here, we use the test statistic found in Step 2 to summarize the ranks and compute the test statistic.

- ***Step 5. Conclusion.***

  The test statistic, which is a summary of the data observed in the sample, is compared to the decision rule to arrive at the conclusion. In the end, one must decide whether to reject the null hypothesis (since it is highly unlikely that the sample data will be observed if the null hypothesis is true) or to accept it (because the sample data are not highly unlikely to be true). (Armitage et al., 2008) (Conover et al., 1999).

9.3. Tests with Two Independent Samples

We discussed methods for comparing the means of two separate samples. It was assumed that the continuous outcome was roughly normally distributed or that the samples were big enough (typically $n_1 > 30$ and $n_2 > 30$) to support the use of the tests described using the Central Limit Theorem. A nonparametric test is suitable when the results are not normally distributed and the samples are small.

The Mann-Whitney U test is a well-liked nonparametric method for comparing results between two independent groups. The Mann-Whitney U test, also known as the Wilcoxon Rank-Sum test or the Mann- Whitney–Wilcoxon test, is used to determine whether two samples are most likely to come from the same population (i.e., that the forms of the two populations are identical). According to some researchers, this test compares the medians of the two groups. Remember that the analogous parametric test contrasts the means of independent groups (H_0: $m_1 = m_2$).

The null and two-sided research hypotheses for the nonparametric test are stated as follows:

- H_0: The two populations are equal.
- H_1: The two populations are not equal.

Instead of defining directionality, the research hypothesis suggests that the populations are not equal because this test is frequently conducted as a two-sided test. If the goal of the research is to identify a change in one population that is greater than the other, then a one-sided research hypothesis is used. The test protocol entails combining the observations from the two samples into a single combined sample, recording the sample from which each observation originates, and then ranking the observations from 1 to $n_1 + n_2$, in that order. Take a look at the following example to see how the process works. To facilitate understanding, we address each of the five steps in the test of hypothesis while providing additional details. In the examples that follow, the five-step process is applied more closely.).

- ***Example 9.1.*** Consider a Phase II clinical trial designed to investigate the effectiveness of a new drug to reduce symptoms of asthma in children. A total of n = 10 participants are randomized to receive either the new drug or a placebo. Participants are asked to record the number of episodes of shortness of breath over a 1-week period following receipt of the assigned treatment. The data are shown below.

Placebo	7	5	6	4	12
New Drug	3	6	4	2	1

The question of interest is whether there is a difference in the number of episodes of shortness of breath over a 1-week period in participants receiving the new drug compared to those receiving the placebo. By inspection, it appears that participants receiving the placebo have more episodes of shortness of breath than those receiving the new drug. The question is whether this observed difference is statistically significant.

In this example, the outcome is a count, and in this sample the data do not follow a normal distribution. In addition, the sample size is small ($n_1 = n_2 = 5$).

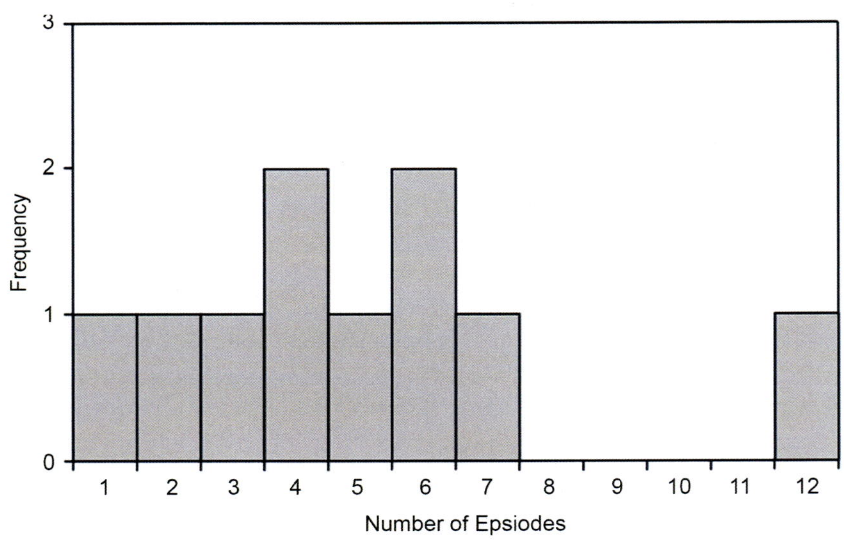

Figure 9.4. *Number of episodes of shortness of breath.*

Source: Lisa M. Sullivan, Essentials of Biostatistics in Public Health Third Edition, ISBN 9781284108194.

Thus, a nonparametric test is appropriate. The hypotheses to be tested are given below, and we run the test at the 5% level of significance (i.e., a = 0.05).

- H_0: The two populations are equal.
- H_1: The two populations are not equal.

Keep in mind that if the null hypothesis is accurate (i.e., Since the two populations are equal, we anticipate that each of the two treatment groups will experience a comparable number of episodes of dyspnoea. To be more precise, we would anticipate that in each of the comparison groups, some participants would report fewer episodes of dyspnoea and others would report more episodes if the number of episodes was the same for those given the new medication and those given the placebo. The observed data does not seem to support this. To ascertain whether the observed data are proof of a statistically significant difference in populations, a hypothesis test is required.

Assigning ranks is the first step, and we do this by arranging the data in the smallest to largest order. As indicated in **Table 9.1**, this is performed on the combined or total sample by combining the data from the two treatment groups and allocating ranks ranging from 1 to 10. Additionally, we must monitor the group assignments for the entire sample (n = 10).

Recall that the lower echelons (e.g., responses in the new drug group are assigned the ranks 1, 2, and 3, whereas the higher ranks (e.g., 9, and 10) correspond to the responses in the group receiving a placebo. Once more, the test's objective is to ascertain whether the observed data are consistent with a distinct response population. Remember that in parametric tests, sample information is summed up in a test statistic and the difference in sample means between two groups is analyzed concerning their variability. Here, a similar strategy is used. In particular, we use the ranks to generate a test statistic.

First, we sum the ranks in each group. In the placebo group the sum of the ranks is 37, and in the new drug group the sum of the ranks is 18. Recall that the sum of the ranks will always equal n(n + 1)/2. As a check on our assignment of ranks, we have n(n + 1)/2 = 10(11)/2 = 55, which is equal to 37 + 18 = 55.

For the test, we call the placebo group 1 and the new drug group 2 (the assignment of groups 1 and 2 is arbitrary—we only need to maintain the group assignments throughout the testing procedure). We let R_1 denote the sum of the ranks in group 1 (i.e., R_1 = 37) and R_2 denote the sum of the ranks in group 2 (i.e., R_2 = 18). If the null hypothesis is true (i.e., if the two populations are equal), we expect R_1 and R_2 to be similar. In this example, the lower values (lower ranks) are clustered in the new drug group (group 2), while the higher values (higher ranks) are clustered in the placebo group (group 1). The question is whether the difference we observe in the sums of the ranks is suggestive of a difference in the populations or is simply due to chance. We now compute a test statistic to summarize the sample information and then compare that test statistic to an appropriate value from a probability distribution corresponding to our selected level of significance.

The test statistic for the Mann-Whitney U test is denoted by U and is the smaller of U_1 and U_2 , defined as follows:

$$U_1 = n_1 n_2 + \frac{n_1(n_1+1)}{2} - R_1$$

$$U_2 = n_1 n_2 + \frac{n_2(n_2+1)}{2} - R_2$$

Table 9.1. *Assigning Ranks*

		Total Sample (Ordered Smallest to Largest)		Ranks	
Placebo	New Drug	Placebo	New Drug	Placebo	New Drug
7	3		1		1
5	6		2		2
6	4		3		3
4	2	4	4	4.5	4.5
12	1	5		6	
		6	6	7.5	7.5
		7		9	
		12		10	

Source: Lisa M. Sullivan, Essentials of Biostatistics in Public Health Third Edition, ISBN 9781284108194.

For this example,

$$U_1 = n_1 n_2 + \frac{n_1(n_1+1)}{2} - R_1 = 5(5) + \frac{5(6)}{2} - 37 = 3$$

$$U_2 = n_1 n_2 + \frac{n_2(n_2+1)}{2} - R_2 = 5(5) + \frac{5(6)}{2} - 18 = 22$$

In example, U = 3. Is this evidence in support of the null hypothesis or the research hypothesis?

Before we address this question, we consider the range of the test statistic U in different situations. First, consider the situation where there is complete separation between the groups. This is a situation where the data most clearly support the research hypothesis (i.e., the two populations are not equal). Specifically, suppose that all of the higher numbers of episodes of shortness of breath, and thus all of the higher ranks, are in the placebo group and all of the lower numbers of episodes of shortness of breath, and thus all of the lower ranks, are in the new-drug group and that there are no ties. Then R_1 = 6 + 7 + 8 + 9 + 10 = 40 and R_2 = 1 + 2 + 3 + 4 + 5 = 15, and $U_1 = 5(5) + \frac{5(6)}{2} - 40 = 0$ and $U_2 = 5(5) + \frac{5(6)}{2} - 15 = 25.$ Thus, when there is a difference in the populations, U = 0.

Consider a second situation where low and high scores are approximately evenly distributed in the placebo and the new-drug groups. This is a situation where the data most clearly support the null hypothesis (i.e., the two populations are equal). Suppose that ranks 2, 4, 6, 8, and 10 are assigned to the number of episodes of shortness of breath reported in the placebo group and ranks 1, 3, 5, 7, and 9 are assigned to the number of episodes of shortness of breath reported in the new drug group. Then R_1 = 2 + 4 + 6 + 8 + 10 = 30 and R_2 = 1 + 3 + 5 + 7 + 9 = 25, and $U_1 = 5(5) + \frac{5(6)}{2} - 30 = 10$ and $U_2 = 5(5) + \frac{5(6)}{2} - 25 = 15$. Thus, when there is no difference between populations, U = 10. Smaller values of U support the research hypothesis and larger values of U support the null hypothesis. In fact, for any test the theoretical range of U is from 0 (complete separation between groups, H_0 most likely false and H_1 most likely true) to $n_1 \times n_2$ (little evidence in support of H_1). In every test, $U_1 + U_2$ is always equal to $n_1 \times n_2$. In our example, U can range from 0 to 25 and smaller values of U support the research hypothesis (i.e., we reject H_0 if U is small). The procedure for determining exactly when to reject H_0 is described next.

We have to decide if the observed U supports the research hypothesis or the null hypothesis in each test. This is carried out using the same methodology as parametric testing. To determine the appropriate critical value, we need the sample sizes ($n_1 = n_2 = 5$) and our two-sided level of significance (a = 0.05). Specifically, we determine a critical value of U such that if the observed value of U is less than or equal to the critical value, we reject H_0 in favor of H1. If the observed value of U exceeds the critical value, we do not reject H_0 dot. In this instance, the decision rule is to reject H_0 if U = 2, and the critical value is 2. As 3 > 2, we do not reject H_0. It is not statistically significant to conclude that the two populations' numbers of episodes of dyspnoea are unequal at a = 0.05. Low power in this instance is probably the reason why statistical significance was not reached. Although the sample sizes may be too small to determine whether there is a statistically significant difference, the sample data would seem to indicate a difference.

- ***Example 9.2.*** A new approach to prenatal care is proposed for pregnant women living in a rural community. The new program involves in-home visits during pregnancy in addition to the usual or regularly scheduled visits. A pilot randomized trial with 15 pregnant women is designed to evaluate whether women who participate in the program deliver healthier babies than women receiving usual care. The outcome is the APGAR score measured 5 minutes after birth. Recall that APGAR scores range from 0 to 10, where a score of 7 or higher is considered normal (healthy), 4–6 is low, and 0–3 is critically low. The data are shown below.

Usual Care	8	7	6	2	5	8	7	3
New Program	9	8	7	8	10	9	6	

Is there statistical evidence of a difference in APGAR scores in women receiving the new and enhanced care versus usual prenatal care? We run the test using the five-step approach.

- ***Step 1. Set up hypotheses and determine the level of significance.***

o H_0 : The two populations are equal.

o H_1 : The two populations are not equal.

$\alpha = 0.05$.

- ***Step 2. Select the appropriate test statistic.***

Because APGAR scores are not normally distributed and the samples are small ($n_1 = 8$ and $n_2 = 7$), we use the Mann–Whitney U test. The test statistic is U, the smaller of $U_1 = n_1 n_2 + \frac{n_1(n_1+1)}{2} - R_1$ and $U_2 = n_1 n_2 + \frac{n_2(n_2+1)}{2} - R_2$ where R_1 and R_2 are the sums of the ranks in groups 1 and 2, respectively.

- ***Step 3. Set up the decision rule.***

To determine the appropriate critical value we need the sample sizes ($n_1 = 8$ and $n_2 = 7$) and our two-sided level of significance ($\alpha = 0.05$.). The critical value for this test is 10, and the decision rule is as follows:

Reject H_0 if $U \leq 10$.

- ***Step 4. Compute the test statistic.***

The first step is to assign ranks of 1 through 15 to the smallest through largest values in the total sample, as shown in Table 9.2. Next, we sum the ranks in each group. In the usual-care group the sum of the ranks is $R_1 = 45.5$ and in the new-program group the sum of the ranks is $R_2 = 74.5$. Recall that the sum of the ranks will always equal n(n + 1)/2. As a check on our assignment of ranks, we have n(n + 1)/2 = 15(16)/2 = 120, which is equal to 45.5 + 74.5

= 120. We now compute U_1 and U_2, as follows:

$$U_1 = n_1 n_2 + \frac{n_1(n_1+1)}{2} - R_1 = 8(7) + \frac{8(9)}{2} - 45.5 = 46.5$$

$$U_2 = n_1 n_2 + \frac{n_2(n_2+1)}{2} - R_2 = 8(7) + \frac{7(8)}{2} - 74.5 = 9.5$$

Thus, the test statistic is U = 9.5.

- ***Step 5. Conclusion.***

  We reject H_0 because 9.5 < 10. We have statistically significant evidence at $\alpha = 0.05$. to show that the populations of APGAR scores are not equal in women receiving usual prenatal care as compared to the new program of prenatal care.

- ***Example 9.3.*** A clinical trial is run to assess the effectiveness of a new antiretroviral therapy for patients with HIV. Patients are randomized to receive a standard antiretroviral therapy (usual care) or the new antiretroviral therapy and are monitored for 3 months. The primary outcome is viral load, which represents the number of HIV copies per milliliter of blood. A total of 30 participants are randomized, and the data are shown below.

Standard Antiretroviral Therapy	7500	8000	2000	550	
	1250	1000	2250	6800	
	3400	6300	9100	970	
	1040	670	400		
New Antiretroviral Therapy	400	250	800	1400	8000
	7400	1020	6000	920	1420
	2700	4200	5200	4100	
	undetectable				

Is there statistical evidence of a difference in viral load in patients receiving the standard therapy versus the new antiretroviral therapy? We run the test using the five-step approach.

Table 9.2. *Assigning Ranks*

		Total Sample (Ordered Smallest to Largest)		Ranks	
Usual Care	**New Program**	**Usual Care**	**New Program**	**Usual Care**	**New Program**
8	9	2		1	
7	8	3		2	
6	7	5		3	
2	8	6	6	4.5	4.5
5	10	7	7	7	7
8	9	7		7	
7	6	8	8	10.5	10.5
3		8	8	10.5	10.5
			9		13.5
			9		13.5
			10		15
				$R_1 = 45.5$	$R_2 = 74.5$

Source: Lisa M. Sullivan, Essentials of Biostatistics in Public Health Third Edition, ISBN 9781284108194.

- ***Step 1. Set up hypotheses and determine the level of significance.***

o H_0: The two populations are equal.

o H_1: The two populations are not equal.

$\alpha = 0.05.$

- ***Step 2. Select the appropriate test statistic.***

Because viral load measures are not normally distributed—generally subject to extreme values or outliers as well as clear limits of detection (e.g., "undetectable")— we use the Mann–Whitney U test. The test statistic is U, the smaller of $U_1 = n_1 n_2 + \frac{n_1(n_1+1)}{2} - R_1$ and $U_2 = n_1 n_2 + \frac{n_2(n_2+1)}{2} - R_2$ where R_1 and R_2 are the sums of the ranks in groups 1 and 2, respectively.

- ***Step 3. Set up the decision rule.***

To determine the appropriate critical value we need the sample sizes ($n_1 = n_2 = 15$) and our two-sided level of significance ($\alpha = 0.05.$).

The critical value for this test is 64, and the decision rule is as follows:

Reject H_0 if $U \leq 64$.

- ***Step 4. Compute the test statistic.***

The first step is to assign ranks of 1 through 30 to the smallest through largest values in the total sample, as shown in Table 9.3. Note that the "undetectable" measurement is listed first in the ordered values (smallest) and assigned a rank of 1.

Next, we sum the ranks in each group. In the standard antiretroviral therapy group, the sum of the ranks is $R_1 = 245$, and in the new antiretroviral therapy group, the sum of the ranks is $R_2 = 220$. Recall that the sum of the ranks will always equal n(n + 1)/2. As a check on our assignment of ranks, we have n(n + 1)/2 = 30(31)/2 = 465, which is equal to 245 + 220 = 465.

We now compute U_1 and U_2, as follows:

$$U_1 = n_1 n_2 + \frac{n_1(n_1+1)}{2} - R_1 = 15(15) + \frac{15(16)}{2} - 245 = 100$$

$$U_2 = n_1 n_2 + \frac{n_2(n_2+1)}{2} - R_2 = 15(15) + \frac{15(16)}{2} - 220 = 125$$

Thus, the test statistic is U = 100.

- ***Step 5. Conclusion.***

We do not reject H_0 because 100 > 64. We do not have statistically significant evidence at $\alpha = 0.05.$ to show that the populations of viral load measures are not equal in patients receiving the standard therapy versus the new antiretroviral therapy.

9.4. Tests with Matched Samples

We now describe nonparametric tests to compare two groups concerning a continuous outcome when the data are collected on matched or paired samples. The parametric procedure was described for the situation in which the continuous outcome followed a normal distribution. Here we consider the situation in which the outcome cannot be assumed to follow a normal distribution.

There are two popular nonparametric tests to compare outcomes between two matched or paired groups. The first is called the Sign test and the second is the Wilcoxon Signed Rank test. We describe both tests here.

Recall that when data are matched or paired, we compute a difference score for each individual and analyze the difference scores. The same approach is followed in nonparametric tests. In parametric tests, the null hypothesis is that the mean difference (μ_d) is zero. In nonparametric tests, the null hypothesis is that the median difference is zero.

- ***Example 9.4.*** Consider a clinical investigation to assess the effectiveness of a new drug designed to reduce repetitive behaviors in children affected with autism. If the drug is effective, children will exhibit fewer repetitive behaviors with treatment as compared with no treatment. A total of 8 children with autism enroll in the study. Each child is observed by the study psychologist for 3 hours both before treatment and then again after treatment, taking the new drug for 1 week. The time that each child is engaged in repetitive behavior during each 3-hour observation period is measured. Repetitive behavior is scored on a scale of 0 to 100, and scores represent the percent of the observation time in which the child is engaged in repetitive behavior. For example, a score of 0 indicates that during the entire observation period the child did not engage in repetitive behavior, while a score of 100 indicates that the child was constantly engaged in repetitive behavior. The data are shown in Table 9.4.

The question of interest is whether there is improvement in repetitive behavior after 1 week of treatment as compared to before treatment. Looking at the data, it appears that some children improve (e.g., Child 5 scored 80 before treatment and 20 after treatment), but some get worse (e.g., Child 3 scored 40 before treatment and 50 after treatment).

Table 9.3. *Assigning Ranks*

		Total Sample (Ordered Smallest to Largest)		Ranks	
Standard Antiretroviral	New Antiretroviral	Standard Antiretroviral	New Antiretroviral	Standard Antiretroviral	New Antiretroviral
7500	400		undetectable		1
8000	250		250		2
2000	800	400	400	3.5	3.5
550	1400	550		5	
1250	8000	670		6	
1000	7400		800		7
2250	1020		920		8
6800	6000	970		9	
3400	920	1000		10	
6300	1420		1020		11
9100	2700	1040		12	
970	4200	1250		13	
1040	5200		1400		14
670	4100		1420		15
400	undetectable	2000		16	
		2250		17	
			2700		18
		3400		19	
			4100		20
			4200		21
			5200		22
			6000		23
		6300		24	
		6800		25	
			7400		26
		7500		27	
		8000	8000	28.5	28.5
		9100		30	
				$R_1 = 245$	$R_2 = 220$

Source: Lisa M. Sullivan, Essentials of Biostatistics in Public Health Third Edition, ISBN 9781284108194.

Because the before- and after-treatment measures are paired, we compute difference scores for each child. In this example, we subtract the assessment of repetitive behaviours measured after treatment from that measured before treatment, so that difference scores represent improvement in repetitive behavior. The question of interest is whether there is significant improvement after treatment. Again, notice that Tests with Matched Samples 233 some children's repetitive behavior gets worse after treatment as compared to before treatment (and thus they have negative improvement).

The differences are shown in **Table 9.5**. In this small sample, the observed difference (or improvement) scores vary widely and are subject to extremes (e.g., the observed difference of 60 is an outlier). Thus, a nonparametric test is appropriate to test whether there is significant improvement in repetitive behavior before versus after treatment.

Table 9.4. *Repetitive Behavior Before and After Treatment*

Child	Before Treatment	After 1 Week of Treatment
1	85	75
2	70	50
3	40	50
4	65	40
5	80	20
6	75	65
7	55	40
8	20	25

Source: Lisa M. Sullivan, Essentials of Biostatistics in Public Health Third Edition, ISBN 9781284108194.

The hypotheses are given below and the test is run at a 5% level of significance.

- H_0 : The median difference is zero.
- H_1 : The median difference is positive.

$\alpha = 0.05$.

Table 9.5. *Differences in Repetitive Behavior*

Child	Before Treatment	After 1 Week of Treatment	Difference (Before – After)
1	85	75	10
2	70	50	20
3	40	50	−10
4	65	40	25
5	80	20	60
6	75	65	10
7	55	40	15
8	20	25	−5

Source: Lisa M. Sullivan, Essentials of Biostatistics in Public Health Third Edition, ISBN 9781284108194.

The null hypothesis, as usual, represents the situation where there is no change or no effect. In this example, the null hypothesis represents the situation where there is no difference in scores before versus after treatment, or no effect of treatment. If the null hypothesis is true, we expect to see some positive differences (improvement) and some negative differences (worsening). If the research hypothesis is true, we expect to see more positive differences, or more children with improvement in repetitive behavior after treatment as compared to before.

Table 9.6. *Signs of the Differences*

Child	Before Treatment	After 1 Week of Treatment	Difference (Before – After)	Sign
1	85	75	10	+
2	70	50	20	+
3	40	50	−10	–
4	65	40	25	+
5	80	20	60	+
6	75	65	10	+
7	55	40	15	+
8	20	25	−5	–

Source: Lisa M. Sullivan, Essentials of Biostatistics in Public Health Third Edition, ISBN 9781284108194.

The Sign test is the simplest nonparametric test for matched or paired data. The approach is to analyze only the signs of the different scores. The signs here are shown in **Table 9.6**. If the null hypothesis is true (i.e., if the median difference is zero), then we expect to see approximately half of the differences as positive and half of the differences as negative. If the research hypothesis is true, we expect to see more positive differences.

The test statistic for the Sign test is the number of positive signs or the number of negative signs, whichever is smaller. In this example, we observe two negative and six positive signs. Is this evidence of significant improvement or simply due to chance?

We again determine whether the observed test statistic (i.e., the number of negative signs in this example) supports the null or research hypothesis. This is done following the same approach used in parametric testing. Specifically, we determine a critical value such that if the smaller of the number of positive or negative signs is less than or equal to that critical value, then we reject H_0 in favor of H_1 , and if the smaller of the number of positive or negative signs is greater than the critical value, then we do not reject H_0 . Notice that this is a one-sided decision rule corresponding to our one sided research hypothesis (the two-sided situation is discussed in the next example).

To determine the appropriate critical value we need the sample size, which is equal to the number of matched pairs (n = 8), and our one-sided level of significance ($\alpha = 0.05.$). For this example, the critical value is 1, and the decision rule is to reject H_0 if the smaller of the number of positive or negative signs is #1. Here we do not reject H_0 because 2 > 1. We do not have statistically significant evidence at $\alpha = 0.05.$ to show that there is improvement in repetitive behavior after treatment as compared to before treatment.

In our usual five-step approach, we set up a decision rule that indicates under what circumstances to reject H_0. For example, with many of our parametric tests, we reject H_0 if the observed test statistic (e.g., Z or t) is more extreme than the critical value. Specifically, we reject H_0 if the test statistic is more extreme than a critical value that comes from a particular probability distribution (e.g., the standard normal distribution) based on a specified level of significance (e.g., $\alpha = 0.05.$). We can use the same approach for the Sign test as illustrated above, or we can consider an alternative approach such as the following.

With the Sign test we can readily compute a p-value based on our observed test statistic and compare that to our stated level of significance (e.g.,$\alpha = 0.05.$). This is analogous to what is done when we run tests of hypothesis with a statistical computing package (e.g., using Excel®). The statistical computing package computes a test statistic and a p-value, and the investigator then compares the p-value to the predetermined level of significance to conclude the hypotheses using the following rule: Reject H0 if $p \leq \alpha$.

The test statistic for the Sign test is the smaller of the number of positive or negative signs, and it follows a binomial distribution with n = the number of subjects in the study and p = 0.5. In this example, n = 8 and p = 0.5. The following probabilities can be computed with either the binomial distribution formula, $P(x\ successes) = \frac{n!}{x!(n-x)!} p^x (1-p)^{n-x}$ or using a statistical computing package such as Excel.

Recall that a p-value is the probability of observing a test statistic as or more extreme than that observed. We observe two negative signs. Thus, the p-value for the test is p = $P(x \leq 2)$. Using **Table 9.7**, $P(x \leq 2)$ = P(0) + P(1) + P(2) = 0.0039 + 0.0313 + 0.1094 = 0.1446.

Because the p-value 0.1446 exceeds the level of significance ($\alpha = 0.05.$), we do not have statistically significant evidence at $\alpha = 0.05.$ to show that there is improvement in repetitive behaviours after treatment compared to before treatment. Notice in the table of binomial probabilities that we would have had to observe at most one negative sign to declare statistical significance using a 5% level of significance.

Table 9.7. *Probabilities Based on the Binomial Distribution Model*

x = Number of Successes	$P(x$ successes)
0	0.0039
1	0.0313
2	0.1094
3	0.2188
4	0.2734
5	0.2188
6	0.1094
7	0.0313
8	0.0039

Source: Lisa M. Sullivan, Essentials of Biostatistics in Public Health Third Edition, ISBN 9781284108194.

In Example 4 we consider a one-sided test (i.e., we hypothesize improvement after treatment). A two-sided test can also be considered, in which we hypothesize a difference in repetitive behavior after treatment compared to before treatment. We can determine a two-sided critical value and again reject H_0 if the smaller of number of positive or negative signs is less than or equal to that of the two-sided critical value. Alternatively, we can compute a two-sided p-value. With a two-sided test, the p-value is the probability of observing many or few positive (or negative) signs. If the research hypothesis is a two-sided alternative (i.e., H_1: The median difference is not zero), then the p-value is computed as p = 2 3 $P(x \leq 2)$. $P(x \geq 6)$ this is equivalent to p = $P(x \leq 2)$ + , representing the situation of few or many successes. Recall that in two-sided tests we reject the null hypothesis if the test statistic is extreme in either direction. Thus, in the Sign test, a two-sided p-value is the probability of observing few or many positive (or negative) signs. Here we observe two negative signs (and thus six positive signs). The opposite situation would be six negative signs (and thus two positive signs, as n = 8). The two-sided p-value is the probability of observing a test statistic as or more extreme in either direction (i.e., $P(x \leq 2)$ + $P(x \geq 6)$ = 0.0039 + 0.0313 + 0.1094 + 0.1094 + 0.0313 + 0.0039 = 2 3 (0.1446) = 0.2892).

There is a special circumstance that needs attention when implementing the Sign test that arises when one or more participants have difference scores of zero (i.e., their paired measurements are identical). If there is just one difference score of zero, some investigators drop that observation and reduce the sample size by 1 (i.e., the sample size for the binomial distribution would be n – 1). This is a reasonable approach if there is just one zero. However, if there are two or more zeros, an alternative approach is preferred. If there is an even number of zeros, we randomly assign them positive or negative signs. If there is an odd number of zeros, we randomly drop one (reduce the sample size by 1) and then randomly assign the remaining observations' positive or negative signs. The following example illustrates the approach.

- ***Example 9.5.*** A new chemotherapy treatment is proposed for patients with breast cancer. Investigators are concerned with patients' ability to tolerate the treatment and, assess their quality of life both before and after receiving the new chemotherapy treatment. Quality of life (QOL) is measured on an ordinal scale and, for analysis purposes, numbers are assigned to each response category as follows: 1 = Poor, 2 = Fair, 3 = Good, 4 = Very Good, 5 = Excellent. The data are shown in Table 9.8. The question of interest is whether there is a difference in QOL after chemotherapy treatment as compared to before.

- ***Step 1. Set up hypotheses and determine the level of significance.***
  - o H_0 : The median difference is zero.
  - o H_1 : The median difference is not zero.

$\alpha = 0.05.$

Table 9.8. *Quality of Life Before and After Chemotherapy Treatment*

Patient	QOL Before Chemotherapy Treatment	QOL After Chemotherapy Treatment
1	3	2
2	2	3
3	3	4
4	2	4
5	1	1
6	3	4
7	2	4
8	3	3
9	2	1
10	1	3
11	3	4
12	2	3

Source: Lisa M. Sullivan, Essentials of Biostatistics in Public Health Third Edition, ISBN 9781284108194.

- ***Step 2. Select the appropriate test statistic.***

  The test statistic for the Sign test is the smaller of the number of positive or negative signs.

- ***Step 3. Set up the decision rule.***

  To determine the appropriate critical value, we need the sample size (or number of matched pairs, n = 12) and our two-sided level of significance ($\alpha = 0.05.$). The critical value for this two-sided test is 2, and the decision rule is as follows:

  Reject H_0 if the smaller of the number of positive or negative signs is ≤ 2.

- ***Step 4. Compute the test statistic.***

  Because the before- and after-treatment measures are paired, we compute difference scores for each patient. In this example, we subtract the QOL measured before treatment from that measured after.

  We now capture the signs of the difference scores. Because there are two zeros, we randomly assign one negative sign (i.e., "–" to patient 5) and one positive sign (i.e., "+" to patient 8), as shown in Table 9.10.

  The test statistic is the number of negative signs, which is equal to 3.

- ***Step 5. Conclusion.***

  We do not reject H_0 because 3 > 2. We do not have statistically significant evidence at $\alpha = 0.05.$ to show that there is a difference in QOL after chemotherapy treatment as compared to before.

  We can also compute the p-value directly using the binomial distribution with n = 12 and p = 0.5. The two-sided p-value for the test is $p = 2 \times P(x \leq 3)$ (which is equivalent to $p = P(x \leq 3) + P(x \geq 9)$). Again, the two-sided p-value is the probability of observing few or many positive (or negative) signs. Here we observe three negative signs (and thus nine positive signs). The opposite situation would be nine negative signs (and thus three positive signs, as n = 12). The two-sided p-value is the probability of observing a test statistic as or more extreme in either direction (i.e., $p = P(x \leq 3) + P(x \geq 9)$) . We can compute the p-value using the binomial formula or a statistical computing package, as follows: $p = 2 \times P(x \leq 3)$ = 2 (P(0) + P(1) + P(2) + P(3)) = 2 3 (0.0002 + 0.0029 + 0.0161 + 0.0537) = 2 3 (0.0729) = 0.1458.

Table 9.9. *Differences in Quality of Life before and After Chemotherapy Treatment*

Patient	QOL Before Chemotherapy Treatment	QOL After Chemotherapy Treatment	Difference (After – Before)
1	3	2	–1
2	2	3	1
3	3	4	1
4	2	4	2
5	1	1	0
6	3	4	1
7	2	4	2
8	3	3	0
9	2	1	–1
10	1	3	2
11	3	4	1
12	2	3	1

Source: Lisa M. Sullivan, Essentials of Biostatistics in Public Health Third Edition, ISBN 9781284108194.

Because the p-value 0.1458 exceeds the level of significance ($\alpha = 0.05.$), we do not have statistically significant evidence at $\alpha = 0.05.$ to show that there is a difference in QOL after chemotherapy treatment compared to before treatment.

In each of the two previous examples, we failed to show statistical significance because the p-value was not less than the stated level of significance. While the test statistic for the Sign test is easy to compute, it does not take much of the information in the sample data into account. All we measure is the difference in each participant's scores, and we do not account for the magnitude of the difference.

Another popular nonparametric test for matched or paired data is called the Wilcoxon Signed Rank Test. Like the Sign test, it is based on difference scores, but in addition to analyzing the signs of the differences, it also takes into account the magnitudes of the observed differences. We now use the Wilcoxon Signed

Rank test to analyze the data in Example 4. In the following example, we address each of the five steps in the test of hypothesis but include more details to promote understanding. (In subsequent examples, the five-step approach is followed more directly.)

- ***Example 6.*** Consider again the clinical investigation to assess the effectiveness of a new drug to reduce repetitive behaviors in children affected with autism. A total of 8 children with autism enrolled in the study, and the amount of time that each child is engaged in repetitive behavior during three-hour observation periods is measured both before treatment and then again after taking the new drug, for 1 week. The data are shown in Table 9.11.

Table 9.10. *Signs of the Differences*

Patient	QOL Before Chemotherapy Treatment	QOL After Chemotherapy Treatment	Difference (After – Before)	Sign
1	3	2	−1	−
2	2	3	1	+
3	3	4	1	+
4	2	4	2	+
5	1	1	0	−
6	3	4	1	+
7	2	4	2	+
8	3	3	0	+
9	2	1	−1	−
10	1	3	2	+
11	3	4	1	+
12	2	3	1	+

Source: Lisa M. Sullivan, Essentials of Biostatistics in Public Health Third Edition, ISBN 9781284108194.

The question of interest is whether there is improvement in repetitive behavior after treatment as compared to before. Again, because the before- and after-treatment measures are paired, we compute different scores for each child (see Table 9.12).

Table 9.11. *Repetitive Behavior Before and After Treatment*

Child	Before Treatment	After 1 Week of Treatment
1	85	75
2	70	50
3	40	50
4	65	40
5	80	20
6	75	65
7	55	40
8	20	25

Source: Lisa M. Sullivan, Essentials of Biostatistics in Public Health Third Edition, ISBN 9781284108194.

Table 9.12. *Differences in Repetitive Behavior*

Child	Before Treatment	After 1 Week of Treatment	Difference (Before – After)
1	85	75	10
2	70	50	20
3	40	50	−10
4	65	40	25
5	80	20	60
6	75	65	10
7	55	40	15
8	20	25	−5

Source: Lisa M. Sullivan, Essentials of Biostatistics in Public Health Third Edition, ISBN 9781284108194.

The next step is to rank the difference scores. In the ranking process, we first order the absolute values of the difference scores and assign ranks using the approach outlined. Specifically, we assign ranks from 1 through n to the smallest through largest absolute values of the difference scores, respectively, and assign the mean rank when there are ties in the absolute values of the difference scores (see **Table 9.13**). The final step is to attach the signs ("+" or "–") of the observed differences to each rank as shown in **Table 9.14**.

Similar to the Sign test, the hypotheses for the Wilcoxon Signed Rank test concern the population median of the difference scores. The research hypothesis can be one- or two-sided. Here we consider a one-sided test.

- H_0: The median difference is zero.
- H_1: The median difference is positive.

$\alpha = 0.05$.

The test statistic for the Wilcoxon Signed Rank test is W, defined as the smaller of W+ and W–, which are the sums of the positive and negative ranks, respectively. If the null hypothesis is true, we expect to see similar numbers of lower and higher ranks that are both positive and negative (i.e., W+ and W– would be similar). If the research hypothesis is true, we expect to see more higher and positive ranks (in this example, more children with substantial improvement in repetitive behavior after treatment as compared to before treatment, i.e., W+ much larger than W–).

In this example, W+ = 32 and W– = 4. Recall that the sum of the ranks (ignoring the signs) will always equal $n(n + 1)/2$. As a check on our assignment of ranks, we have $n (n + 1)/2 = 8(9)/2 = 36$, which is equal to 32 + 4. The test statistic is W = 4.

Table 9.13. *Ranking the Absolute Values of the Differences*

Observed Differences	Ordered Absolute Values of Differences	Ranks
10	–5	1
20	10	3
–10	–10	3
25	10	3
60	15	5
10	20	6
15	25	7
–5	60	8

Source: Lisa M. Sullivan, Essentials of Biostatistics in Public Health Third Edition, ISBN 9781284108194.

Table 9.14. *Attaching Signs to the Ranks*

Observed Differences	Ordered Absolute Values of Difference Scores	Ranks	Signed Ranks
10	–5	1	–1
20	10	3	3
–10	–10	3	–3
25	10	3	3
60	15	5	5
10	20	6	6
15	25	7	7
–5	60	8	8

Source: Lisa M. Sullivan, Essentials of Biostatistics in Public Health Third Edition, ISBN 9781284108194.

Next we must determine whether the observed test statistic W supports the null or the research hypothesis. This is done following the same approach used in parametric testing. Specifically, we determine a critical value of W such that if the observed value of W is less than or equal to the critical value, we reject H_0 in favor of H_1, and if the observed value of W exceeds the critical value, we do not reject H_0. To determine the appropriate one-sided critical value, we need the sample size (n = 8) and our one-sided level of significance (a = 0.05). For this example, the critical value of W is 6, and the decision rule is to reject H_0 if $W \leq 6$. Thus, we reject H_0 because 4 < 6. We have statistically significant evidence at $\alpha = 0.05$. to show that the median difference is positive (i.e., that there is significant improvement in repetitive behavior in children affected with autism after treatment as compared to before treatment).

Notice that when we analyzed the data presented in Example 4 using the Sign test, we failed to find statistical significance. However, when we use the Wilcoxon Signed Rank test (Example 6), we conclude that there is statistically significant evidence at $\alpha = 0.05$. to show that the median difference is positive (i.e., that there is significant improvement in repetitive behavior in children affected with autism after treatment as compared to before). The discrepant results are due to the fact that the Sign test uses very little information in the data and is a less powerful test (i.e., can fail to reject H_0 when in fact it is false).

- ***Example 9.7.*** A study is run to evaluate the effectiveness of an exercise program in reducing systolic blood pressure in patients with prehypertension (defined as a systolic blood pressure between 120 mmHg and 139 mmHg or a diastolic blood pressure between 80 mmHg and 89 mmHg). A total of 15 patients with prehypertension enroll in the study, and their systolic blood pressures are measured. Each patient then participates in an exercise training program where they learn proper techniques and execution of a series of exercises. Patients are instructed to do the exercise program 3 times per week for 6 weeks. After 6 weeks, systolic blood pressures are again measured. The data are shown in **Table 9.15**.

Table 9.15. *Systolic Blood Pressure Before and After Exercise Program*

Patient	Systolic Blood Pressure Before Exercise Program	Systolic Blood Pressure After Exercise Program
1	125	118
2	132	134
3	138	130
4	120	124
5	125	105
6	127	130
7	136	130
8	139	132
9	131	123
10	132	128
11	135	126
12	136	140
13	128	135
14	127	126
15	130	132

Source: Lisa M. Sullivan, Essentials of Biostatistics in Public Health Third Edition, ISBN 9781284108194.

The question of interest is whether there is a difference in systolic blood pressure after participating in the exercise program compared to before participating in the exercise program.

- ***Step1. Set up hypotheses and determine the level of significance.***
  - o H_0: The median difference is zero.
  - o H_1: The median difference is not zero. $\alpha = 0.05$.
- ***Step 2. Select the appropriate test statistic.***

The test statistic for the Wilcoxon Signed Rank test is W, defined as the smaller of W+ and W–, which are the sums of the positive and negative ranks, respectively.

- ***Step 3. Set up the decision rule.***

The critical value of W can be found. We need the sample size (n = 15) and our two-sided level of significance ($\alpha = 0.05.$). The critical value for this two-sided test is 25, and the decision rule is as follows:

$$\text{Reject } H_0 \text{ if } W \leq 25.$$

- ***Step 4. Compute the test statistic.***

Because the before- and after-systolic blood pressure measures are paired, we compute difference scores for each patient (see **Table 9.16**).

The next step is to rank the ordered absolute values of the difference scores using the approach outlined in Section 10.1. Specifically, we assign ranks from 1 through n to the smallest through largest absolute values of the difference scores, respectively, and assign the mean rank when there are ties in the absolute values of the difference scores (see **Table 9.17**).

The final step is to attach the signs ("+" or "–") of the observed differences to each rank as shown in **Table 9.18**.

In this example, W+ = 89 and W– = 31. Recall that the sum of the ranks (ignoring the signs) will always equal n(n + 1)/2. As a check on our assignment of ranks, we have n (n + 1)/2 = 15(16)/2 = 120, which is equal to 89 + 31. The test statistic is W = 31.

Table 9.16. *Differences in Systolic Blood Pressure Before and After Exercise Program*

Patient	Systolic Blood Pressure Before Exercise Program	Systolic Blood Pressure After Exercise Program	Difference (Before – After)
1	125	118	7
2	132	134	–2
3	138	130	8
4	120	124	–4
5	125	105	20
6	127	130	–3
7	136	130	6
8	139	132	7
9	131	123	8
10	132	128	4
11	135	126	9
12	136	140	–4
13	128	135	–7
14	127	126	1
15	130	132	–2

Source: *Lisa M. Sullivan, Essentials of Biostatistics in Public Health Third Edition, ISBN 9781284108194.*

Table 9.17. *Ranking the Absolute Values of the Differences*

Observed Differences	Ordered Absolute Values of Differences	Ranks
7	1	1
−2	−2	2.5
8	−2	2.5
−4	−3	4
20	−4	6
−3	−4	6
6	4	6
7	6	8
8	−7	10
4	7	10
9	7	10
−4	8	12.5
−7	8	12.5
1	9	14
−2	20	15

Source: Lisa M. Sullivan, Essentials of Biostatistics in Public Health Third Edition, ISBN 9781284108194.

Table 9.18. *Attaching Signs to the Ranks*

Observed Differences	Ordered Absolute Values of Differences	Ranks	Signed Ranks
7	1	1	1
−2	−2	2.5	−2.5
8	−2	2.5	−2.5
−4	−3	4	−4
20	−4	6	−6
−3	−4	6	−6
6	4	6	6
7	6	8	8
8	−7	10	−10
4	7	10	10
9	7	10	10
−4	8	12.5	12.5
−7	8	12.5	12.5
1	9	14	14
−2	20	15	15

Source: Lisa M. Sullivan, Essentials of Biostatistics in Public Health Third Edition, ISBN 9781284108194.

- ***Step 5. Conclusion.***

  We do not reject H_0 because 31 > 25. We do not have statistically significant evidence at $\alpha = 0.05$. to show that the median difference in systolic blood pressure is not zero (i.e., that there is a significant difference in systolic blood pressure after the exercise program as compared to before the exercise program). (Higgins et al., 2011) (Lehmann et al., 2005).

9.5. Tests with More than Two Independent Samples

We presented techniques for testing the equality of means in more than two independent samples using analysis of variance (ANOVA). An underlying assumption for the appropriate use of ANOVA was that the continuous outcome was approximately normally distributed or that the samples were sufficiently large (usually n_j > 30, where j = 1, 2, ..., k and k denotes the number of independent comparison groups). An additional assumption for the appropriate use of ANOVA is the equality of variances in the k comparison groups. ANOVA is generally robust when the sample sizes are small but equal. When the outcome is not normally distributed and the samples are small, a nonparametric test is appropriate. A popular nonparametric test to compare outcomes among more than two independent groups is the Kruskal- Wallis test. The Kruskal–Wallis test is used to compare medians among k comparison groups (k > 2) and is sometimes described as an ANOVA with the data replaced by their ranks. The null and research hypotheses for the Kruskal–Wallis nonparametric test are stated as follows:

- H_0: The k population medians are equal.
- H_1: The k population medians are not all equal.

The procedure for the test involves pooling the observations from the k samples into one combined sample, keeping track of which sample each observation comes from, and then ranking lowest to highest from 1 to N, where $N = n_1 + n_2 + ... + n_k$. To illustrate the procedure, we consider the following example, addressing each of the five steps in the test of hypothesis including more details to promote understanding. (In the subsequent example, the five-step approach is followed more directly.)

- ***Example 9.8.*** A clinical study is designed to assess differences in albumin levels in adults following different low-protein diets. Albumin is measured in grams per deciliter(g/dL) of blood, and low-protein diets are often prescribed for patients with kidney disease. Clinically, albumin is also used to assess whether patients get sufficient protein in their diets. Three diets are compared, ranging from 5% to 15% protein, and the 15% protein diet represents a typical American diet. The albumin levels of participants following each diet are shown in Table 9.19.

Table 9.19. *Albumin levels in Three Different Diets*

5% Protein	10% Protein	15% Protein
3.1	3.8	4.0
2.6	4.1	5.5
2.9	2.9	5.0
	3.4	4.8
	4.2	

Source: Lisa M. Sullivan, Essentials of Biostatistics in Public Health Third Edition, ISBN 9781284108194.

The question of interest is whether there is a difference in albumin levels among the three different diets. For reference, normal albumin levels are generally between 3.4 g/dL and 5.4 g/dL. By inspection, it appears that participants following the 15% protein diet have higher albumin levels than those following the 5% protein diet. The issue is whether this observed difference is statistically significant.

In this example, the outcome is continuous, but the sample sizes are small and not equal across comparison groups ($n_1 = 3$, $n_2 = 5$, $n_3 = 4$). Thus, a nonparametric test is appropriate. The hypotheses to be tested are given below and we run the test at the 5% level of significance (i.e., $\alpha = 0.05.$).

- H_0: The three population medians are equal.
- H_1: The three population medians are not all equal.

To conduct the test we assign ranks using the procedures. The first step in assigning ranks is to order the data from smallest to largest. This is done on the combined or total sample, pooling the data from the three comparison groups, and assigning ranks from 1 to 12, as shown in Table 9.20. We also need to keep track of the group assignments in the total sample (n = 12).

Notice that the lower ranks (e.g., 1, 2.5, and 4) are assigned to the 5% protein diet group, while the higher ranks (e.g., 10, 11, and 12) are assigned to the 15% protein diet group. Again, the goal of the test is to determine whether the observed data support a difference in the three population medians. Recall that in the parametric tests, discussed in Chapter 7, when comparing means among more than two groups, we analyze the differences among the sample means (mean square between treatments) relative to their within-group variability and summarize the sample information in a test statistic (F statistic). In the Kruskal–Wallis test we again summarize the sample information in a test statistic, one based on the ranks.

Table 9.20. *Assigning Ranks*

			Total Sample (Ordered Smallest to Largest)			Ranks		
5% Protein	10% Protein	15% Protein	5% Protein	10% Protein	15% Protein	5% Protein	10% Protein	15% Protein
3.1	3.8	4.0	2.6			1		
2.6	4.1	5.5	2.9	2.9		2.5	2.5	
2.9	2.9	5.0	3.1			4		
	3.4	4.8		3.4			5	
	4.2			3.8			6	
					4.0			7
				4.1			8	
				4.2			9	
					4.8			10
					5.0			11
					5.5			12

Source: Lisa M. Sullivan, Essentials of Biostatistics in Public Health Third Edition, ISBN 9781284108194.

The test statistic for the Kruskal–Wallis test is denoted H and is defined as follows:

$$H=\left(\frac{12}{N(N+1)}\sum_{j=1}^{k}\frac{R_j^2}{n_j}\right)-3(N+1),$$

where k = the number of comparison groups, N = the total sample size, n_j is the sample size in the jth group, and R_j is the sum of the ranks in the jth group.

In this example R_1 = 7.5, R_2 = 30.5, and R_3 = 40. Recall that the sum of the ranks will always equal n(n + 1)/2. As a check on our assignment of ranks, we have n(n + 1)/2 = 12(13)/2 = 78, which is equal to 7.5 + 30.5 + 40 = 78.

In this example,

$$H=\left(\frac{12}{N(N+1)}\sum_{j=1}^{k}\frac{R_j^2}{n_j}\right)-3(N+1)=$$

$$\frac{12}{12(13)}\left(\frac{7.5^2}{3}+\frac{30.5^2}{5}+\frac{40^2}{4}\right)-3(13)=7.52.$$

In every test, we must determine whether the observed test statistic H supports the null or the research hypothesis. This is done following the same approach used in parametric testing. Specifically, we determine a critical value of H such that if the observed value of H is greater than or equal to the critical value, we reject H_0 in favor of H_1, and if the observed value of H is less than the critical value, we do not reject H_0. To determine the appropriate critical value, we need the sample sizes (n_1 = 3, n_2 = 5, and n3 = 4) and our level of significance ($\alpha = 0.05.$). For this example the critical value is 5.656; thus we reject H_0 because 7.52 > 5.656. We have statistically significant evidence at $\alpha = 0.05.$ to show that there is a difference in median albumin levels among the three different diets.

Notice the critical values for the Kruskal–Wallis test for tests comparing three, four, or five groups with small sample sizes. If there are three or more comparison groups and five or more observations in each of the comparison groups, it can be shown that the test statistic H approximates a χ2 distribution with df = k – 1. Thus, in a Kruskal–Wallis test with three or more comparison groups and five or more observations in each group, the critical value for the test can be found:

Critical Values of the χ2 Distribution. The following example illustrates this situation.

- ***Example 9.9.*** A personal trainer is interested in comparing the anaerobic thresholds of elite athletes. The anaerobic threshold is defined as the point at which the muscles cannot get more oxygen to sustain activity or the upper limit of aerobic exercise. It is a measure that is also related to maximum heart rate. The data in Table 9.21 are anaerobic thresholds for distance runners, distance cyclists, distance swimmers, and cross-country skiers. The question of interest is whether there is a difference in anaerobic thresholds among the different groups of elite athletes.
- ***Step 1. Set up hypotheses and determine the level of significance.***

o H_0: The four population medians are equal.

o H_1: The four population medians are not all equal.

$\alpha = 0.05.$

- ***Step 2. Select the appropriate test statistic.***

The test statistic for the Kruskal–Wallis test is denoted H and is defined as follows:

$$H = \left(\frac{12}{N(N+1)} \sum_{j=1}^{k} \frac{R_j^2}{n_j} \right) - 3(N+1),$$

where k = the number of comparison groups, N = the total sample size, n_j is the sample size in the jth group, and R_j is the sum of the ranks in the jth group.

- ***Step 3. Set up the decision rule.***

Because there are four comparison groups and five observations in each of the comparison groups, we find the critical value for df = k – 1 = 4 – 1 = 3 and a = 0.05. The critical value is 7.81, and the decision rule is to reject H_0 if $H \geq 7.81$.

Table 9.21. *Anaerobic Thresholds*

Distance Runners	Distance Cyclists	Distance Swimmers	Cross-Country Skiers
185	190	166	201
179	209	159	195
192	182	170	180
165	178	183	187
174	181	160	215

Source: *Lisa M. Sullivan, Essentials of Biostatistics in Public Health Third Edition, ISBN 9781284108194.*

- ***Step 4. Compute the test statistic.***

To conduct the test we assign ranks using the procedures outlined. The first step in assigning ranks is to order the data from smallest to largest. This is done on the combined or total sample, pooling the data from the four comparison groups, and assigning ranks from 1 to 20. We also need to keep track of the group assignments in the total sample (n = 20). Table 9.22 shows the ordered data.

We next assign the ranks to the ordered values and sum the ranks in each group (Table 9.23).

Recall that the sum of the ranks will always equal n(n + 1)/2. As a check on our assignment of ranks, we have n(n + 1)/2 = 20(21)/2 = 210, which is equal to 46 + 62 + 24 + 78 = 210.

Table 9.22. *Ordering the Anaerobic Thresholds*

				Total Sample (Ordered Smallest to Largest)			
Distance Runners	**Distance Cyclists**	**Distance Swimmers**	**Cross-Country Skiers**	**Distance Runners**	**Distance Cyclists**	**Distance Swimmers**	**Cross-Country Skiers**
185	190	166	201			159	
179	209	159	195			160	
192	182	170	180	165			
165	178	183	187			166	
174	181	160	215			170	
				174			
					178		
				179			
							180
					181		
					182		
						183	
				185			
							187
					190		
				192			
							195
							201
					209		
							215

Source: Lisa M. Sullivan, Essentials of Biostatistics in Public Health Third Edition, ISBN 9781284108194.

In this example,

$$H = \left(\frac{12}{N(N+1)} \sum_{j=1}^{k} \frac{R_j^2}{n_j} \right) - 3(N+1) =$$

$$\frac{12}{20(21)} \left(\frac{46^2}{5} + \frac{62^2}{5} + \frac{24^2}{5} \frac{78^2}{5} \right) - 3(21) = 9.11.$$

- ***Step 5. Conclusion.***

  Reject H_0 because 9.11 > 7.81. We have statistically significant evidence at $\alpha = 0.05.$ to show that there is a difference in median anaerobic thresholds among the four different groups of elite athletes.

Notice that in this example the anaerobic thresholds of the distance runners, cyclists, and cross-country skiers are comparable (looking only at the raw data). The distance swimmers appear to be the athletes that differ from the others in terms of anaerobic thresholds. Recall, similar to the analysis of variance tests, that we reject the null hypothesis in favor of the alternative hypothesis if any two of the medians are not equal. (Siegel et al., 1988) (Zar et al., 2010).

Table 9.23. *Assigning Ranks*

Total Sample (Ordered Smallest to Largest)				Ranks			
Distance Runners	Distance Cyclists	Distance Swimmers	Cross-Country Skiers	Distance Runners	Distance Cyclists	Distance Swimmers	Cross-Country Skiers
		159				1	
		160				2	
165				3			
		166				4	
		170				5	
174				6			
	178				7		
179				8			
			180				9
	181				10		
	182				11		
		183				12	
185				13			
			187				14
	190				15		
192				16			
			195				17
			201				18
	209				19		
			215				20
				$R_1 = 46$	$R_2 = 62$	$R_3 = 24$	$R_4 = 78$

Source: Lisa M. Sullivan, Essentials of Biostatistics in Public Health Third Edition, ISBN 9781284108194.

A Closer Look

Mann-Whitney U Test

The Mann-Whitney U test, also known as the Wilcoxon rank-sum test, is a nonparametric statistical method used to compare the central tendencies of two independent groups. It is particularly useful when the assumptions of parametric tests, such as the t-test, are not met, such as when the data are not normally distributed or when the sample sizes are small. Here's an overview of the Mann-Whitney U test in 300 words:

The Mann-Whitney U test begins by combining the data from both groups and ranking them from smallest to largest, regardless of group membership. Ranks are assigned based on the combined order, with ties resolved by assigning the average rank. The test statistic, U, is then calculated as the sum of ranks for one of the groups.

Under the null hypothesis of no difference between the groups, the distribution of ranks should be similar in both groups. Therefore, the expected value of U under the null hypothesis is calculated. If the observed U value is significantly smaller or larger than expected, it suggests that one group tends to have higher or lower ranks, indicating a difference between the groups.

The significance of the observed U value is typically determined using critical values from the Mann-Whitney U distribution or by comparing it to p-values obtained from large-sample approximations or Monte Carlo simulations. If the p-value is below a predetermined significance level (e.g., 0.05), the null hypothesis is rejected, indicating a statistically significant difference between the groups.

Advantages of the Mann-Whitney U test include its robustness to violations of normality assumptions, its ability to analyze ordinal or non-normally distributed continuous data, and its efficiency in estimating differences in central tendencies between groups. However, it is less powerful than parametric tests when data meet the assumptions of parametric tests, and it assumes that the shapes of the distributions in both groups are similar.

The Mann-Whitney U test is a valuable tool for comparing two independent groups in public health research when parametric assumptions are not met. It allows researchers to make valid statistical inferences about group differences without relying on stringent distributional assumptions.

Summary

- Nonparametric tests in biostatistics play a vital role in public health research by providing robust statistical methods for analyzing data when certain assumptions of traditional parametric tests are not met or when dealing with non-normal distributions.
- Parametric tests are based on certain assumptions for their appropriate use. For example, when running tests of hypothesis for means of continuous outcomes, all parametric tests assume that the outcome is approximately normally distributed in the population.
- The test statistic is a single number that summarizes the sample information. In nonparametric tests, the observed data are converted into ranks and then the ranks are summarized into a test statistic.
- There are two popular nonparametric tests to compare outcomes between two matched or paired groups. The first is called the Sign test and the second is the Wilcoxon Signed Rank test.
- Another popular nonparametric test for matched or paired data is called the Wilcoxon Signed Rank Test. Like the Sign test, it is based on difference scores, but in addition to analyzing the signs of the differences, it also takes into account the magnitudes of the observed differences.
- A popular nonparametric test to compare outcomes among more than two independent groups is the Kruskal– Wallis test. The Kruskal–Wallis test is used to compare medians among k comparison groups (k > 2) and is sometimes described as an ANOVA with the data replaced by their ranks.

References

1. Armitage, P., Berry, G., & Matthews, J. N. S. (2008). *Statistical Methods in Medical Research* (4th ed.). Wiley-Blackwell.
2. Conover, W. J. (1999). *Practical Nonparametric Statistics* (3rd ed.). Wiley.
3. Day, S. J., & Graham, D. F. (2017). *Sample Size and Power for Nonparametric Tests in Biomedical Research*. Boca Raton, FL: CRC Press.
4. Higgins, J. P. T., & Green, S. (Eds.). (2011). *Cochrane Handbook for Systematic Reviews of Interventions*. Wiley.
5. Lehmann, E. L., & Romano, J. P. (2005). *Testing Statistical Hypotheses* (3rd ed.). Springer.
6. Rosner, B. (2015). *Fundamentals of Biostatistics* (8th ed.). Cengage Learning.
7. Siegel, S., & Castellan, N. J. (1988). *Nonparametric Statistics for the Behavioral Sciences* (2nd ed.). McGraw-Hill.
8. Zar, J. H. (2010). *Biostatistical Analysis* (5th ed.). Pearson.

Chapter 10

SURVIVAL ANALYSIS AND DATA VISUALIZATION

Contents

Introduction 277
10.1. Survival Analysis 279
10.2. Data Visualization 293
Summary 316
References 316

Introduction

In evidence-based medicine, survival analysis is frequently utilized to look at the time-to-event series. Time-to-event series can show the duration of any dichotomous event and are frequently used for survival/death events. Examples include the length of time a patient must receive treatment before entering remission, the severity of their illness, and the number of hours they must stay in the hospital before being discharged. This technique allows for the comparison of individual patients or groups of patients. Nonparametric methods such as log-rank tests and Kaplan-Meier estimations can be used to analyze relationships between multiple groups. Researchers can use Cox proportional hazard models to quantify the impact of the comparison or comparisons. Although survival analysis techniques were initially applied in medical research, they are now widely used in engineering and financial services, among other fields. Complex medical statistics are represented graphically in a way that is easy to understand through data visualization. Even without highly developed math skills, it enables users to quickly and easily obtain qualitative insights, changes, patterns, and trends while drawing insightful conclusions.

Orientation and Directional Terms

Term	Definition	Illustration
Censoring	Survival Analysis often encounters censoring, where the event of interest has not occurred by the end of the study or is not observed for some other reason. Censored data poses challenges but is a common occurrence in longitudinal studies.	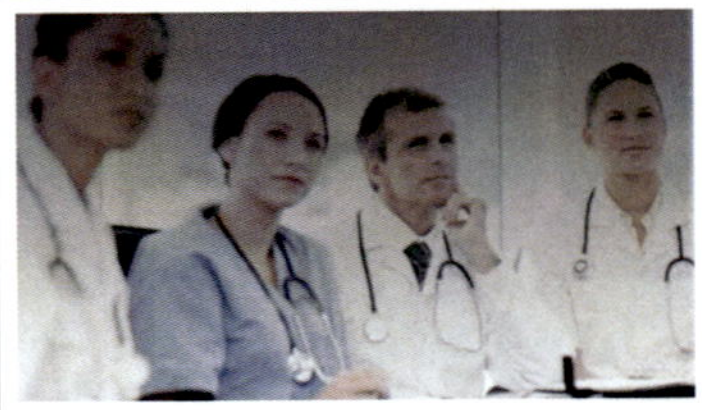
Cox Proportional-Hazards Model	The Cox model is a widely employed semi-parametric model that allows for the examination of the impact of covariates on the hazard rate. It assumes that the hazard ratio remains constant over time.	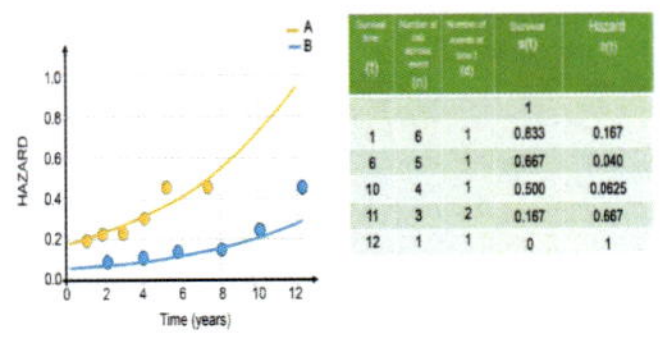
Data Visualization	Data visualization can help doctors identify patterns, anomalies, and diseases, and improve patient care. It can also help with transparency, fraud detection, and patient outcomes.	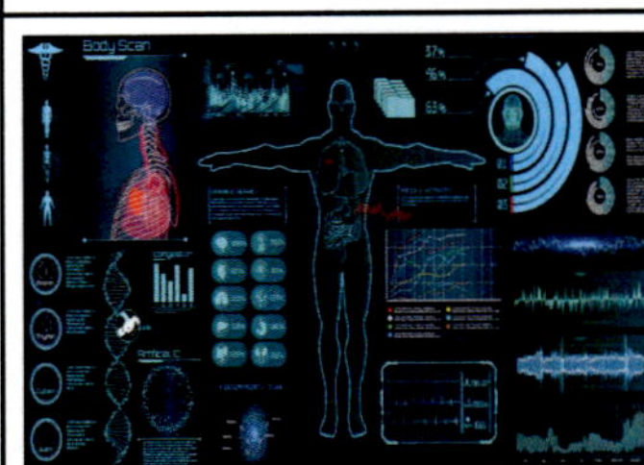
Kaplan-Meier Estimator	The Kaplan-Meier estimator is a non-parametric method used to estimate the survival function from censored data. It provides a step-function approximation of the survival curve and is particularly useful for visualizing survival probabilities over time.	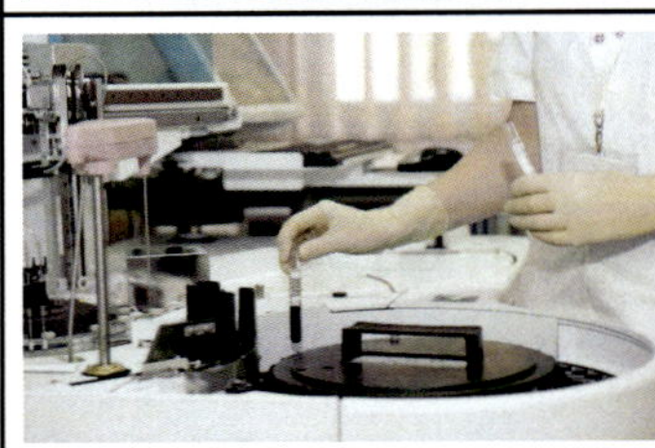
Medical Research	Survival Analysis is extensively used in clinical trials to assess the efficacy of treatments and estimate the survival probabilities of patients with specific conditions.	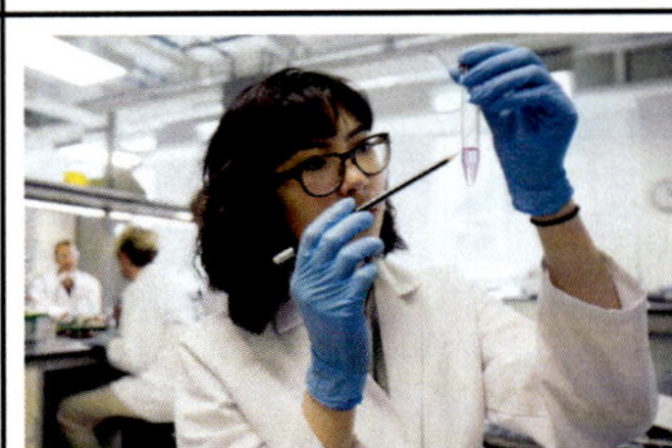
Survival analysis	Survival analysis is a statistical technique that uses time-to-event data to analyze the time until an event occurs.	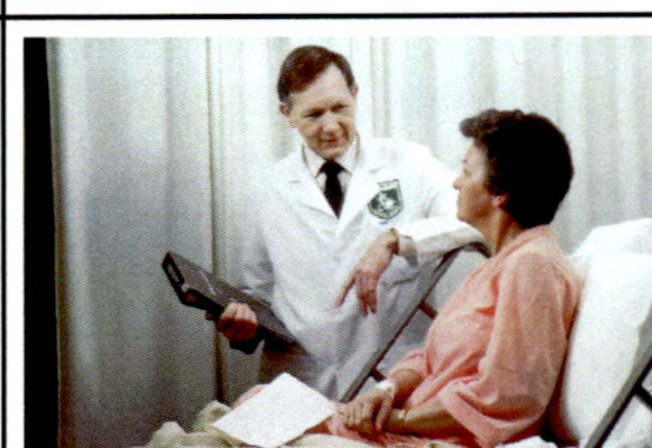

10.1. Survival Analysis

Now, we look at a distinct kind of outcome variable known as a time-to-event variable. The amount of time that passes before a participant experiences an interesting event (e.g., heart attack, cancer that has remitted, or demise). Due to the particular characteristics of time-to-event variables, statistical analysis of these variables necessitates the use of different methods than those previously discussed for other kinds of outcomes. Even though death is not always the result, statistical analysis of these variables is known as time-to-event analysis or survival analysis. The following types of questions are relevant to survival analysis: What is the likelihood that a participant will live for five years? Are there variations in survival among groups (e.g., between patients receiving a new medication and those receiving a standard medication in a clinical trial)? How do specific behavioral, clinical, or personal traits impact participants' chances of surviving?

Time-to-event variables have many special characteristics. First, the distributions of times to events are frequently skewed and are always positive. For example, most events (relapses) may happen early in the follow-up, with very few occurring later, in a study measuring the time to relapse in high-risk patients. However, the majority of events (deaths) may happen later in the follow-up in a study on time to death in a community-based sample. Conventional statistical techniques that presume distributions are normal do not apply. The use of nonparametric procedures is possible, but there are further problems. To be more precise, not all study participants have complete data—that is, actual time-to-event data—available to researchers. Many studies enrol participants over a period of time (months or years), with the study coming to an end on a designated date in the calendar. As a result, those who enrol later are monitored for a shorter amount of time than those who enrol sooner. Certain participants may withdraw from the study prior to its conclusion (by moving away or showing disinterest, for example), and some may pass away during the follow-up period (provided that the death is not the outcome of interest). For each of these cases, our follow-up data is not complete. The reason why the true survival time, also referred to as failure time, is unknown is because the study either ends or a participant withdraws before the event occurs. We do know that the participant's survival time has elapsed longer than the time of the last follow-up observation. We refer to these periods as "censored times."

Censorship takes many different forms. The most prevalent kind of censoring is known as "right censoring," which happens when a participant's last observed follow-up time is less than the time to event because they did not experience the event of interest during the study. This may happen if a participant withdraws from the study before it is finished or if they are event-free after the observation period. First, the participant's observed time is shorter than the follow-up period; second, the participant's observed time is equal to the follow-up period. The following examples serve as illustrations of these issues.

Example 10.1.

A 10-year follow-up of 10 participants in a small prospective study is conducted to monitor the development of myocardial infarction, also known as a heart attack. Over two years, study participants are recruited, and they may be tracked for up to ten years. **Figure 10.1a** illustrates the experiences of the participants. Be aware that some participants enrol in the study after the deadline (some by as much as two years), and that they may be monitored for up to ten years following their enrolment. Three participants experience myocardial infarction (MI) during the study period; one participant passes away; two participants discontinue the study (for unclear reasons); and four participants finish the 10-year follow-up without experiencing MI. The identical data are shown in Figure 10.1b, but survival time is shown beginning at a shared time zero (i.e., as though everyone took part in the study at the same moment).

What is the probability that a participant will experience a MI over ten years based on the data presented in Figure 10.1b? Three out of ten participants experienced an MI during follow-up, but the 30 percent figure is likely an underestimate of the actual percentage because two participants left the study early and may have experienced an MI had they been followed for the entire ten years. They have censored their observed times. Furthermore, one participant passes away following a three-year follow-up. If we exclude all three, the estimate of the likelihood that a participant suffers an MI is 3/7 = 43 percent, which is significantly higher than the initial estimate of 30 percent. Should these three people be included in the analysis, and if so, how? Survival data is distinct because it frequently does not include all participants who are tracked for the duration of the follow-up period. In this brief instance, Participant 4 has been under observation for 4 years and has not experienced a MI during that time. After two years of observation, participant 7 has not experienced an MI. Even though they are not affected by the noteworthy event, they nonetheless provide valuable information. This data is used by survival analysis techniques to estimate the probability of an event. It is assumed that the censored data will be used appropriately. To be more precise, we take it that censorship has nothing to do with whether the event of interest is likely to occur or not. This type of censoring, known as non-informative censoring, works on the fundamental premise that, in the event that the participants whose data are censored were actually observed, their failure times (or times to event) would be distributed similarly.

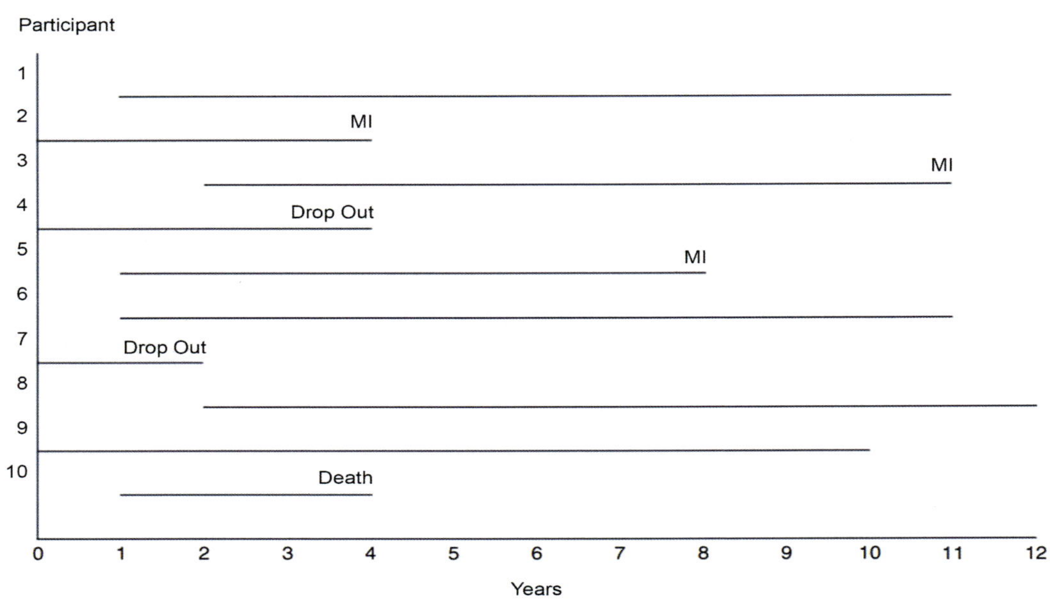

(a)

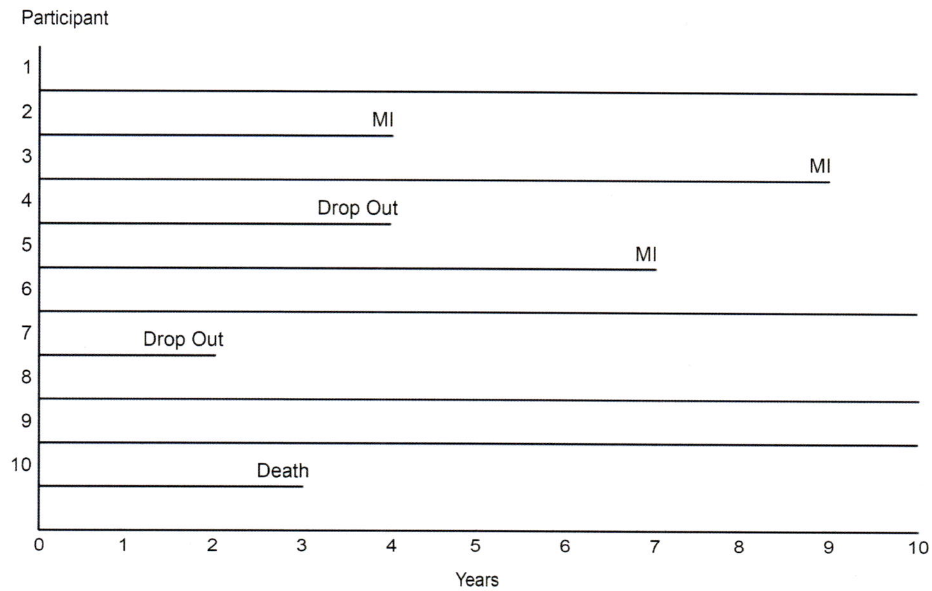

(b)

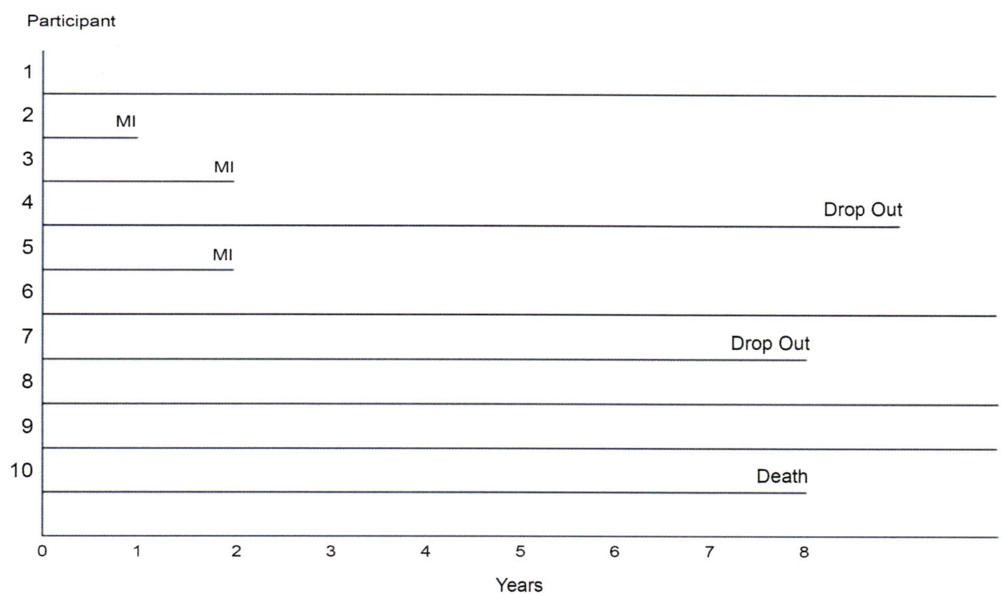

(c)

Figure 10.1. *Participants' experiences in a 10-year study of myocardial infarction.*

Source: Lisa M. Sullivan. Essentials of Biostatistics in Public Health, Third Edition. Jones & Bartlett Learning.

Examine the same study and ten distinct participants' experiences, as shown in **Figure 10.1c**. Observe that in **Figure 10.1c**, three participants experience MI once more, one passes away, two discontinue the study, and four survive the 10-year follow-up without experiencing MI. But in the course of follow-up, the events (MIs) happen much earlier, and the drop-outs and deaths happen later. When estimating the probability of a participant suffering an MI over ten years, should the variations in the experiences of the participants depicted in Figure 10.1c versus Figure 10.1b have an impact? In survival analysis, we examine not only the number of participants experiencing the event of interest, which is a binary indicator of event status but also the timing of the events.

10.1.1. Survival Data

We measure two critical pieces of information in survival analysis. First, we assess if a participant experiences the relevant event(s) during the study period. An indicator or dichotomous variable that is frequently coded as 1 for an event that occurred or 0 for an event that did not occur during the study observation period reflects this. We additionally track follow-up times for every participant. The moment at which participants are thought to be at risk for the outcome of interest is known as time zero, or the time origin. Time at risk is often measured from the outset of the study (i.e., during enrolment). Because the risk of stroke is very low before the age of 55, researchers may choose to enrol participants in a prospective cohort study assessing the time to incident stroke who are 55 years of age or older. A prospective cohort study assessing the time to incident cardiovascular disease may include individuals 35 years of age and above in its participant pool. A minimum age may be stated as a requirement for participation in each of these studies. The follow-up period is calculated starting at time zero, which can be either the study's beginning or the moment the participant is deemed to be at risk. It continues until one of three things happens: the event, the study's conclusion, or the participant's loss. The time origin in a clinical trial is typically regarded as the randomization time.

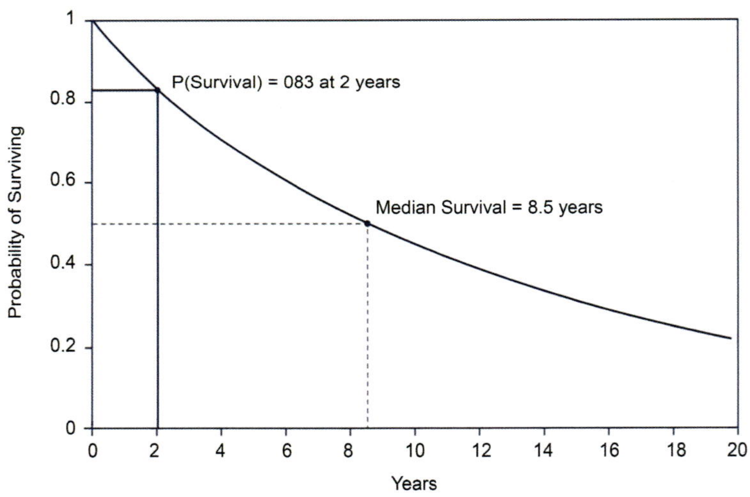

Figure 10.2. *Sample survival curve.*

Source: Lisa M. Sullivan. Essentials of Biostatistics in Public Health, Third Edition. Jones & Bartlett Learning.

Cohort studies and clinical trials frequently involve the enrolment or recruitment of patients over several months or years. To precisely measure the follow-up time, it is crucial to document the entry time. Once more, the time to event is of interest to us, but for different reasons (e.g., the study participant withdraws, or the study observation period expires), it is not always possible to determine the time to event. We measure follow-up time, which is less than the time to the event, and censor these follow-up times for participants who do not experience the event of interest.

In survival analysis, we estimate a survival function based on event status and follow-up time data. The survival function, which is a function of time, shows the likelihood that an individual will live past a specific point in time. Examine a 20-year prospective study on the prognosis of myocardial infarction patients. The survival function, also known as the survival curve, may resemble the one displayed in **Figure 10.2** because the study's outcome is all-cause mortality.

The vertical axis displays the percentage of people who survive or the probability of survival, while the horizontal axis represents time in years. The survival probability at time zero is 1, meaning that all participants are alive. The likelihood of survival at two years is roughly 0.83, or 83 percent (refer to the solid lines in **Figure 10.2**). The chance of surviving at ten years is roughly 0.47, or 47 percent. Estimating the median survival, or the point in the study at which 50% of the participants are still alive, is frequently interesting. The median survival in **Figure 10.2** is roughly 8.05 years (**Figure 10.2** dashed lines).

The survival curve is flat (i.e., a survival curve that remains near 1) denotes excellent survival, while one that falls sharply toward 0 denotes poor survival. The survival function is represented as a smooth curve in **Figure 10.2**. The survival function is displayed as a step function rather than a smooth curve in the majority of applications.

10.1.2. Estimating the Survival Function

One can estimate a survival function or survival curve in a number of ways. Many well-known parametric techniques are available for modelling survival data, and they vary in what is assumed about the distribution of survival times within the population. The exponential, Weibull, Gompertz, and log-normal distributions are a few common distributions. The exponential model, which is arguably the most well-liked, makes the assumption that a participant's chance of experiencing the relevant event is unrelated to the length of their event-free period. Different assumptions are made by other distributions regarding the likelihood that an individual will develop the event (i.e., it might grow, shrink, or alter over time). For additional information on parametric survival analysis techniques, see Lee and Wang and Hosmer and Lemeshow.

Here, we concentrate on two nonparametric techniques that don't make any assumptions about how an individual's probability of developing the event changes over time. We estimate and plot the survival distribution, also known as the survival curve, using nonparametric techniques. Plotting survival curves as step functions is common, as **Figure 10.3** illustrates. The x-axis displays time, and the y-axis displays survival (as a percentage or proportion of those who are at risk). Be aware that the percentage of participants "surviving" (represented by the y-axis) may also represent the percentage of participants free of another outcome event, such as the percentage free of cardiovascular disease or MI, rather than the percentage of participants who are alive (which assumes that the outcome of interest is death). It can also be used to show the proportion of participants who do not have a positive outcome (e.g., cancer remission). Observe that after two years, the survival probability decreases to 90% from 100%. Nine years is the median survival (i.e., 50% of the population survives past nine years; dashed lines indicate this).

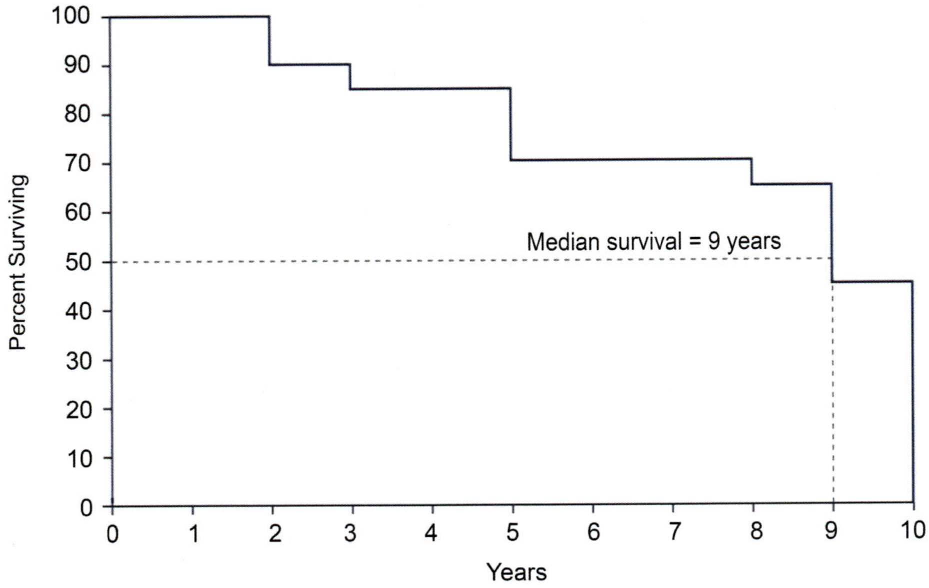

Figure 10.3. *Survival function.*

Source: Lisa M. Sullivan. Essentials of Biostatistics in Public Health, Third Edition. Jones & Bartlett Learning.

Example 10.2.

Examine a small prospective cohort study that aims to investigate death time. Participants in the study who are 65 years of age or older will be monitored for a maximum of 24 years. Twenty participants are enrolled in the study over five years, and they will be monitored until they pass away, the study concludes, or they withdraw from the study (lost to follow-up). Please take note that a participant's maximum follow-up period is less than 24 years if they enrol after the study's launch. For instance, a participant's maximum follow-up period is 22 years if they enrol two years after the study starts. All biostatistical analyses require high-quality data. It is crucial for survival analysis applications that the study start and end dates, as well as the event of interest, are precisely defined and measured. In **Table 10.1**, the data are displayed.

Three participants in the study have received full follow-up, while six deaths have occurred (i.e., 24 years old). Due to delayed enrolment or loss to follow-up, the remaining 11 have fewer than 24 years of follow-up.

An actuarial table, also known as a life table, can be used to summarize the participant experiences. Life tables come in a variety of common forms and applications. For example, some are used to calculate life expectancy, while others are employed by the insurance sector to determine rates. We concentrate on a specific kind of life table known as a cohort life table or follow-up life table that is frequently used in bio-statistical analysis. The experiences of participants in a cohort study or clinical trial are summarized in a follow-up life table over a predetermined period, either until the time of the event of interest or until the end of the study, whichever comes first.

Table 10.1. *Year of Death or Year of Last Contact*

Participant Identification Number	Year of Death	Year of Last Contact
1		24
2	3	
3		11
4		19
5		24
6		13
7	14	
8		2
9		18
10		17
11		24
12		21
13		12
14	1	
15		10
16	23	
17		6
18	5	
19		9
20	17	

Source: Lisa M. Sullivan. Essentials of Biostatistics in Public Health, Third Edition. Jones & Bartlett Learning.

We first divide the follow-up times into intervals that are equally spaced in order to create a life table. Example 10.2 considers 5-year intervals of 0–4 years, 5–9 years, 10–14 years, 15–19 years, and 20–24 years, with a maximum follow-up of 24 years. The number of participants who are still alive at the start of each interval, the number who pass away, and the number who are censored are added together (refer to **Table 10.2**).

The notation we employ in our life-table analysis is as follows. To create the life table for the data in Example 10.2, we first define the notation.

Table 10.2. *Number Alive, Number of Deaths, and Number Censored in Each Interval*

Interval in Years	Number Alive at Beginning of Interval	Number of Deaths During Interval	Number Censored
0–4	20	2	1
5–9	17	1	2
10–14	14	1	4
15–19	9	1	3
20–24	5	1	4

Source: Lisa M. Sullivan. Essentials of Biostatistics in Public Health, Third Edition. Jones & Bartlett Learning.

- N_t = number of participants who are event-free and considered at risk during interval t (e.g., in this example, the number alive, as our outcome of interest is death)
- D_t = number of participants who die (or suffer the event of interest) during interval t
- C_t = number of participants who are censored during interval t
- N_{t*} = the average number of participants at risk during interval t

In constructing actuarial life tables, the following assumptions are often made: First, the events of interest (e.g., deaths) are assumed to occur at the end of the interval, and censored events are assumed to occur uniformly (or evenly) throughout the interval. Therefore, an adjustment is often made to N_t to reflect the average number of participants at risk during the interval, N_{t*}, which is computed as follows: $N_{t*} = N_t - C_t /2$ (i.e., we subtract half of the censored events).

- q_t = proportion dying (or suffering event) during interval t, $q_t = D_t /N_{t*}$
- p_t = proportion surviving (remaining event-free) during interval t, $p_t = 1 - q_t$

- S_t = proportion surviving (remaining event-free) past interval t

S_t is the proportion surviving (or remaining event-free) past interval t, sometimes called the cumulative survival probability. It is computed as follows: First, the proportion of participants surviving past time 0 (the starting time) is defined as $S_0 = 1$ (all participants are alive or event-free at time zero or the start of the study).

To be more precise, $S_1 = p_1$ represents the likelihood that a participant will survive past interval 1. The probability that a participant survives past interval 2 means that they had to survive past interval 1 and through interval 2: S_2 = P(survive past interval 2) = P(survive through interval 2) × P(survive past interval 1), or $S_2 = p_2 \times S_1$. In general, $S_{t+1} = p_{t+1} \times S_t$. Table 10.3 displays the follow-up life table format. The table's columns contain the intervals, participant counts at risk, the count of individuals experiencing the event of interest (e.g., die), how many participants are lost to follow-up or censored, the percentages of participants who experience the event of interest and those who do not, and the likelihood of survival. There are twenty participants alive or at risk at time 0, which is the beginning of the first interval (0–4 years). One participant is censored, and two participants pass away during the intermission. To get $N_{t*} = N_t - C_t/2 = 20 - (1/2) = 19.5$, we apply the correction for the number of participants censored during that interval. Table 10.3 for the first interval lists the calculations for the remaining life table elements.

Table 10.3. *Constructing The Life Table—First Interval*

Interval in Years	Number at Risk During Interval, N_t	Average Number at Risk During Interval, N_{t^*}	Number of Deaths During Interval, D_t	Lost to Follow-Up, C_t	Proportion Dying During Interval, q_t	Proportion Surviving Interval, p_t	Survival Probability, S_t
0–4	20	20 – (1/2) = 19.5	2	1	2/19.5 = 0.103	1 – 0.103 = 0.897	1(0.897) = 0.897

Source: Lisa M. Sullivan. Essentials of Biostatistics in Public Health, Third Edition. Jones & Bartlett Learning.

Table 10.4. *Constructing the Life Table—Second Interval*

Interval in Years	Number at Risk During Interval, N_t	Average Number at Risk During Interval, N_{t^*}	Number of Deaths During Interval, D_t	Lost to Follow-Up, C_t	Proportion Dying During Interval, q_t	Among Those at Risk, Proportion Surviving Interval, p_t	Survival Probability, S_t
0–4	20	20 – (1/2) = 19.5	2	1	2/19.5 = 0.103	1 – 0.103 = 0.897	1(0.897) = 0.897
5–9	17	17 – (2/2) = 16.0	1	2	1/16 = 0.063	1 – 0.063 = 0.937	(0.937)(0.897) = 0.840

Source: Lisa M. Sullivan. Essentials of Biostatistics in Public Health, Third Edition. Jones & Bartlett Learning.

The second interval, which is 5–9 years, is now added (see Table 10.4). The number at risk is equal to that of the previous interval (0–4 years) minus the number of censored and deceased individuals (i.e., $N_t = N_{t-1} - D_{t-1} - C_{t-1} = 20 - 2 - 1 = 17$). $S_4 = p_4 = 0.897$ is the probability that a participant will live past four years, or the first interval if the upper limit of the interval is used to define the time. The formula for calculating survival probabilities is $S_{t+1} = p_{t+1} \times S_t$. A participant's likelihood of surviving for nine years is $S_9 = p_9 \times S_4 = 0.937\ 3\ 0.897 = 0.840$.

The whole follow-up life table for the data in Example 10.2 is found in **Table 10.5**. The follow-up life table in **Table 10.5** is created using the actuarial method, with time being divided into equally spaced intervals. This approach has a drawback in that, especially with small samples, the survival probabilities can vary depending on how the intervals are arranged. This problem is addressed by the widely used Kaplan–Meier approach, also known as the product-limit approach, which re-estimates the survival probability each time an event occurs (in Example 10.2, each time a death occurs). The Kaplan–Meier approach can be used appropriately under a few presumptions. More specifically, we assume that survival probabilities for participants recruited early and later in the study are similar and that censoring occurs regardless of the chance of developing the event of interest. These presumptions must hold for each comparison group when comparing multiple groups, for example, to ensure that censoring is not more common in one group than the other.

Table 10.5. *Life Table for Data in Example 10.2*

Interval in Years	Number at Risk During Interval, N_t	Average Number at Risk During Interval, N_{t^*}	Number of Deaths During Interval, D_t	Lost to Follow-Up, C_t	Proportion Dying During Interval, q_t	Among Those at Risk, Proportion Surviving Interval, p_t	Survival Probability, S_t
0–4	20	19.5	2	1	0.103	0.897	0.897
5–9	17	16.0	1	2	0.063	0.937	0.840
10–14	14	12.0	1	4	0.083	0.917	0.770
15–19	9	7.5	1	3	0.133	0.867	0.688
20–24	5	3.0	1	4	0.333	0.667	0.446

Source: Lisa M. Sullivan. Essentials of Biostatistics in Public Health, Third Edition. Jones & Bartlett Learning.

Using the Kaplan–Meier method, **Table 10.6** displays the life table for the data in Example 10.2. The times when events or censoring take place, the number of participants at risk (N_t), the number of deaths (D_t), the number censored (C_t), and the survival probability (S_t) are listed in **Table 10.6**. Keep in mind that the table's initial values are time = 0 and survival probability = 1. All participants are at risk at time = 0 (baseline, or the beginning of the study), and the survival probability is 1 (or 100%). $S_{t+1} = S_t \times ((N_{t+1} - D_{t+1})/N_{t+1})$ is used to calculate the survival probability with the data layout shown in **Table 10.6**. The table's initial rows provide a detailed breakdown of the survival probability calculations. It is significant to remember that the actuarial life-table approach and the Kaplan-Meier approach calculations are comparable. The primary distinction is in the time intervals: the Kaplan–Meier approach uses observed event times and censoring times, whereas the actuarial life-table approach considers equally spaced intervals.

These calculations can be laborious when dealing with big datasets. But a lot of computer programs can produce the analyses quickly (e.g., SAS®). After the data are arranged according to time and the number of events and censored times are summed up, Microsoft Excel® can also be used to calculate the survival probabilities.

We can create a Kaplan-Meier survival curve using the life table. Figure 10.4 displays the Kaplan-Meier survival curve for the data in Example 10.2. The symbols in Figure 10.4's survival curve stand for each event time, which can be either a censored or a death. By finding the year 10 on the x-axis and reading up and over to the y-axis, we can also calculate the probability that a participant will survive for an additional ten years using the survival curve. Eighty-four percent of participants have survived for a decade or more (dashed lines in Figure 10.4). Similarly, 68% of participants have survived for more than 20 years. Finding 0.5 on the y-axis and reading down to the x-axis yields the median survival. It is estimated that the median survival is 23 years. Point estimates are what these estimates of the median survival time and the survival probabilities at particular times are, and you should treat them as such. Standard errors and confidence interval estimates of survival probabilities can be computed using various statistical computing packages and formulas. The Greenwood formula, also known as the survival standard error formula, is a widely used formula that can be calculated as follows:

Table 10.6. *Life Table for Data in Example 10.2 Using the Kaplan–Meier Approach*

Time, years	Number at Risk, N_t	Number of Deaths, D_t	Number Censored, C_t	Survival Probability, $S_{t+1} = S_t \times ((N_{t+1} - D_{t+1})/N_{t+1})$
0	20			1†
1	20	1		$1 \times [(20 - 1)/20] = 0.950$
2	19		1	$0.950 \times [(19 - 0)/19] = 0.950$
3	18	1		$0.950 \times [(18 - 1)/18] = 0.897$
5	17	1		$0.897 \times [(17 - 1)/17] = 0.844$
6	16		1	0.844
9	15		1	0.844
10	14		1	0.844
11	13		1	0.844
12	12		1	0.844
13	11		1	0.844
14	10	1		0.760
17	9	1	1	0.676
18	7		1	0.676
19	6		1	0.676
21	5		1	0.676
23	4	1		0.507
24	3		3	0.507

†Recall that $S_0 = 1$.

Source: Lisa M. Sullivan. Essentials of Biostatistics in Public Health, Third Edition. Jones & Bartlett Learning.

$$\mathrm{SE}(S_t) = S_t\sqrt{\Sigma\frac{D_t}{N_t(N_t - D_t)}}.$$

The quantity

$$\frac{D_t}{N_t(N_t - D_t)}$$

is added for the number of deaths (D_t) and the number of people at risk (N_t) that occur during the relevant period (i.e., cumulative over all periods preceding the period of interest). **Table 10.7** provides a summary of the standard errors that were calculated for the survival estimates based on the data in Example 10.2. Keep in mind that the margin of error, or 1.96 × SE(S_t), is displayed in the final column and is utilized to calculate the 95 percent confidence interval estimates (i.e., S_t ± 1.96 × SE(S_t)).

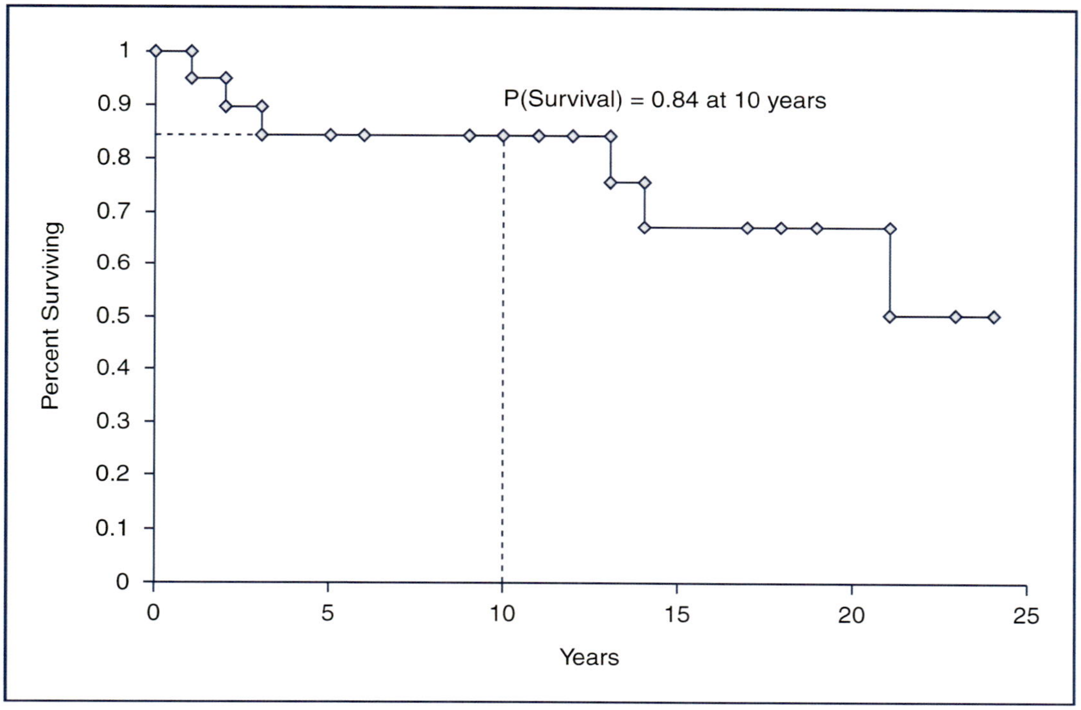

Figure 10.4. *Kaplan-Meier survival curve for data in example 10.2.*

Source: Lisa M. Sullivan. Essentials of Biostatistics in Public Health, Third Edition. Jones & Bartlett Learning.

A few researchers would rather create cumulative incidence curves than survival curves, which display the cumulative odds of encountering the event of interest. The Kaplan-Meier method makes it simple to calculate cumulative incidence, also known as cumulative failure probability, from the life table. It is calculated as 1 – St. The cumulative failure probabilities for the data in Example 10.2 are displayed in **Table 10.8**. The cumulative incidence of death for study participants enrolled in the experiment detailed in Example 10.2 is displayed in **Figure 10.6**. We can calculate the probability that a participant will pass away by a specific time point using **Figure 10.6**. For instance, at 15 years, the likelihood of dying is roughly 33% (dashed lines).

Table 10.7. *Standard Errors of Survival Estimate for the Data in Example 10.2*

Time, years	Number at Risk, N_t	Number of Deaths, D_t	Survival Probability, S_t	$\frac{D_t}{N_t(N_t - D_t)}$	$\sum\frac{D_t}{N_t(N_t - D_t)}$	$S_t\sqrt{\sum\frac{D_t}{N_t(N_t - D_t)}}$	$1.96 \times SE(S_t)$
0	20		1				
1	20	1	0.950	0.003	0.003	0.049	0.096
2	19		0.950	0.000	0.003	0.049	0.096
3	18	1	0.897	0.003	0.006	0.069	0.135
5	17	1	0.844	0.004	0.010	0.083	0.162
6	16		0.844	0.000	0.010	0.083	0.162
9	15		0.844	0.000	0.010	0.083	0.162
10	14		0.844	0.000	0.010	0.083	0.162
11	13		0.844	0.000	0.010	0.083	0.162
12	12		0.844	0.000	0.010	0.083	0.162
13	11		0.844	0.000	0.010	0.083	0.162
14	10	1	0.760	0.011	0.021	0.109	0.214
17	9	1	0.676	0.014	0.035	0.126	0.246
18	7		0.676	0.000	0.035	0.126	0.246
19	6		0.676	0.000	0.035	0.126	0.246
21	5		0.676	0.000	0.035	0.126	0.246
23	4	1	0.507	0.083	0.118	0.174	0.341
24	3		0.507	0.000	0.118	0.174	0.341

Source: Lisa M. Sullivan. Essentials of Biostatistics in Public Health, Third Edition. Jones & Bartlett Learning.

Figure 10.5 displays the Kaplan-Meier survival curve (represented as a solid line) and the 95 percent confidence limits (represented as .ted lines) for the survival probability estimates.

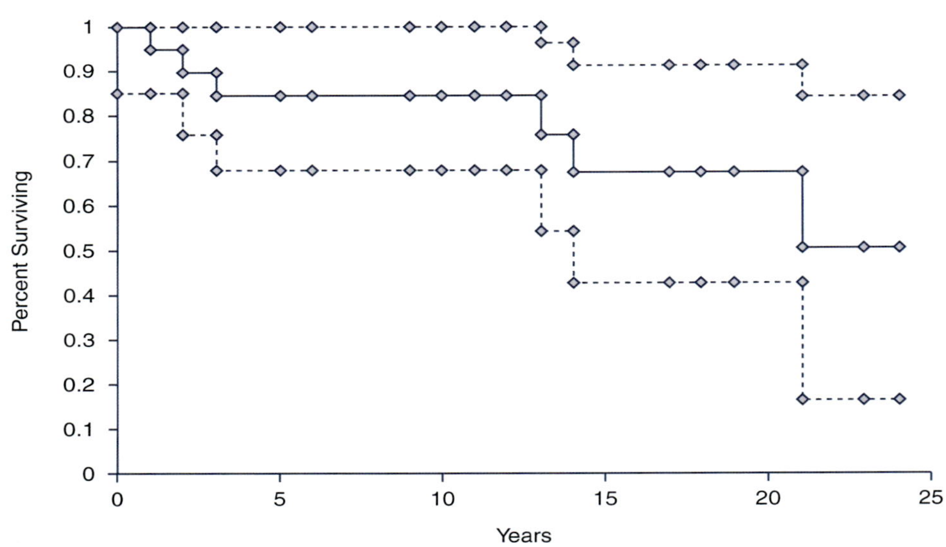

Figure 10.5. *Kaplan–Meier survival curve with confidence intervals for data in example 10.2.*

Source: *Lisa M. Sullivan. Essentials of Biostatistics in Public Health, Third Edition. Jones & Bartlett Learning.*

Table 10.8. *Life Table with Cumulative Failure Probabilities for Data in Example 10.2*

Time, years	Number at Risk, N_t	Number of Deaths, D_t	Number Censored, C_t	Survival Probability, S_t	Failure Probability, $1 - S_t$
0	20			1	0
1	20	1		0.950	0.050
2	19		1	0.950	0.050
3	18	1		0.897	0.103
5	17	1		0.844	0.156
6	16		1	0.844	0.156
9	15		1	0.844	0.156
10	14		1	0.844	0.156
11	13		1	0.844	0.156
12	12		1	0.844	0.156
13	11		1	0.844	0.156
14	10	1		0.760	0.240
17	9	1	1	0.676	0.324
18	7		1	0.676	0.324
19	6		1	0.676	0.324
21	5		1	0.676	0.324
23	4	1		0.507	0.493
24	3		3	0.507	0.493

Source: Lisa M. Sullivan. Essentials of Biostatistics in Public Health, Third Edition. Jones & Bartlett Learning.

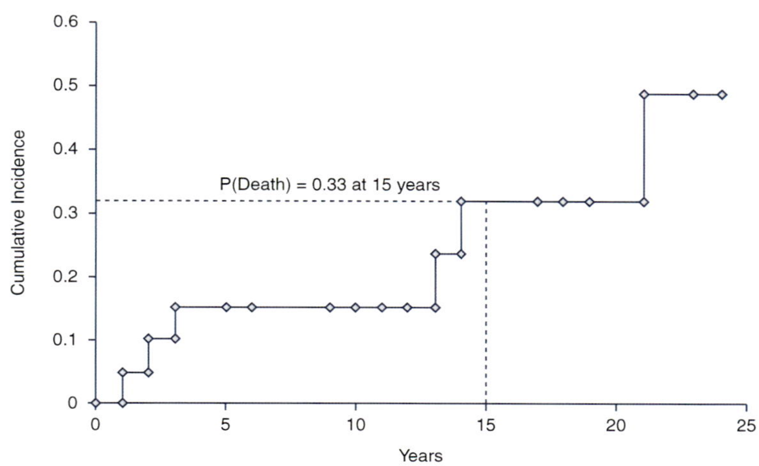

Figure 10.6. *Cumulative incidence curve for data in example 10.2.*

Source: Lisa M. Sullivan. Essentials of Biostatistics in Public Health, Third Edition. Jones & Bartlett Learning.

10.1.3. Issues of Concern

Because survival analysis is used so frequently in medical literature, healthcare professionals need to be familiar with the basic ideas and analyses that go along with these methods. These include log-rank tests, Kaplan-Meier, and Cox proportional hazards models. When there is a binary or dichotomous outcome of interest, survival analysis is employed. Usually, comparisons are made between multiple groups; for instance, one group might receive treatment A while another might receive treatment B. The likelihood of surviving (or not experiencing an event) until a given time point is known as the survival function, while the rate at which the event occurs within a given time frame is known as the hazard rate. Knowing the times of the initial event at the origin and the last event is necessary to calculate survival time. Truncation is useful in limiting bias when selecting a sample for survival analysis; investigators should avoid selecting subjects for whom they know the likelihood of an event occurring or not to validate their theories.

10.1.3.1. Censoring

An essential subject in survival analysis is censorship. Subjects who were censored never encountered the desired result within the allotted study period. It is inappropriate to link the occurrence of an event to the censorship of an individual. Right censoring happens when someone did not experience the event within the allotted timeframe (occurred after, or unsure if and when the incident occurred). Left censoring occurs when someone experienced the event before origin. Censoring essentially means that the study's findings cannot be used to determine the subject's desired outcome. The time before a person or group encounters the relevant event or result, or until it is censored, is examined by survival analysis. Results would be skewed if censored subjects were ignored or excluded. While the researchers have no control over certain aspects of the study, censoring can be minimized by selecting study participants who exhibit traits associated with improved retention in the study.

10.1.3.2. Life Tables

Unlike other survival analysis techniques, life tables (also called actuarial life tables) classify the observation outputs into discrete time events. The outputs of life tables display whether the case happened if the person was censored, and when it happened. A life table can be used to ascertain the percentage of patients who experience an event (e.g., passing away) during which time the result happened. Additionally, life tables can show who was and wasn't censored (experienced the event in the timeframe). One should presume that experiencing an event at different intervals remains constant within these life tables. For instance, patients with breast cancer may be less likely to die if they are given a second medication midway through their treatment, which could invalidate the results. Although life tables are still helpful, a new approach was suggested by Kaplan and Meier in 1958 that did away with the need for a pre-determined time interval. Their approach allows for the assessment of events and outcomes of interest in real-time, independent of time intervals.

10.1.3.3. Kaplan-Meier Method

The Kaplan-Meier (KM) approach is one of the survival analysis techniques that is most commonly utilized. The likelihood of survival is estimated using the KM method. A KM survival curve is frequently used in this method to symbolize the survival function. The KM curves, like life tables, make the assumption that the people who were censored would have had comparable results and that the people who were recruited later in the study had the same odds as the people recruited earlier. If the majority of the observations are uncensored, the KM plots a survival curve that frequently reports the median survival time(s), a reliable estimate. To give a range of potential values for the population based on the sample, one can compute confidence intervals (CIs) for KM probabilities and plot CIs in the survival curves.

The significance of the difference between the groups is not indicated by the curve itself. The log-rank test can be used to accomplish this.

10.1.3.4. Log-rank

A non-parametric test for comparing the survival distributions of two or more groups is the log-rank test. This test investigates the null hypothesis (that there are no differences in distribution between the groups), assuming that censoring has no bearing on prognosis. To put it another way, scientists can ascertain whether curves comparing two distinct groups were statistically significant, i.e., if one group's event rate is continuously greater than the other's over time. When a data set contains censored observations, log-rank tests are used; in the absence of censored cases, the Wilcoxon rank-sum test can be used to compare survival times. Researchers who report log-rank tests ought to include the full distribution under test rather than just a subset of it. In contrast to a Cox proportional hazard model, which can ascertain an estimate of the difference between groups, the log-rank test itself has limitations.

10.1.3.5. Cox Proportional Hazard Model

A semiparametric regression model that enables researchers to investigate the effects of various variables on survival curves is the Cox proportional hazards model. Semiparametric refers to the approach's assumption of a relationship between the covariates and outcome but lacks the need for a particular survival function distribution. Hazard ratios (HR) represent the Cox model's output.

The likelihood that an event or outcome will occur within a unit of time, presuming the subject has survived up to that point, is known as the hazard or hazard function. The ratio between the two distinct treatment groups is represented by the hazard ratio (HR). The risk for the event connected to that variable rises as the value above 1. As HR falls below 1, there is less risk. The Cox proportional hazards model creates HRs by examining the relationships between the predictors in these analyses.

The Cox model makes the crucial assumption that the proportionate hazards between the variables don't change over time. Researchers can create relative risk (RR) for an individual to experience an event based on risk factors by adjusting for confounders using Cox hazard models.

10.1.4. Clinical Significance

Log-rank tests, hazard regressions, and KM survival curves can all be computed with software. There are other survival analyses available; this article focuses on the three that are most frequently used in the medical literature. Healthcare practitioners can appropriately evaluate survival analysis techniques in literature to make evidence-based decisions in practice or their own clinical studies by having a basic understanding of the frequently used survival analyses covered here.

10.2. Data Visualization

To direct changes that will enhance population health, solid evidence is required. Effective study design, meticulous data collection and organization, and accurate and clear reporting of findings are all necessary.

It is crucial to communicate data and statistical findings understandably, and there are numerous ways to do this. Text, tables, and figures are among the available options. Depending on how we interpret the data and findings, the significance of the findings, the message we want to get across, and the target audience for the message, the best format will vary (i.e., the viewers). On the other hand, poorly written text and poorly designed tables and figures can confuse. Written text and well-designed tables and figures can improve understanding. To present results as clearly as possible, text, tables, and figures should be used in conjunction with one another. Consistency and synergy between the different formats are also necessary to best serve information consumers and readers. While some results work better when presented textually, others work better when tabulated. Only if figures and graphical displays are of the highest caliber and are meticulously crafted can they effectively convey complex relationships concisely, show patterns, and trends, shorten the length of a report or publication, and improve the reader's comprehension of the findings.

Any statistical analysis must include effective communication of statistical results, which calls for the author to execute the process with skill. The American Statistical Association created "Ethical Guidelines for Statistical Practice," which include eight broad topic areas and ethical considerations for each, to help researchers report their findings. In addition to obligations to "report sufficient information to give readers, including other practitioners, a clear understanding of the intent of the work, how and by whom it was performed, and any limitations on its validity," the guidelines also address professionalism and obligations to human subjects. When sharing data and statistical findings, 15 key points need to be taken into account, according to the reporting guidelines. As a result, transparent, equitable, and consistent reporting of data and statistical findings is essential to ethical statistical practice.

To ensure that results are reproducible, statisticians must not only effectively communicate data and statistical results to other statisticians. Perhaps even more crucially, however, is to communicate with non-statisticians as colleagues and collaborators, as they are frequently in a position to make changes based on empirical evidence that will improve population health.

10.2.1. Design Principles

If we are presenting results orally to an audience, we need to move quickly to conclusions. Before we get into specific design principles for effective tables and figures, we need to think about one of the several important questions that directs our process: How will we engage with our audience? Audience members must comprehend the question of interest, its significance, and our method of analysis; they cannot absorb every nuance or stage of an analysis during an oral presentation. These presentations have a larger, more expansive frame. In contrast, since readers can go through the information at their own pace when reading a written report of the results, we can include a lot more detail. Nevertheless, we still need to stay on target and avoid providing readers with too much irrelevant information. Simultaneously, we have to give readers enough information to enable them to draw reliable conclusions and make relevant comparisons. We next turn our attention to the details after we have a general strategy in mind.

A multitude of first-rate resources are at one's disposal to assist in the creation of impactful tables and figures. These resources, which are arguably the most well-known, are from Edward E. Tufte, who provides a wealth of online resources in addition to having written multiple books on the subject. Tufte advocates for a number of guidelines that are primarily focused on the creation of figures or graphical displays, but they are also relevant to the creation of tables. To pique readers' or customers' curiosity and inspire them to want to spread the word about the content, he exhorts the developer to "provoke thought about the subject at hand." The significance of the data or statistical findings must be made abundantly clear to readers or consumers. They must be motivated to interact and show an interest in what is being presented. When creating tables or figures to provide a narrative by summarizing data and statistical findings, we must begin with a broad overview of the situation before delving deeper into specifics.

Tufte advocates for clarity of presentation and honesty in data visualization. Cutting down on what he refers to as "chart junk" is one way to accomplish this. "Chart junk" is the term used to describe superfluous elements in a table or figure that serve no purpose. According to Tufte, chart junk obscures the primary point being made by the table or figure. On the other hand, he supports data presentations that specifically encourage comparison as a way to interact with the data and statistical findings. Tables and figures must be arranged to give readers or consumers the appropriate information in enough detail to enable them to draw valid comparisons and find meaning as they examine the data or statistical findings to encourage this kind of interaction.

The CONVINCE principles for effective data visualization are another set of guidelines that is intended for graphical displays but can also be used for tabular displays. Consistent with Tufte's ideas, the CONVINCE principles emphasize important points and are made simple to recall by their clever acronym:

- **Convey meaning:** with clear labeling of titles, axes, legends, variables, rows, and columns.
- **Objectivity in presentation:** which is maximized with fair scaling of axes so that data and statistical results are not hidden or exaggerated.
- **Necessity of all table and figure elements:** that is, avoiding clutter and unnecessary items in tables and figures that detract from the message at hand, consistent with Tufte's recommendation to minimize chart junk.
- **Visual honesty:** again calling for appropriate use of specific table and chart types, along with scaling and labeling that present data in a fair and balanced way.
- **Imagining the audience:** reinforcing the notion that we, as the developers of tables and figures, must know our audience, what they need to know, and how we might best meet their needs through our delivery.
- **Nimble:** a specific principle that perhaps is most salient to graphical displays, through which readers or consumers are able to access more data or additional levels of detail should they need or wish to delve deeper. This is perhaps best achieved through interactive graphics.
- **Context:** a principle that overlaps with Tufte's principles, urging us to provide readers or consumers with sufficient background to understand the question of interest and its importance, and then appropriate data and statistical results so that they may draw valid conclusions
- **Encourage interaction:** engaging readers and consumers to care about the data, and to explore more deeply.

Steven Few offers eight fundamental ideas or principles for data visualization as a third set of guidelines. Once more, Few's guidelines pertain to figures but are generally applicable to tables as well. He exhorts us to do the following.

- ***Simplify data and statistical results for presentation.*** This is always a delicate balance, as we never want to oversimplify data so that important nuances are lost, but rather find the point at which those nuances are clear and the data are digestible

- ***Ask.*** Few encourage us to create tables and figures that encourage the reader to want to know more, to ask where the data come from, to consider why we are investigating this particular question or issue, and ideally to think about which actions might be taken based on what we communicate.
- ***Compare.*** We must develop tables and figures that allow readers to make valid comparisons so that they can interpret differences, effects, and impact.
- ***Explore.*** We must develop tables and figures that allow readers to explore the data and to discover things on their own.
- ***Attend.*** To communicate our findings as effectively as possible, this principle states that we must comprehend the readers or consumers of the data or statistical results. To effectively communicate our findings to our audience, we need to consider what our audience needs to see to understand the data or statistical results. We also need to make sure that the most important messages are not obscured by cluttered tables or overly complex figures.
- ***Ensure diversity.*** Few recommend that data be presented in a variety of ways to promote a range of interpretations. This is a goal that is probably easiest to accomplish with interactive graphical displays rather than tabular displays, but it is still something that should be considered in all data and statistical result presentations. We must make data and statistical findings easily comprehensible to a wide range of viewers. We have to take into account our audience's varying viewpoints, educational backgrounds, and literacy levels. When creating tables or figures for a research article versus a presentation to a community group, we might, for instance, proceed differently.
- ***Be skeptical.*** As both creators and consumers of data and statistical results, we should question what we see. Where did the data come from? Which inferences are appropriate? What are the limitations of the data?
- ***Respond.*** This idea has to do with sharing statistics and data. As biostatisticians, gathering, organizing, and analyzing data is undoubtedly our primary concern. A crucial and necessary extra component of our work is results communication. Actually, we disseminate the findings by the "Ethical Guidelines for Statistical Practice."

Before we go any further into creating powerful tables and figures, there are a few important points that should be emphasized again. We must argue why the data and statistical findings are significant, or why the reader should care, regardless of the format in which we present our data and findings. To make sure that the reader or consumer can concentrate on the most crucial parts of the data and statistical results, we must draw attention to the most significant components and be transparent about our process (the steps we took and why). Making sure that our message is precise, understandable, and memorable is our ultimate goal.

10.2.2. When and How to Use Text, Tables, and Figures

The audience and our intended method of interaction with them must be taken into account before determining the most effective way to convey the results. To find the most effective method for sharing data and statistical results, it is important to think about the following: will we provide a stand-alone document or report summarizing the results, or will we have the opportunity to present and discuss the results and if so, how much time, space, and flexibility will we have? What do they need to know? How will they use the information? How can we best reach them?

Based on Velany Rodriguez's "Tips on Effective Use of Tables and Figures in Research Papers," this section provides some broad guidelines for selecting text, tables, figures, or graphical displays. We must be consistent in our language and terminology usage, regardless of the format that is used to present the data—and we frequently use multiple formats within a single presentation or report.

Text formats work well for simple, constrained results, like three or four numbers. It is best to report data in text format if putting it in a table would only result in a table with a small number of rows and columns. Reporting findings that are not essential to the investigation's primary goals is another reason to use text rather than a table or figure. Since many readers scan papers and reports first, before reading the text, the results of the primary analysis should usually be presented in a table or figure. Text summaries of ancillary data, or information that broadens the reader's perspective or points them toward more resources, are recommended.

Generally speaking, when numbers less than 10 are given in the text as integers (whole numbers), they should be expressed in words (e.g., "nine") and all numbers greater than 10 ought to be expressed as integers (e.g., "14"). The precision and purpose of the measure should be taken into consideration when determining the number of digits or decimal places to present. Summaries are typically displayed with one extra decimal place than the measured values. As an illustration, let's say that each participant in a research of a novel weight-loss intervention has their weight measured in pounds, with measurements made to the nearest pound (integer values). We may give the mean weight and the standard deviation of the weights in the study sample to provide an overview. To the closest tenth of a place, these data would be displayed (e.g., $\overline{X}$ = 146.2 pounds, and s = 9.7 pounds). Whenever feasible, all variables displayed in the same table should have the same number of decimal places. For instance, in this same study, we may state that the participants' average age (e.g., $\overline{X}$ = 53.7 years) in addition to a few fundamental clinical parameters like their mean total serum cholesterol levels and their mean systolic and diastolic blood pressures. In this instance, all summary statistics ought to be reported to one decimal place, or the tenth place. The exception might be a mean of 0.003, in which case we would report 0.003 rather than 0.0 for consistency's sake.

Generally speaking, it is best to provide a point estimate (e.g., relative risk, mean, proportion, and difference in means) combined with a variability measure (e.g., confidence interval, standard deviation, and standard error). Assuming that there are no outliers, the sample mean and standard deviation are helpful when summarizing the distribution of a continuous measure. The median and interquartile range are appropriate if there are outliers. The standard deviation provides insight into the measure's variability within the study sample when there are no outliers. For instance, we could report a mean systolic blood pressure (SBP) of 123.4 mm Hg and a standard deviation of 14.3 mm Hg if we measure SBP in millimetres of mercury (mm Hg) in a sample of n = 75 patients. We could report a point estimate of 123.4 mm Hg and a standard error of $14.3/\sqrt{75} = 1.7$ mm Hg, if we want to estimate the mean SBP in a population or generalize our findings based on our sample of n = 75 patients. The standard error is a way to gauge the uncertainty of the estimate, which in this instance is the sample mean. It is also known as a measure of sampling variability. In certain studies and documents, summary statistics for a continuous variable like SBP may be shown as 123.4 ± 14.3 mm Hg or 123.4 ± 1.7 mm Hg. However, since different people sometimes show different measures after the "±" sign, it is clearer to indicate what is presented in words rather than by using the sign. The presentation's interpretability is not improved by the usage of the plus and minus signs. However, the statistics that are being presented must be made clear if this or any other symbol is used in the text (or in a table) (e.g., mean ± std dev, 123.4 ± 14.3 mm Hg).

Writing that is clear and succinct is crucial when presenting data and statistical findings. Writing is a crucial skill that can be developed via practice and feedback. It involves planning, drafting, editing, and proofreading. Writing that conveys statistical results, along with other types of technical writing, calls for a certain set of abilities, such as conciseness, consistency, and clarity. Technical writing is concerned with making sure that technical details are clear; it is not reflective or creative writing. Technical details must be explained in detail, and any jargon or acronyms must be used sparingly, carefully, and thoughtfully.

When we need to present a large number of results or statistics and their precise values are crucial, tables are a suitable format. Tables can succinctly summarize a lot of data (e.g., sets of numbers spanning several groups). When arranged effectively, a table can facilitate appropriate comparisons and information digestion for the reader or consumer, particularly for data that would be challenging to condense into a text summary. Consider the following scenario: let's say we are interested in tracking the weight gain (or growth) of babies born to mothers from various racial and ethnic backgrounds. Weights at birth and at 1, 2, 3, 4, 5, and 6 months of age are measured in grams. There are numerous weights to show, and understanding the precise values of these weights is crucial to understanding potential disparities between racial and ethnic groupings. Depending on whether the objective is to quantify the variability of the estimates of the mean weights in each group or to summarize the distribution of weights in each group, weights for each racial/ethnic group at each time point could be presented in a table with mean weights and standard deviations or standard errors.

Tables are also helpful for showing dichotomous variables (the presence or absence of particular qualities or circumstances, some of which are uncommon). For instance, we may want to report on co-occurring disorders in a group of individuals taking part in a novel behavioral intervention for addiction. The sample might include n = 65 young adults between the ages of 20 and 39 years. We would like to give a brief description of the participants and their medical histories before assessing the intervention's effectiveness. We find that a small percentage of participants had comorbid conditions like high blood pressure, high cholesterol, diabetes, heart disease, and cancer, given their ages. Even though these conditions are uncommon, it's crucial to know how much of an impact they have on participants. However, the tiny percentages would be difficult to read in a text and would be obscured by a figure. It is crucial to include both the absolute numbers of participants impacted and the percentages when presenting these data in a table—not just the percentages on their own. As an illustration, we may state that 4/65 (6.2%) of the subjects have elevated cholesterol levels (e.g., serum cholesterol levels above 240 mg/dL overall).

Every table ought to have a message to convey. Tables can be divided or joined as needed to improve readability. Whatever is on it, every table needs to be built with a specific purpose in mind (e.g., to characterize the research sample, to contrast groups based on the main result, and to enumerate the risk variables connected to a result). Every table's primary point—or points, for that matter—should be cited in the paper or report in which it appears. This also applies to figures. If not, there's no reason to include the table (or figure).

As was previously mentioned, before reading a paper or report's entire text, readers frequently consult the tables and figures. To make sure that tables and figures are self-explanatory, they must be properly labelled and annotated. For the table to function independently, it must be labelled with clarity and conciseness. Both the variables and the units of measurement in the table should have clear definitions. The table should include the answers to the questions of what, where, when, and how the variables were measured. Last but not least, if a table (or figure) has been modified from another source, it must be cited.

When we want to show trends or regional variations, or complex relationships between variables that cannot be shown with tables or text, figures are appropriate. There are numerous varieties of figures that can be created, from extremely simple figures (e.g., bar charts, histograms, box-whisker plots) to interactive infographics that are frequently seen in emails, news reports, social media posts, and websites.

The author should take great care when creating figures, making sure they are clear and concise. Axes should be properly labelled, all figures should have descriptive titles and important points should be strategically highlighted with lines, markers, and legends. The utilization of figures can prove to be highly advantageous when comparing groups, interventions, or both. In addition to considering which comparisons to make, we also need to consider how the reader or consumer will interpret the figures.

Assume, for instance, that we carry out a clinical trial to assess if a nonsteroidal anti-inflammatory drug (NSAID) can effectively reduce pain intensity in n = 80 patients with lower back pain when compared to a placebo. At baseline (the start of the study), the level of pain experienced by each patient is measured on a scale from 0 to 10, where 0 represents no pain and 10 represents excruciating pain. After four weeks on the prescribed treatment, patients are randomized in equal numbers to receive either the NSAID or a placebo, and their level of pain is assessed once more. Assume that patients taking NSAIDs experience a change in pain intensity of 1.3 units, with a standard error of $3.7/\sqrt{40} = 0.6$ unit, as measured by deducting the pain intensity at 4 weeks from the baseline pain intensity. The change in pain intensity for patients receiving the placebo is 0.2 units, with a standard error of $4.6/\sqrt{40} = 0.7$ unit. Patients who received an NSAID compared to those who received a placebo had a mean change in pain intensity of 1.1 units, with a 95% confidence interval of -0.7 to 2.9 units. Over 4 weeks, there is no statistically significant difference in pain intensity between patients receiving an NSAID and those receiving a placebo.

Let's say that the researchers used a stratified randomization scheme to balance the groups according to patient sex because they anticipated that there might be a difference in the effectiveness of the NSAID. One effective way to communicate the results could be to create a graphical display that compares the changes in pain intensity over 4 weeks in men and women receiving NSAIDs versus placebo. Two distinct ways to view the information are shown in Figures 10.9 and 10.10. Which works better?

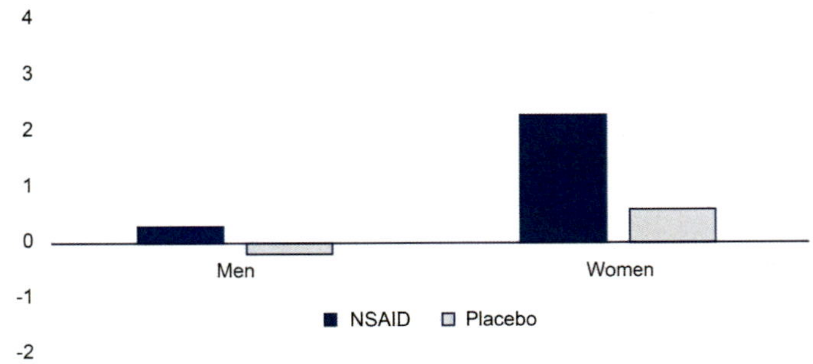

(a)

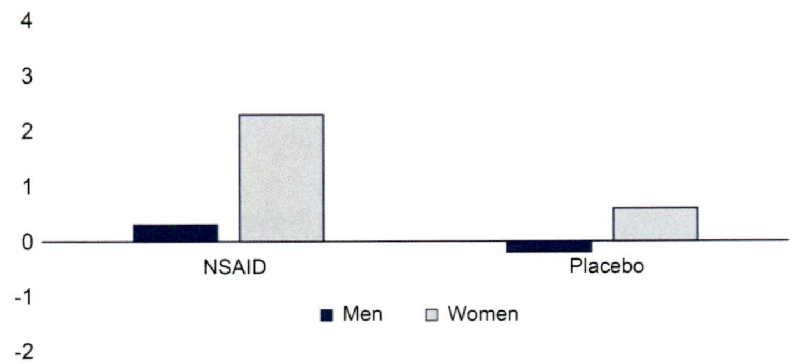

(b)

Figure 10.7. *Mean change in pain intensity over 4 weeks.*

Source: Lisa M. Sullivan. Essentials of Biostatistics in Public Health, Third Edition. Jones & Bartlett Learning.

Figure 10.7a demonstrates that while the change in pain intensity among men who received an NSAID versus placebo was not significantly different (leftmost set of bars), the change in pain intensity among women who received an NSAID versus placebo was significantly different (rightmost set of bars). To facilitate the comparison of men and women receiving different treatments, Figure 10.7b presents the exact same data in a different format. The NSAID-using patients' pain intensity changes more in women than in men, as the leftmost set of bars in Figure 10.1b illustrates. Figure 10.7b's rightmost set of bars illustrates how little the pain intensity changed for both men and women who received a placebo. While Figure 10.7b makes it simpler to compare the responses of the two sexes within treatments, Figure 10.7a makes it easier to compare the various treatments within the two sexes.

Comparing bars that are closer together is simpler for readers than bars that are farther apart. Because they determine the figure's format, we must take these comparisons into account when creating figures. As an illustration, Figure 10.8 shows the percentage response at 24 and 48 hours after treatment for each of the four comparison groups. Which comparison is the simplest to draw, considering the layout of the figure (i.e., does the display make it easier to compare responses between groups over time or at particular points in time within groups)?

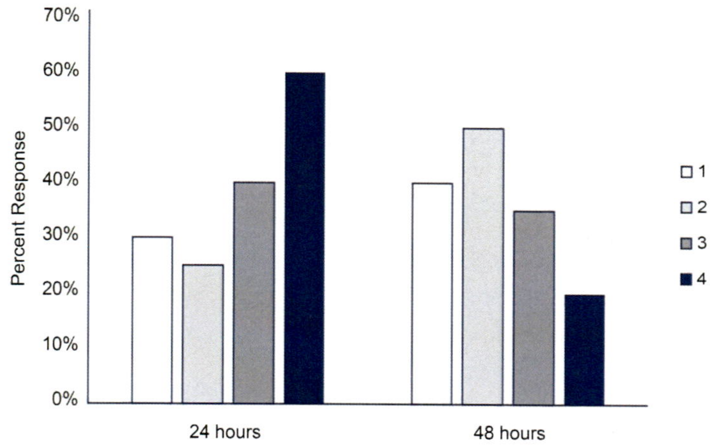

Figure 10.8. *Response to treatment by group and time.*

Source: Lisa M. Sullivan. Essentials of Biostatistics in Public Health, Third Edition. Jones & Bartlett Learning.

We must first choose what we want to communicate and to whom, regardless of the format we use to communicate data and statistical results. Then, keeping in mind the fundamentals of excellent design at all times, we can select the format that most effectively reaches the intended audience.

10.2.3. Resenting Data and Statistical Results in Tables

The needs of the readers or consumers must come first when creating tables, and we must think about how to best serve their needs while communicating data and statistical findings. A smart first step is to consider the narrative we want to present. The narrative starts with the question of interest, which is typically best answered in text form: Why did we conduct this study or investigation? What is known about the subject and where are the gaps in the body of knowledge? On occasion, though, there might be a significant background or context that needs to be summed up, and to do so, we can compile the most important results from earlier research. We can go into greater detail about the particular sample we examined, what we measured, how we measured it, and what we discovered once the question or purpose has been clearly stated and any pertinent background information has been provided. It is important to consider the message that each table in a presentation, paper, or report will convey as we arrange them. The presentation, paper, or report should flow logically from the broad overview to the finer points, and the tables should function as a single, coherent whole. Each table should, however, be able to stand alone and present a distinct argument. Tables are useful tools for accurately displaying data and enabling comparisons. Which statistics are presented and how the tables are arranged depend on the particular comparisons that are of interest.

When presenting data and statistical findings to our audience through tables, we need to consider the situation, time, location, and context. When setting up tables for a presentation, it is important to think about how the audience will interact with it, whether it will be interactive or if questions will be asked until the end, what the audience expects, whether it will be delivered online or in person, how the room will be set up if it is in person, and how close the audience will be to the screen. We want to avoid adding more obstacles to the already difficult task of communicating with an audience by being mindful of how we build our tables.

When preparing tables to summarize data and statistical results, we must always adhere to the style guides and requirements of the journals, websites, publishers, and clients we submit abstracts, papers, reports, and posters. Articles in a variety of formats, such as original research, commentary, essays, opinions, and systematic reviews, are published in journals. For tables (and figures) in a given type of paper, there are requirements that must be met in order for the paper to be accepted for publication. For instance, the majority of journals give authors access to thorough style guides and guidelines for getting their manuscripts ready for submission. This is a summary of some of the pertinent style manuals for the publications that we could work on. It should be noted that while some of these resources apply to multiple journals, others are endorsed by particular professional organizations and are unique to a single journal.

- The style guide for the American Journal of Public Health outlines the components of a manuscript along with specific requirements for each.
- The style guide endorsed by the American Statistical Association applies to its family of journals and includes manuscript components and specific style requirements and guidelines for each.
- A style guide that offers direction to writers wishing to publish in numerous medical journals is supported by the American Medical Association, though certain medical and biomedical journals have their particular guidelines. For instance, the International Committee of Medical Journal Editors' "Recommendations for the Conduct, Reporting, Editing and Publication of Scholarly Work in Medical Journals" are mandatory reading for writers submitting work to the New England Journal of Medicine and Circulation, the official journal of the American Heart Association.
- The American Psychological Association (APA) style is commonly used in the social sciences, and there are several online and for-purchase resources available from APA for potential authors.

These guidelines capture some general principles that are in line with the concepts discussed in the previous section on design principles, but they also lay out some very specific requirements.

10.2.3.1. Components of a Table

We first go over the elements of a table before getting into particular table types and their contents. Recall that it is generally not advised to split larger tables or combine smaller ones because doing so could muddle the message in the former scenario and lose it in the latter.

Clear and succinct titles are a sign of a good table. The title should make it obvious enough for the reader to know what the table is showing without having to read the text again. What is being shown and among whom should be explained in the title (i.e., important comparative groups) and when. It is typically displayed at the top of the table and should typically consist of no more than two lines. In a paper or report, tables ought to be numbered according to the sequence in which they are mentioned. Tables should be included in the paper or report close to where the data or statistical results are discussed, rather than at the end, which could make it difficult for the reader to refer to them while reading the text, unless the journal, website, or client recommends otherwise. Longer tables with more specific information may be moved to an online supplement or appendix, if available.

When organizing a paper or report, the logical flow of the tables should be taken into account. Secondary or ancillary data or results should never come before the primary findings. A description of the study participants or other background information is frequently included in the first table to set the scene for the main findings, which are presented shortly after.

The table's body is made up of data, which includes sample sizes, means, percentages, and the outcomes of statistical tests. The table's columns are frequently arranged to highlight the most significant data comparisons. When assembling a table's structure, also referred to as its table shell, we need to take the relevant comparisons into account. If at all possible, the data to be compared should be shown in adjacent columns. To illustrate the difference in performance on a standardized test before and after an educational intervention, for instance, the measurements obtained prior to and following the intervention ought to be arranged in adjacent columns to enable easy comparison.

A distinct heading for each column in the table is also necessary. The column headings ought to be brief enough to not need more than one line. Each column only needs one heading because multiple headings can be confusing. Above the column headings is a column spanner that describes the grouping variable (e.g., "Treatment"). In certain cases, a column spanner is required to make the meaning clear, but at other times the column headings are adequate to describe and differentiate the groups. See Example 10.3 for an example of how we tabulate the results of a regression analysis. The column spanner can also be used to describe the statistics that will be displayed in the columns.

A table's rows frequently display different variables. Units of measurement and variable names need to be stated precisely and with clarity. The measurement units are very significant. To enable readers and consumers to make meaningful comparisons, it is imperative that the precise units used be reported for certain clinical and laboratory measures, as they may be measured and reported using different scales regularly. Clinical and laboratory measures have specific guidelines that should be consulted when reporting data, just as journals have style guides for reporting data and statistical results in tables and figures. Certain publications, websites, or customers may favor metric measurements (e.g., grams, and meters) to U. S. units (e.g., feet, pounds), and when applicable, adhere to their conventions. The amount of rounding that is appropriate for the data is usually two decimal places.

They can make it more difficult to read the data in a table. Gridlines, which are frequently seen in spreadsheets, are superfluous in tables. The table's body should contain minimal, if any, lines. To enable relevant comparisons, the table's columns should have uniform spacing and be reasonably close to one another. A table's white space, both inside and outside, can be used to draw attention to particular features of the data and statistical findings. Clarity is the aim; this is achieved by designing a table that enables the reader or customer to quickly identify the most important takeaways from the data and statistical findings.

Figure 10.9 displays a table's components.

Table number. Table title

Description of what follows	**Column spanner**		
	Heading 1	Heading 2 . . .	Heading x
Rows (variables and units)	Data		

Note: Footnotes, references

Figure 10.9. *Components of a table.*

Source: Lisa M. Sullivan. Essentials of Biostatistics in Public Health, Third Edition. Jones & Bartlett Learning.

Example 10.3

Logistic regression analysis is used to evaluate the associations between body mass index (BMI) categories—normal (BMI ≤ 25.0), overweight (25.0 < BMI < 30.0), and obese (BMI ≥ 30.0)—and three outcomes— incident myocardial infarction, incident cardiovascular disease, and incident stroke, which are considered separately.

The relationships between the three BMI categories (normal weight, overweight, and obesity) are compiled in **Table 10.9**, which also includes odds ratios and their 95 percent confidence intervals.

Table 10.9. *Association Between BMI Categories and Incident Cardiovascular Disease After Adjustment for Clinical Risk Factors*

	Odds Ratio* (OR) (95% Confidence Interval)		
	Normal Weight	**Overweight**	**Obese**
Incident myocardial infarction	1.00 (Reference)	1.01 (0.69–1.29)	1.14 (1.01–1.50)
Incident cardiovascular disease	1.00 (Reference)	1.21 (0.89–1.37)	1.36 (1.13–2.54)
Incident stroke	1.00 (Reference)	0.99 (0.82–1.08)	1.18 (1.09–1.23)

Source: Lisa M. Sullivan. Essentials of Biostatistics in Public Health, Third Edition. Jones & Bartlett Learning.

If more information is required to understand the data or statistical findings shown in the table, it can be found in the footnotes, which can be found at the bottom of Tables 10.9. Such justifications ought to be excluded from the title and column headings since they could make the results more difficult to interpret. The footnotes provide definitions for all symbols and abbreviations. The footnotes explain the acronyms. The audience will determine whether or not to use abbreviations. The audience can encourage readability if they are aware of the acronyms. It takes more effort for the audience to find definitions if they are not familiar with the abbreviations.

Drafting table shells, or templates, prior to starting a statistical analysis is a good practice. What will be shown in tables and how are described in the table shells? The table shells aid in the author's mental organization as they craft a coherent and understandable account of the study's findings. An example of a table shell that can be used to summarize participant background characteristics in a study that compares an intervention group to a control group is **Table 10.10**. Observe that variable names and units are specified in the table shell (first column). The summary statistics that will be displayed are listed, and in certain instances, the precise number of decimal places that will be displayed is also mentioned (p-values are reported in the last column). **Table 10.10** displays the title at the top of the table, with the various intervention groups serving as the main comparison groups represented by the columns.

Table 10.10. *Example of a Table Shell*

	Treatment		
Characteristic	**Intervention Group (n = xx)**	**Control Group (n = xx)**	***p*-value***
Age, years	$\overline{X}(s)$	$\overline{X}(s)$	x.xx
Years lived in United States, years	$\overline{X}(s)$	$\overline{X}(s)$	x.xx
English proficiency			x.xx
No practical proficiency	n (%)	n (%)	
Elementary proficiency	n (%)	n (%)	
Limited proficiency	n (%)	n (%)	
Full proficiency	n (%)	n (%)	
Native or bilingual proficiency	n (%)	n (%)	

Source: Lisa M. Sullivan. Essentials of Biostatistics in Public Health, Third Edition. Jones & Bartlett Learning.

It is recommended that tables stick to a single font style and use enhancements like boldface, italics, and other styles sparingly, if at all. Table designers occasionally worry about whether the reader or customer will locate the important information or draw important conclusions, but if the table is organized properly, these should be obvious. There are some exceptions. For instance, using boldface to highlight particular data points may be beneficial when there is a lot of information to process. The same data are displayed in Tables 10.13 and 10.14, both with and without improvements. Are the improvements useful? Keep in mind that some might be, but others might just add extra clutter.

The comparison groups in a paper or report that have multiple tables with the same groups must be arranged consistently among the tables. It is never appropriate to rearrange the groups or change the direction of the tables (i.e., flip between rows and columns).

Table 10.11. *Impact of High Intake of Grains and Incident Cardiovascular Disease and Cancer*

Grain	Odds Ratio (95% Confidence Interval)
Incident Cardiovascular Disease	
Whole-grain bread	0.85 (0.72, 0.97)
Whole-grain cereal	0.71 (0.63, 0.84)
Refined grain	1.05 (0.87, 1.36)
White bread	1.10 (0.95, 1.30)
Rice (white and brown)	0.99 (0.92, 1.04)
Total grains	1.03 (0.91, 1.24)
Incident Cancer	
Whole-grain bread	0.91 (0.77, 0.99)
Whole-grain cereal	0.91 (0.86, 0.97)
Refined grain	0.97 (0.84, 1.06)
White bread	1.01 (0.95, 1.13)
Rice (white and brown)	0.94 (0.87, 1.02)
Total grains	0.95 (0.86, 1.11)

Source: Lisa M. Sullivan. Essentials of Biostatistics in Public Health, Third Edition. Jones & Bartlett Learning.

10.2.3.2. Tabulating Summary Statistics

The first table describing the participants is a common feature of professional reports and scientific papers that describe clinical research. To help readers assess the generalizability of the findings and any potential limitations to the conclusions that might be made, it is best practice to include a summary of the study participants. We carefully define each variable, characteristic, and the units in which each was measured before arranging them in a table to summarize the characteristics of the study sample.

Proportions are typically more difficult to understand than percentages when reporting dichotomous, categorical, and ordinal variables. Nevertheless, to enable readers and customers to arrange the data differently should they choose to investigate further, we should consistently provide the numbers of participants in each response category along with the percentages. Unless there are anomalies or missing data, the total sample percentages should add up to 100%. To make sure that the table is self-explanatory, the latter possibility should be covered in both the text and a footnote.

Example 10.4

Let's say we look into how three behavioral interventions—self-help, group therapy, and individual therapy—affect n = 270 senior citizens who live in assisted living facilities in terms of reducing their cigarette smoking. Before summarizing the primary conclusions, which are predicated on particular metrics of cigarette smoking (e.g., cigarettes smoked daily), we start by listing the participants' demographic details who were allocated to the three behavioral intervention groups. Table 10.12 may be how the final table appears.

Please take note that, in order to make it easier to compare variables between intervention groups, we have included column percentages (percentages that add up to 100 percent within columns) for each characteristic in Table 10.12. The outputs of statistical computing packages frequently include frequencies, row percentages, and column percentages when summarizing dichotomous, categorical, and ordinal variables. Selecting the most appropriate data is a necessary step in creating tables for presentation. Take a look at the example below, where data is displayed as frequencies initially, followed by row and column percentages. Which data presentation is the most helpful?

Table 10.12. *Background Characteristics of Study Participants by Intervention Group*

Characteristic*	Intervention Group		
	Self-Help (n = 100)	Group Therapy (n = 90)	Individual Therapy (n = 80)
Age, years	78.2 (6.2)	79.6 (5.9)	81.4 (5.7)
Male sex, n (%)	46 (46%)	38 (42%)	28 (35%)
Education, years	9.3 (4.2)	10.7 (3.9)	8.6 (4.1)
Marital status			
Single, never married, n (%)	9 (9%)	11 (12%)	5 (6%)
Married or domestic partnership, n (%)	36 (36%)	36 (40%)	23 (29%)
Widowed, n (%)	43 (43%)	33 (37%)	43 (54%)
Divorced or separated, n (%)	12 (12%)	10 (11%)	9 (11%)

Source: Lisa M. Sullivan. Essentials of Biostatistics in Public Health, Third Edition. Jones & Bartlett Learning.

Example 10.5

We want to compare the prevalence of obesity and overweight in men and women who took part in the 1980s Framingham Heart Study offspring examination. The percentage of men and women who are overweight (25.0 < BMI < 30.0), obese (BMI ≥ 30.0), and normal weight (BMI ≤ 25.0) is displayed in Table 10.13.

Table 10.13. *Numbers of Men and Women by BMI Category*

Normal weight	631	1289	1920
Overweight	925	452	1377
Obese	312	253	565

* BMI is body mass index = $\text{weight}_{kg}/\text{height}_m^2$; normal weight (BMI ≤ 25.0), overweight (25.0 < BMI < 30.0), and obese (BMI ≥ 30.0).

Source: Lisa M. Sullivan. Essentials of Biostatistics in Public Health, Third Edition. Jones & Bartlett Learning.

565 participants meet the criteria for obesity: 312 men and 253 women. What is the extent of obesity in the study sample? Is the extent of obesity different in men versus women? It is challenging to summarize results to make the appropriate comparison when all that is known about each BMI category is the frequencies or numbers of participants. The same data are displayed in Table 10.14 along with row percentages.

Table 10.14. *Distribution of Men and Women in Normal, Overweight, and Obese Categories of BMI*

BMI* Category	Men (*n* = 1868, 48%)	Women (*n* = 1994, 52%)	Total (*n* = 3862)
Normal weight	631 (33%)	1289 (67%)	1920
Overweight	925 (67%)	452 (33%)	1377
Obese	312 (55%)	253 (45%)	565

* BMI is body mass index = $weight_{kg}/height_m^2$; normal weight (BMI ≤ 25.0), overweight (25.0 < BMI < 30.0), and obese (BMI ≥ 30.0).

Source: Lisa M. Sullivan. Essentials of Biostatistics in Public Health, Third Edition. Jones & Bartlett Learning.

The row percentages, or the percentages that add up to 100 percent in each row of the table, are not useful in addressing the pertinent questions. What is the level of obesity in the study sample? Is the level of obesity different in men versus women? On the other hand, Table 10.14 provides useful information in response to a different query: What proportion of participants are female? The data in the top row of the table indicates that 52% of participants (1994) are female. 253 (45 percent) of the 565 participants who meet the criteria for obesity are women. What is the percentage of women among the obese participants? The same data are displayed in Table 10.15 along with column percentages, or percentages that add up to 100% for each column.

Table 10.15. *Distribution of BMI Categories in Men and Women*

BMI* Category	Men (*n* = 1868)	Women (*n* = 1994)	Total (*n* = 3862)
Normal weight	631 (34%)	1289 (65%)	1920 (50%)
Overweight	925 (49%)	452 (23%)	1377 (36%)
Obese	312 (17%)	253 (13%)	565 (14%)

* BMI is body mass index = $weight_{kg}/height_m^2$; normal weight (BMI ≤ 25.0), overweight (25.0 < BMI < 30.0), and obese (BMI ≥ 30.0).

Source: Lisa M. Sullivan. Essentials of Biostatistics in Public Health, Third Edition. Jones & Bartlett Learning.

The information provided in Table 10.15 enables us to respond to the queries. What percentage of the study sample is obese? 565 participants, or 14%, meet the criteria for obesity. Does the percentage of men and women who meet the criteria for obesity differ from one another? About 17% of men and 13% of women are considered obese.

The standard deviation or interquartile range is typically reported to summarize variability and the mean or median is typically used to summarize central tendency when summarizing continuous variables. Whether or not there are outliers in the sample will determine which particular statistics are used. Organizing the continuous variable into categories is an additional option for characterizing the study sample in a table of a paper or report. We present BMI as a continuous variable in three ordinal categories (normal, overweight, and obese) in Tables 10.16 through 10.18. When categorizing a continuous measure for presentation, three to ten categories are typically thought to be suitable. Less than three categories may lead to excessive aggregation, which obscures the data's details. When additional collapsing is required, results with more than ten categories may be challenging to understand. It is best to use any natural or recognized cut-points, like the BMI and SBP cut-points, that define clinically meaningful categories of variables. Unless the clinically relevant categories yield more interpretable results, we can still use the continuous variable in statistical analysis to capture the full extent of variability in the measure even if we choose to summarize it using ordinal categories in a table.

It is recommended to include measures of variability, such as standard errors or confidence limits, when presenting summary statistics in tables, such as means, proportions, odds ratios, relative risks, differences in means, and regression coefficients. In certain contexts, different measures of variability make sense. For instance, means and standard errors may be appropriate if we are presenting the means of an outcome measured in each of the four comparison groups (e.g., in an analysis where analysis of variance [ANOVA] is used to test for a statistically significant difference in means). The estimated odds ratios along with the 95 percent confidence intervals may be appropriate if we are presenting odds ratios that quantify the associations between a set of dichotomous risk factors and a dichotomous outcome.

10.2.3.3. Tabulating Statistical Significance

P-values, or statistical significance levels, should be reported in tables under the guidelines provided by the particular journal or report. For instance, certain journals limit p-values to two or three decimal places and demand precise significance levels in tables and the text (e.g., $p = 0.03$ or $p = 0.032$). The majority of journals advise against using symbols like "NS" to denote non-significance when a p-value is higher than a typical cut-off (e.g., $p > 0.05$). They would rather that authors report the observed p-value, $p = 0.27$, instead. Last but not least, reporting "$p < 0.001$" rather than the precise value is typically sufficient if a p-value is less than 0.001. P-values are almost always taken to be two-sided. Should a test be administered in a biased manner, this decision needs to be made explicit and supported.

We must exercise caution to avoid using too much scientific jargon when communicating statistical significance to a non-technical audience. To help readers or consumers understand how to interpret the results being presented, we need to define statistical significance.

Interestingly, when discussing the background or baseline features of subjects in a parallel-group randomized controlled trial (e.g., comparing an experimental treatment to an active control or a placebo), we could create a table like **Table 10.16**, where the columns stand for the two treatments (experimental versus placebo) that are being contrasted. Conducting statistical tests comparing background or baseline characteristics of participants in a randomized controlled trial is not necessary, despite some variability in practice. Although statistical tests are not required for this purpose, it is always important to carefully review background or baseline characteristics to make sure that groups are balanced. Examine the information that **Table 10.16** summarizes. Seem to be the treatment groups in balance?

Table 10.16. *Characteristics of Participants at Baseline*

	Treatment	
Characteristic*	**Experimental (n = 636)**	**Placebo (n = 640)**
Age, years	45.7 (6.4)	45.9 (6.2)
Male sex, n (%)	292 (46%)	289 (45%)
Systolic blood pressure, mm Hg	128.2 (14.7)	127.9 (14.4)
Diastolic blood pressure, mm Hg	78.3 (9.1)	76.9 (8.6)
Total cholesterol, mg/dL	201.5 (42.7)	209.3 (44.5)
Body mass index, kg/m^2	26.4 (3.9)	25.9 (4.1)

* Values are means (standard deviations) for continuous characteristics and n (%) for categorical measures.

Source: Lisa M. Sullivan. Essentials of Biostatistics in Public Health, Third Edition. Jones & Bartlett Learning.

10.2.3.4. Tabulating Regression Results

In tabulating the outcomes of the linear regression analysis, the regression coefficients and a measure of the estimated regression coefficients' variability (e.g., the estimated regression coefficients' standard errors or 95 percent confidence intervals). The regression coefficients are typically exponentiated to generate odds ratios and hazards ratios, respectively, when tabulating the results of a logistic or Cox proportional hazards regression analysis. Along with the estimated odds and hazard ratios, the 95 percent confidence intervals are typically provided to help assess statistical significance and provide an indication of the accuracy—or lack thereof—of the effect estimates.

Example 10.6

To compare birth weights and preterm birth rates among mothers from diverse racial/ethnic backgrounds, a cohort study is conducted. n = 453 moms who identify as white, black, or Hispanic take part in the study in total. In the beginning of the study, mothers provide their ages in years. They are then followed to delivery when the baby's birth weight and gestational age are measured. Births that occur before 37 weeks of pregnancy are classified as preterm births. An analysis of multiple linear regressions linking birth weight to gestational age, mother age, and race/ethnicity is presented in Table 10.17. The hold-out or reference group is the white race, and other racial/ethnic groups are modelled as dummy variables. A multiple logistic regression analysis linking maternal age and racial/ethnic background to preterm birth is summarized in Table 10.18. It is not required to include the regression coefficients in Table 10.18 in addition to the odds ratios. In general, odds ratios provide a more comprehensible summary of the relationships.

The units of the independent variable must be included when reporting regression coefficients because the regression coefficient's interpretation is dependent on these units. The change in the outcome (Y) concerning a one-unit change in the predictor (X) is represented by the regression coefficient (b_i). A one-unit change for some predictors is not clinically meaningful, so we may want to report the outcome change concerning a larger, more significant change.

Table 10.17. *Association Between Racial/Ethnic Background, Maternal Age, Gestational Age, and Birth Weight*

Characteristic	Regression Coefficient*	Standard Error	*p*-Value
Intercept	−4366.5	188.3	<0.01
Racial/ethnic group			
White	Reference	—	
Black	−46.0	47.0	0.33
Hispanic	46.7	47.6	0.32
Maternal age, years	−0.27*	2.8	0.92
Gestational age, weeks	193.6*	4.7	<0.01

* Regression coefficients are based on multiple linear regression analysis and are relative to a one-year change in maternal age and a one-week change in gestational age.

Source: Lisa M. Sullivan. Essentials of Biostatistics in Public Health, Third Edition. Jones & Bartlett Learning.

Table 10.18. *Association Between Racial/Ethnic Background, Maternal Age, and Preterm Birth*

Characteristic	Regression Coefficient*	Odds Ratio (OR)	95% Confidence Interval for OR
Intercept	0.37	—	—
Racial/ethnic group			
White	Reference	—	—
Black	−0.16	0.85	(0.50, 1.47)
Hispanic	0.13	1.14	(0.65, 2.01)
Maternal age, years	0.03*	1.03	(1.00, 1.06)

* Regression coefficients are based on multiple logistic regression analysis and are relative to a one-year change in maternal age.

Source: Lisa M. Sullivan. Essentials of Biostatistics in Public Health, Third Edition. Jones & Bartlett Learning.

Think about Example 10.6 once more. When the mother's racial/ethnic background and the neonate's gestational age are taken into account, the regression coefficient linked to maternal age in Table 10.17 calculates the expected change in birth weight with a 1-year change in mother age. Similarly, after controlling for the mother's age and racial/ethnic background, the regression coefficient linked to gestational age measures the predicted change in birth weight associated with a 1-week change in gestational age. A birth weight difference of about 0.27 grams is linked to a 1-year difference in the mother's age. Estimating the expected difference in birth weight associated with a 5-year difference in maternal age, for instance, might be more instructive. This difference is $-0.27 * 5 = -1.35$ grams.

Observe that when we alter the effect about a 1-year change versus a 5-year change, the standard error of the estimate remains unchanged. By making the necessary adjustments to the odds ratio and 95 percent confidence interval, we could demonstrate a comparable impact of maternal age (5 years) on preterm birth. To generate odds ratios, we exponentiate regression coefficients obtained from a logistic regression analysis [e.g., $\exp(0.03) = 1.03$]. After adjusting for racial/ethnic background, an older mother (by 1 year) has a 1.03 times higher chance of having a preterm birth than a younger mother. To compute the odds ratio relative to a 5-year difference in maternal age, we use $\exp(c \times b_1)$, where c = the number of units (here, $c = 5$). When controlling for the mother's race/ethnic background, the odds of preterm birth are $\exp(5 \times 0.03) = 1.16$ times higher for the older mother compared to a 5-year difference in maternal age.

The confidence interval for an odds ratio relative to a 1-year difference in a predictor is computed as follows. First, we estimate the logistic regression equation and obtain the regression coefficient (e.g., b_1) and its standard error [e.g., $SE(b_1)$]. Assuming we have a sufficient sample size, the lower 95% confidence limit is computed as $\exp[b_1 - 1.96 \times SE(b_1)]$ and the upper 95% confidence limit is computed as $\exp[b_1 + 1.96 \times SE(b_1)]$. These formulas produce confidence intervals for the odds ratio relative to a one-unit change in the predictor. If we wish to estimate the confidence interval relative to a c-unit change in the predictor, we use the following expression: $\exp[c \times b_1 \pm 1.96 \times c \times SE(b_1)]$. In our example, the confidence interval relative to a 5-year difference in maternal age is $\exp(5 \times 0.03 \pm 1.96 \times 5 \times 0.017)$, where 0.017 is the standard error of the estimated regression coefficient. This is equivalent to $\exp(0.15 \pm 0.17)$, or $\exp(-0.02, 0.32) = (0.98, 1.38)$. Thus, an older mother (by 5 years) has 1.16 times the odds of preterm birth as compared to a younger mother, adjusted for racial/ethnic background, with a 95% confidence interval for the odds ratio of (0.98, 1.38).

Greek letters (β, for example) should not be used as column headers in the tables because they usually relate to unknown population parameters rather than sample estimates. When tabulating regression results, it is usually clearer to use text such as "odds ratio" or "regression coefficient" in the column headings.

It's crucial to include all of the data when presenting regression analysis results. To give the reader the full set of results, it is crucial to include the estimate of the y-intercept. However, there are some situations in which it could make sense to display only a portion of the results in the main table (i.e., a table incorporated into the text) and comprehensive findings in an online supplement or appendix. For instance, the regression coefficient linked to the outcome is primary if the relationship of interest is primarily the correlation between a specific risk factor and the outcome. To maintain the focus of the main point, the regression coefficients and y-intercept for the other variables in the model (e.g., confounders) can be displayed in comprehensive detail in an online supplement or appendix.

Example 10.7

Assume for the moment that we wish to assess the relationship between moderate to heavy drinking—that is, more than one drink for women and more than two for men—and hypertension. A systolic blood pressure of 140 mm Hg or higher, or a diastolic blood pressure of 90 mm Hg or higher, is considered hypertension. An observational study with $n = 2500$ participants yields data. Initially, the researchers employed a basic logistic regression model that connected the status of hypertension with the indicator of moderate to heavy drinking. After that, they estimate a number of models taking into account extra confounding factors. All of the data for each model is compiled in **Table 10.19**, which is more than could be required in a paper or report's body.

The relationship between moderate to heavy drinking and hypertension is the main area of interest. However, the primary comparison is obscured because the table summarizes a great deal of other associations.

Generally speaking, we want to keep the amount of unnecessary information or features in tables to a minimum so that the reader can concentrate on the important stuff. Hence, numerous horizontal or vertical lines should not be present in tables as they are usually regarded as unnecessary to the primary focus of the table, which is the data or statistics being displayed. When presenting data and statistical findings visually, precision and clarity of presentation are the main objectives Benítez et al., 2011; Cabral et al., 2008).

Table 10.19. *Association Between Moderate to Heavy Drinking and Hypertension*

	Odds Ratio* (95% Confidence Intervals for Odds Ratios)		
Characteristic	**Unadjusted Model**	**Age- and Sex-Adjusted Model**	**Fully Adjusted Model***
Intercept			
Moderate to heavy drinking	1.18 (0.90, 1.53)	1.44 (1.10, 1.90)	1.43 (1.08, 1.89)
Age, years		1.05 (1.04,1.07)	1.06 (1.04, 1.07)
Male sex		0.92 (0.75, 1.20)	0.92 (0.74, 1.43)
Current smoker			0.93 (0.60, 1.43)
Body mass index, kg/m^2			1.02 (0.99, 1.04)
Moderate to heavy physical activity, hours per week			0.99 (0.94, 1.03)
Lives alone			0.96 (0.63, 1.14)
Diabetes			0.85 (0.63, 1.14)

* Odds ratios are based on multiple logistic regression analysis and are relative to a one-unit change in each predictor, adjusted for other variables in the model.

Source: Lisa M. Sullivan. Essentials of Biostatistics in Public Health, Third Edition. Jones & Bartlett Learning.

A Closer Look

Cure Rate Models

Cure rate models are statistical tools used to analyze survival data that includes individuals who have long-term survival. They are part of survival analysis and involve censored subjects, so a sufficient knowledge of survival analysis is required to analyze them.

For cure rate models, a positive probability of a cure is assumed. So the cumulative survival curve for a cure rate model converges to $p > 0$ as time goes to infinity, where p is called the cure probability, cure fraction, or cure rate. Often the goal in these models is to estimate p.

For nonparametric methods such as the Kaplan – Meier approach, p is difficult to detect. It would be the asymptotic limit as t gets larger, but the Kaplan – Meier curve gives us no information about the behavior of the survival curve beyond the last event time or censoring time (whichever is last). So estimating the cure rate requires a parametric mixture model.

The mixture model for cure rates was first introduced by Berkson and Gage (1952). The general model is given by the following equation:

$$S(t) = p + (1 - p)S_1(t)$$

where p is the cure probability, and $S_1(t)$ is the survival curve for those who are not cured. $S_1(t)$ is the conditional survival curve given the patient is not cured. The conditional survival curve can be estimated by parametric or nonparametric methods. For an extensive treatment of cure rate models using the frequentist approach, see Maller and Zhou (1996). The Bayesian approach to cure rate models can be found in Ibrahim et al. (2001).

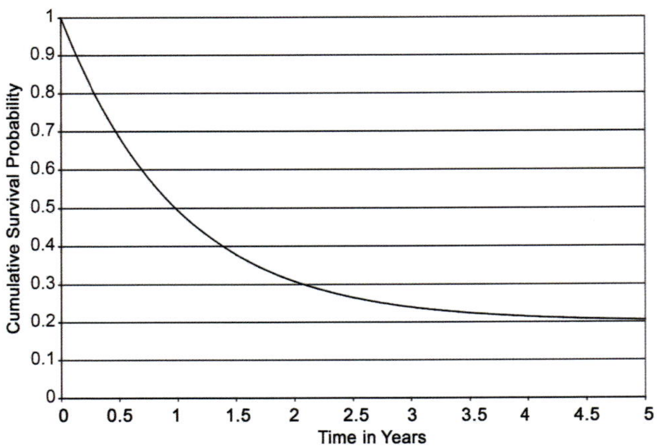

Figure 10.10. *Exponential cure rate model with cure rate p = 0.20 and exponential rate parameter λ = 1.*

Source: *Michael R. Chernick. The Essentials of Biostatistics for Physicians, Nurses, and Clinicians. John Wiley & Sons, Inc.*

We illustrate a parametric mixture survival curve with an exponential survival curve with rate parameter $\lambda = 1$, for the conditional survival curve $S_1(t)$ and with survival probability $p = 0.2$. This curve is shown in **Figure 10.10**.

Although cure rate modelling began with Berkson and Gage in the 1950s, much of the literature came about in the 1990s when computing became much faster and the EM algorithm for the frequency approach and MCMC methods for Bayesian approaches became easy to implement. Until recently, the free software WinBUGS was the main option for doing MCMC methods for the Bayesian modelling approach. However, very recently in SAS Version 9.2, MCMC methods have been added as a procedure in SAS/STAT. Users of SAS software may find this more convenient.

Summary

- Survival analysis is widely used in evidence-based medicine to examine the time-to-event series. Often used for survival/death events, time-to-event series can illustrate time to any dichotomous event.
- Data visualization is the representation of complex medical stats in a digestible graphical format. It allows users to easily obtain qualitative insights, changes, patterns, and trends while drawing valuable conclusions...even without developed math skills.
- Censoring is an important topic in survival analysis. Censored subjects never experienced the outcome of interest during the study's specified timeframe. Whether or not an individual is censored should not be associated with whether or not the event occurred. Left censoring occurs when an individual experienced the event before origin; right censoring occurs when an individual did not experience the event during the specified timeframe (occurred after, or unsure if and when the incident occurred).
- Life tables (also known as actuarial life tables) differ from other methods of survival analysis in that the observation outputs are categorized into distinct time events. Life tables present outputs that show whether the case occurred, whether the individual was censored, and the time of that event. When examining a life table, one can determine the proportion of patients experiencing an event (e.g., dying) during which interval the outcome occurred.
- One of the most frequently used methods of survival analysis is the Kaplan-Meier (KM) approach. The KM method estimates the likelihood of survival. This approach often utilizes a KM survival curve to represent the survival function.
- The log-rank test is a non-parametric test that compares two or more groups' survival distributions. This test, which assumes censoring is unrelated to prognosis, examines the null hypothesis (that there are no differences in distribution between the groups).
- The Cox proportional hazards model is a semiparametric regression model that allows researchers to examine the effects of multiple variables on survival curves. Semiparametric means that the method does not require a specific distribution of the survival function; however, it does assume a relationship between the covariates and outcome. The output of the Cox model is presented in hazard ratios (HR).
- Strong evidence is needed to guide changes that will improve population health. We must design studies efficiently, collect and organize data carefully, and report findings clearly and accurately.

References

1. Benítez-Parejo, N., Rodríguez del Águila, M. M., & Pérez-Vicente, S. (2011). Survival analysis and Cox regression. *Allergologia et Immunopathologia, 39*(6), 362–373.
2. Cabral, J. (2008). Statistical primer for cardiovascular research: Multiple comparisons procedures. *Circulation, 117*, 698–701.
3. Crawley, M. J. (2005). *Statistics: An Introduction Using R.* New York: John Wiley & Sons.

4. Des Jarlais, D. C., Lyles, C., Crepaz, N., & TREND Group. (2004). Improving the reporting quality of nonrandomized evaluations of behavioral and public health interventions: The TREND statement. *American Journal of Public Health, 94*, 361–366.
5. Flynn, R. (2012). Survival analysis. *Journal of Clinical Nursing, 21*(19-20), 2789–2797.
6. Gelman, A., & Unwin, A. (2014). Infovis and statistical graphics: Different goals, different looks. Retrieved from http://www.stat.columbia.edu/~gelman/research/published/vis14.pdf
7. George, B., Seals, S., & Aban, I. (2014). Survival analysis and regression models. *Journal of Nuclear Cardiology, 21*(4), 686–694.
8. Hoven, N. (2016). Steven Few on data visualization: 8 core principles. Tableau. Retrieved from http://www.tableau.com/blog/stephen-few-data-visualization
9. Isson, J. P., & Harriott, J. (2012). *Win with Advanced Business Analytics: Creating Business Value from Your Data*. Hoboken, NJ: John Wiley & Sons.
10. Kalbfleisch, J. D., & Prentice, R. L. (2002). *The Statistical Analysis of Failure Time Data* (2nd ed.). New York: Wiley.
11. Kleinbaum, D. G., & Klein, M. (2005). *Survival Analysis: A Self-Learning Text*. New York: Springer Science + Business Media.
12. Koletsi, D., & Pandis, N. (2017). Survival analysis, part 2: Kaplan-Meier method and the log-rank test. *American Journal of Orthodontics and Dentofacial Orthopedics, 152*(4), 569–571.
13. Lee, E. T., & Wang, J. W. (2003). *Statistical Methods for Survival Data Analysis* (3rd ed.). New York: John Wiley & Sons.
14. Rodrigues, V. (2015). Tips on effective use of tables and figures in research papers. Editage Insights. Retrieved from http://www.editage.com/insights/tips-on-effective-use-of-tables-and-figures-in-research-papers
15. Schober, P., & Vetter, T. R. (2018). Survival analysis and interpretation of time-to-event data: The tortoise and the hare. *Anesthesia & Analgesia, 127*(3), 792–798.
16. Schultz, K. F., Altman, D. G., & Moher, D. (2010). CONSORT 2010 statement: Updated guidelines for reporting parallel group randomized trials. *British Medical Journal, 340*(7748), 698–702.
17. Thuijs, D. J. F. M., Hickey, G. L., & Osnabrugge, R. L. J. (2018). Statistical primer: Basics of survival analysis for the cardiothoracic surgeon. *Interactive Cardiovascular and Thoracic Surgery, 27*(1), 1–4.
18. Tufte, E. R. (2001). *The Visual Display of Quantitative Information* (2nd ed.). Cheshire, CT: Graphics Press.
19. Tufte, E. R. (2016). The work of Edward Tufte and Graphics Press. Retrieved from http://www.edwardtufte.com/tufte/
20. Watanabe, H. (2012). Applications of statistics to medical science, IV survival analysis. *Journal of Nippon Medical School, 79*(3), 176–181.

INDEX

A

Acquired immune deficiency syndrome (AIDS) 8
Adequate numbers 10
Advanced modeling techniques 137
Alcohol consumption 132
Alternative hypotheses 169, 191, 206, 207, 249
Alzheimer's disease 39, 41
American Statistical Association (ASA) 175
Analytic epidemiology 44

B

Bar chart 65
Bayesian regression model 133
Bayes Theorem 120
Benford's Law 115
Binomial distribution 110, 111, 112, 114, 115, 180, 260, 261, 262
Binomial random variable 112, 114, 124
Biochemistry 66
Biomedical research 23, 175
Biomedical science 23
Biostatistics 1, 3, 4, 9, 10, 23, 24, 25, 27, 28, 29, 30, 31, 33, 50, 52, 53, 54, 57, 60, 161, 162, 228, 229, 230, 232, 233, 234, 248, 249, 252, 254, 256, 258, 259, 261, 262, 263, 264, 265, 266, 267, 268, 269, 270, 271, 272, 273, 275, 281, 282, 284, 285, 286, 287, 288, 289, 290, 291, 300, 301, 304, 305, 306, 307, 308, 310, 311, 313, 314
Blood group 76
Blood pressure 2, 13, 18, 39, 40, 88, 89, 90, 91, 92, 93, 149, 167, 168, 190, 195, 197, 198, 210, 215, 266, 267, 268, 297, 298, 312
Blood samples 18
Body mass index 13, 91, 92, 304
Bootstrap sampling 87, 96
Breast cancer 40
Bronchial cancer 39

C

Cancer 39, 40, 48, 57, 215, 306
cardiovascular disease 2, 4, 5, 6, 8, 10, 11, 13, 18, 50, 51, 56, 57, 209, 282, 283, 304
Case-control studies 12
Case studies 66, 153
Cauchy distribution 110
Center for Disease Control 24
Child mortality 133, 137
Chi-square tests 164
Cholesterol 2, 6, 7, 11, 13, 16, 18, 88, 90, 92, 93, 98, 149, 200, 201, 209, 297, 298
Chronic disease 39
Chronic kidney diseases (CKD) 39
Chronic Obstructive Pulmonary Disease 39
Civil registration 129
Clinical exams 66
Clinical medicine 120, 122
Clinical trial 7, 16

Cluster sampling 86, 97
Cohort study 8, 9, 10, 13, 18, 33, 50, 53, 57, 149, 282, 284, 310
Colon cancer 40
Communicable or Infectious Disease 41
Comparative Risk Assessment 130
Complex curve 133
Confidence intervals 127, 128, 140, 176, 191, 192, 196
Control group 16, 19, 21, 27, 56, 145, 190, 200, 210, 305
Coverage errors 135, 186
COVID-19 pandemic 28, 29
Criminal justice systems 132
Crossover trial 16, 17, 18, 33, 139, 202, 203
Crude analysis 21
Cumulative distribution 34, 113
Cumulative frequencies 75
Cumulative incidence (CI) 51, 58

D

Data analysis 23, 24, 28, 47, 97, 102, 146, 156, 168, 176, 177, 180, 210
Data collection 8, 13, 20, 24, 25, 27, 28, 30, 31, 48, 66, 69, 86, 170, 177, 183, 185, 186, 187, 293
Data distribution 76, 77, 96
Data management 20, 24
Decision-making sequence 116
Degrees of freedom (DF) 181
Diarrheal diseases 39
Dichotomous variables 87, 88, 89, 298
Disability-Adjusted Life Years (DALYs) 36
Discrete distributions 110, 113, 124
Disease burden 36
Disjoint events 102

E

Efficient communication 29
Empirical data 130, 137, 173
Environmental factors 26, 45
Environmental variables 38
Epidemiologic triangle 37
Epidemiology 5, 27, 30, 31, 41, 42, 44, 61, 163, 191, 240
Experimental treatment 7, 14, 15, 16, 17, 19, 21, 22, 247, 309

F

Focus group discussions (FGD) 66
Food and Drug Administration (FDA) 7, 21, 32
Foodborne diseases (FBD) 48
Frequency distribution 65, 72, 73, 74, 75, 76, 79, 81, 88, 90
Frequency polygon 82
Frequency polygons 34, 78
Frequentist statistical modeling 132

G

Gastric cancer 40
Genomic data 27
Global health issues 132
Government publications 68
Guidelines for Accurate and Transparent Health Estimates Reporting (GATHER) 135

H

Harm patients 119
Healthcare industry 163
Healthcare professionals 26, 175, 177
Health management information systems 129
Health policy 36
Health statistics 136
Heart failure 18, 162
High response rates 68
Hippocrates 43
Histogram 65, 82
Homogeneous 12
Human immunodeficiency virus 40
Human populations 5, 27, 33
Hypertension 40, 57, 59, 90, 313
Hypertensive Heart Disease 40, 41

I

Immunological status 38
Incidence density (ID) 52, 61
Incidence rate 36

Infection transmission 46
Infectious diseases 24, 30, 31, 32, 37, 40, 130
Infectious microorganism 38, 61
Influence illness 45
Institute for Health Metrics and Evaluation (IHME) 49
Intent to Treat (ITT) 21
Internal Revenue Service (IRS) 83
International agencies 129
International Classification of Disease 48
International databases 48
International rankings 136
International scale 30
International statistics 136
Interquartile ranges 153

J

Joint probability 105

L

Least squares method 224, 228
LINCS (Learning Information Network Communication System) 28
Liver Cirrhosis 41
Lower true limit (LTL) 75
L-tryptophan 38

M

Mathematical models 3, 31, 130
Mathematical relations 31
Maximum tolerated dose (MTD) 22
Mean difference (MD) 148, 149
Measurement errors 135
Medical records 10, 23, 33, 204
Medication history 18
Meta-analysis 26, 131, 139, 140, 141, 144, 146, 147, 148, 149, 150, 153, 156, 157, 161
Microscopes 66
Model covariates 135
Monte Carlo 87, 274
Morbidity 27, 36, 47, 49, 158
Mortality rate 165
Motivation 67, 69
Multicenter trials 15
Multilevel modeling 132, 133
Mutually exclusive events 102, 105
Mycobacterium tuberculosis 39
Myocardial infarctions (MIs) 155

N

National Center for Emerging and Zoonotic Infectious Diseases (NCEZID) 24
National death registrations 129
Neonatal conditions 39
Neurological diseases 41
New Drug Application (NDA) 23, 32
Nominal group techniques 66
Non-communicable 27, 41
Non-communicable diseases (NCDs) 40
Non-hierarchical regression models 133
Non-parametric tests 164
Non-profit organizations 26
Non-response error 188
Normal pregnancy 204
Null hypothesis 165, 184
Numerical data 75

O

Observational studies 7, 14, 23, 164
Odds ratio 56, 57, 58, 137, 138, 141, 142, 144, 145, 146, 147, 154, 155, 159, 160, 236, 311, 312

P

Parameter uncertainty 135
Patient symptoms 122
Peripheral artery disease 18
Per Protocol analysis 21
Personal hygiene 38
Pharmaceutical trials 14
Point prevalence (PP) 50, 58
Population-attributable risk (PAR) 55
Population distribution 87, 171
Population mean 84, 86, 169, 187, 190, 196, 208, 227, 228, 241
Population surveys 129
Potential hazards 25
Potential risks 20

Pretest probability 119, 120
Primary data 68
Probability densities 110
Probability distributions 107, 109, 110, 124, 132, 246
Probability education 120
Probability model 100, 103, 124
Probability theory 84, 115
Programming computers 116
Public health education 2
Public health policies 24, 27
Public health surveillance 28, 43

Q

Qualitative Variable 218
Quality control 20, 72, 117, 189, 190

R

Radiography 66
Random assignment 7, 14, 17
Random error 128
Randomized controlled trial (RCT) 14, 33
Random sample 83, 84, 85, 86, 87, 169, 171, 182, 191
Random sampling 65, 84, 86, 87, 97, 166, 181, 195, 223
Ratio of means (RoM) 149
Rectal cancer 40
Regression analysis 30, 132, 141, 164, 178, 217, 218, 225, 236, 240, 241, 242, 303, 304, 310, 311, 312
Regression Analysis 218, 242
Regression line 223, 224, 225, 228, 229, 241
Regression mean squares 227
Relative risk (RR) 56, 61, 293
Representative system 47
Research questions (RQs) 174
Respiratory diseases 40
Respiratory tract infection (RTI) 39
Risk ratio 56, 61, 137, 138, 141, 142, 144, 145, 146, 147, 160
Road injuries 39

S

Safety monitoring data 22
Sampling errors 135, 185, 186
Scatter Diagram 218, 219
Secondary data 68
Self-administered interviews 66
Self-Harm 40, 41
Sensitivity analysis 136, 155
Simple Random Sampling 65, 84
Simpson's Paradox 115
Social groups 46
Socio-economic 67
Socioeconomic 38, 42, 45, 46, 61
Standard deviation (SD) 148, 151, 153
Standardized mean difference (SMD) 148
Statistical analysis 3, 23
Statistical inference 87, 100, 102, 162, 175, 197
Statistical methodology 24
Statistical model 26, 134, 136
Statistical modelling 3
Statistical procedures 24, 136
Statistical research 7
Stomach cancer 40
Student's t distribution 110
Summary measures of population health (SMPH) 48
Surveillance system 28
Survival analysis 156, 164, 277, 279, 280, 282, 283, 284, 291, 292, 293, 314, 316, 317
Sustainable Development Goals 129, 160
Systematic biases 129, 135
Systematic sampling 65, 85

T

Telephone interviews 66, 67
Test hypotheses 25, 87
Tuberculosis (TB) 39

U

Under-five mortality rate (U5MR) 133
Uniform distribution 110, 113, 114
UN Interagency Group on Mortality Estimation (UN-IGME) 133

Univariable analysis 217
Upper true limit (UTL) 75

V

Vaccination rates 24
Venn diagrams 102, 105, 124
Vital signs 18

W

Waiting Time Paradox 115
World Health Organization (WHO) 24

Y

Years Lived with Disability (YLDs) 36, 47
Years of Life Lost (YLLs) 47

Z

Zero probability 109

FSC
www.fsc.org
MIX
Papier | Fördert gute Waldnutzung
FSC® C083411

Kolibri 360 GmbH
Ferdinand-Jühlke-Straße 7
99095 Erfurt, Deutschland
produktsicherheit@kolibri360.de